Physical
Assi
Examinati

Fourth

Physical Therapist Assistant Examination Review

Fourth Edition

Theresa Meyer, PT

SLACK
INCORPORATED

an innovative information, education, and management company

6900 Grove Road   Thorofare, NJ 08086

The material in this book has been compiled to help the student review and prepare for the certification exam. The author and the publisher are not responsible for errors or omissions, or for consequences from application of the book, and makes no warranty, expressed or implied, in regard to the contents of the book.

ISBN 1-55642-589-9 (alk. paper).

Printed in the United States of America.

Published by: SLACK Incorporated
               6900 Grove Road
               Thorofare, NJ 08086-9447 USA
               Telephone: 856-848-1000
               Fax: 856-853-5991
               www.slackbooks.com

This book is also available with computer testing software in a two-volume format (ISBN 1-55642-475-2). The information presented here is the same as in the alternate format, except for any small errors that have been corrected in this version. Contact SLACK Incorporated for more information on the two-volume set with software option.

Contact SLACK Incorporated for more information about other books in this field or about the availability of our books from distributors outside the United States.

DEDICATION

To my niece, Kelsey Marie Crabtree, and my godson, Alexander Justin Madruga,
with all my love.

CONTENTS

ABOUT THE AUTHOR

Theresa Meyer, BS, PT received her physical therapy degree from Thomas Jefferson College of Allied Health in 1986. She also received a BA degree in health and physical education from Messiah College in 1984.

Theresa started her career as a traveling physical therapist for Pro Therapy of America. This experience allowed her to gain valuable insight into a wide variety of health care settings, including home health, long-term care, outpatient facilities, as well as acute and rehabilitation hospitals. This also provided exposure to many health care systems throughout the United States.

She attended the World Physical Therapy Conference in Sydney, Australia in 1986 to further her education of physical therapy and research internationally. At this time, she wrote the most widely used physical therapy review books for the board licensure examination. This project was born out of a desire to assist with the stress and time constraints that physical therapy students undergo in preparation for the national board licensure examination. Theresa Meyer's *Review Book for the Physical Therapy Licensing Exam*, was the first book on the market to assist the student in exam preparation. She also wrote the *Review Book for the Physical Therapist Assistant*, which offered a multipurpose approach to assist physical therapist assistant students in studying for the board exam and comprehensive finals. Both books are best-sellers and have been used as textbooks in the United States and internationally. The books evolved through many updates and revisions to become two-volume sets with the addition of a software program to simulate computer examination testing in the current examination format.

In 1987, Theresa Meyer founded, and is the owner of, Midwest Hi-Tech Publishers. In 1988, Pro Therapy promoted her to Director of Rehabilitation at Three Rivers Area Hospital in Michigan. She developed cardiac rehabilitation, sports medicine, and fitness programs for the hospital while managing both inpatient and outpatient programs. She also served as their Regional Director for Southwest Michigan. She intertwined her responsibilities at the hospital with a consultant position to additional hospitals and outpatient facilities in the areas of new program development, clinic management, personnel hiring, staff education and preparation for JCAHO and Medicare reviews.

At this time, Theresa was attending many American Physical Therapy conventions to accelerate her learning in physical therapy. Her next career step was cofounding Physical Therapy and Sports Medicine Centers, a private practice that grew from one clinic in 1990 to 10 clinics. The private practices provided Michigan communities with state-of-the-art facilities and highly trained staff. She wrote a *Guide to Evaluation with Forms for the Physical Therapist* to provide physical therapists a succinct and easy method to perform comprehensive examinations of patients. She also worked as an educator for Pro Exam Source, teaching review workshops for the licensing examination to physical therapists and physical therapist assistants.

She sold her private practices to a national corporation in 1997 and retired. In 1998, she was a cofounder in Outpatient Certification Consultants. She and her partner wrote a new manual for Medicare certification, *Outpatient Policy and Procedure Manual*, to assist clinics in preparing for Medicare certification and meeting health care guidelines. Currently, she resides in Michigan and is working as a consultant and author.

PREFACE

The *Physical Therapist Assistant Examination Review* book was developed to provide comprehensive review for aiding the physical therapist assistant in passing the state licensing examination or school test and comprehensive finals. The book highlights the significant study areas in physical therapy. This book will provide a condensed and organized method of learning. The goal of the review book is to provide a database of key concepts in physical therapy that will provide the student with a strong foundation for answering multiple questions on the same information while using different contexts or formats. The goal is not simple memory recall, but an integration of the learning material.

The advantage to utilizing the review book is in providing more effective utilization of study time. Answering many sample questions to develop an analysis of your strengths and weaknesses is necessary prior to taking the actual examination. Each question has an explanation for the correct and incorrect answers to facilitate further learning. The student will be able to apply the information to a wide variety of questions on the same topic by studying the chapters of information and sample questions. The chapters are organized to maximize the learning experience and include charts, graphs, narrative, and outline formats.

The recommend utilization of the review book for studying is to study the chapters of information, then proceed to the sample test questions. If the passing rate on the sample questions is less than 75%, it is recommended that you restudy prior to taking the examination. If you have an area of concern that you already know prior to taking the test, I recommend reviewing your class notes at the same time as that chapter in the review book. For example, if pediatrics is an area of concern, pull your pediatric class notes and review both at the same time. This will further strengthen your comprehension of the subject.

It is also recommended that the student utilize class notes, previous examinations, and the bibliography for further study. Many factors go into preparing for the examination, including adequate preparation time, educational foundation, study habits, adequate rest, and proper nutrition. The student needs to realize that studying the book alone does not guarantee passing the test. Please prepare by being aware of all the factors necessary for proper test preparation.

Preparing for the Examination and Instructions for Use of the Review Book

1. Passing exam scores will vary by state. Be sure to check with the state in which you are taking your exam, or plan on working in, for their guidelines on passing scores. Some states will also require a jurisprudence examination on the rules, laws, and regulations governing physical therapy in that state, a test of English language proficiency, AIDS training, credential evaluation, and a supervised practice period. Check with the state you will be practicing in to determine what is necessary for licensure.

2. Study ahead of time systematically utilizing the review book as follows:
   - Study one chapter at a time.
   - Do not skip from mid-chapter to another. You may study chapters in the order that best fits your needs. For example, reviewing areas of strength first and proceeding to areas that require more time.
   - If you have class notes that you feel are pertinent and the information is not included in the book, then integrate them into these chapters.

3. After studying all the chapters, proceed to the sample test questions at the end of the book.

4. If several questions are missed in one area, further research is recommended utilizing the bibliography list or restudying the review book chapters.

5. Visit the site of the examination prior to the test to become acquainted with its location and parking.

6. Recheck for all documents necessary to take the exam: identification, ID with photo, and signature on identification.

7. Please note this review book is intended to assist in preparing for the state licensure exam. Since many factors (eg, adequate preparation time, educational foundation, study habits, etc) contribute to passing the exam/finals, studying the review book alone does not guarantee passing the examination/finals.

8. Do not cram for the exam the night before but get a good night's rest instead. On the morning of the exam, eat a healthy breakfast and plan to leave so you arrive at the site 15 to 20 minutes early. Think positively and good luck!

CHAPTER 1

Gross Anatomy

MUSCLE ACTIONS

Shoulder

Flexion
Deltoid—anterior
Biceps
Pectoralis major
Coracobrachialis

Extension
Deltoid—posterior
Triceps—long head
Teres major
Latissimus dorsi

Abduction
Deltoid—middle
Supraspinatus
Biceps—long head

Adduction
Pectoralis major
Teres major
Biceps—short head
Coracobrachialis
Latissimus dorsi
Triceps—long head

Lateral Rotation
Infraspinatus
Teres minor
Deltoid—posterior
Pectoralis major

Medial Rotation
Subscapularis
Teres major
Deltoid—anterior

Elbow

Flexion
Biceps
Brachialis
Brachioradialis
Extensor carpi radialis longus
Pronator teres
Palmar longus
Flexor carpi radialis
Flexor carpi ulnaris

Extension
Triceps
Anconeus

Forearm

Pronation
Brachioradialis
Pronator teres
Pronator quadratus
Flexor carpi radialis

Supination
Biceps
Brachioradialis
Supinator

Wrist

Extension	Flexion	Abduction	Adduction
Extensor carpi radialis longus	Flexor carpi radialis	Extensor carpi radialis longus	Extensor carpi ulnaris
Extensor carpi radialis brevis	Flexor pollicis longus	Extensor carpi radialis brevis	Flexor carpi ulnaris
Extensor carpi ulnaris	Flexor carpi ulnaris	Extensor pollicis brevis	
Extensor digitorum	Abductor pollicis longus	Extensor pollicis longus	
Extensor pollicis longus	Palmaris longus	Extensor digitorum	
	Flexor digitorum superficialis	Flexor carpi radialis	
	Flexor digitorum profundus	Abductor pollicis longus	

Scapula

Elevation	Depression	Abduction	Adduction
Upper trapezius	Lower trapezius	Serratus anterior	Middle trapezius
Serratus anterior —upper	Serratus anterior —lower		Rhomboids
Rhomboids			
Levator scapulae			

Lateral Rotation Upward	Medial Rotation Downward
Trapezius	Levator scapulae
Serratus anterior	Rhomboids

Finger Digits

Thumb extension	Extensor pollicis longus/brevis
Metacarpophalangeal (MCP) abduction	Abduction pollicis longus
Thumb adduction	Adduction pollicis
Thumb abduction	Abduction pollicis brevis
MCP flexion	Flexor pollicis brevis
Interphalangeal (IP) flexion	Flexor pollicis longus
Opposition	Opponens pollicis
2nd to 5th digit	Flexor digitorum sublimis
proximal interphalangeal (PIP) flexion	Flexor digitorum profundus
	Lumbricales
2nd to 3rd digit distal interphalangeal (DIP) flexion	Extensor digitorum communis
2nd to 3rd MCP flexion	Extensor digiti quintiproprius
2nd to 3rd digit MCP with IP extension	

Neck

Flexion	Extension	Lateral Flexion
Sternocleidomastoid	Upper trapezius	Longus colli
	Semispinalis capitis	Obliquus capitis superior

Longus capitis
Longus colli
Scalenus anterior
Rectus capitis
anterior
Platysma

Splenius capitis
Splenius cervicis
Longissimus capitis
Longissimus cervicis

Rectus capitis lateralis
Splenius cervicis
Scalenus anterior
Splenius capitis
Scalenus medius
Upper trapezius
Scalenus posterior
Longissimus capitis
Sternocleidomastoid
Iliocostalis—cervical

**Rotation—
Same Side**
Longus colli
Longus capitis
Rectus capitis
anterior
Rectus capitis
posterior
Obliquus capitis
inferior
Splenius cervicis
Splenius capitis
Longissimus
capitis

**Rotation—
Opposite Side**
Sternocleidomastoid
Scalenus anterior
Scalenus posterior
Scalenus medius
Upper trapezius
Semispinalis cervicis
Cervical multifidus
Cervical rotators

Temporomandibular Joint (TMJ)

Protraction
Pterygoideus
medialis (internus)
Pterygoideus
lateralis (externus)

Elevation
Masseter temporalis
(pterygoideus medialis internus)

Trunk/Back

Flexion
Rectus abdominis
Internal oblique
External oblique
Iliocostalis lumborum

Extension
Erector spinae
Longissimus thoracis
Quadratus lumborum
Semispinalis

Rotation
External oblique
Latissimus dorsi
Internal oblique
Ilicostalis lumborum
Intercostal (8-12)
Multifidus
Iliohypogastric
Rotators
Rectus abdominis

Elevation of the Pelvis
Internal oblique
External oblique
Quadratus lumborum

Hip

Flexion
Psoas major
Iliacus
Sartorius
Rectus femoris
Tensor fasciae latae
Gluteus minimus
Pectineus

Extension
Semimembranosus
Semitendinosus
Biceps femoris—
long head
Piriformis
Adductor magnus—
posterior

Medial Rotators
Adductor longus
Adductor brevis
Gluteus minimus
Gluteus medius—anterior
Semimembranosus
Semitendinosus
Tensor fasciae latae

Lateral Rotators
Psoas major
Iliacus
Sartorius
Internal obturator
External obturator
Gluteus medius—
posterior

Adductor magnus
—anterior
Adductor brevis
Adductor longus

Gluteus medius—
posterior
Gluteus maximus

Gluteus maximus
Gemellus—superior
Gemellus—inferior
Quadratus femoris
Biceps femoris—long head
Piriformis

Abduction
Tensor fasciae latae
Gluteus minimus
Gluteus medius
Gemelli—inferior
Gemelli—superior
Obturator—internal
Piriformis
Iliacus
Sartorius
Psoas major

Adduction
Adductor longus
Adductor brevis
Adductor magnus
Pectineus
Gracilis
Gluteus maximus—lower
Obturator—external

Knee

Flexion
Semimembranosus
Semitendinosus
Biceps femoris
Sartorius
Gracilis
Popliteus
Plantaris
Gastrocnemius

Extension
Rectus femoris
Vastus lateralis
Vastus intermedius
Vastus medialis

Medial Rotation
Sartorius
Gracilis
Popliteus
Semimembranosus
Semitendinosus

Lateral Rotation
Biceps femoris

Ankle

Inversion
Tibialis—anterior
Tibialis—posterior
Flexor hallucis
longus
Flexor digitorum
longus
Extensor hallucis
longus

Eversion
Peroneus brevis
Peroneus longus
Peroneus tertius
Extensor digitorum longus

Dorsiflexion
Tibialis anterior
Peroneus tertius
Extensor digitorum longus
Extensor hallucis longus

Plantar Flexion
Tibialis posterior
Peroneus brevis
Peroneus longus
Plantaris
Soleus
Gastrocnemius
Flexor digitorum longus
Flexor hallucis longus

Toes

Great toe MIP
extension
Great toe IP flexion
Great toe MIP
flexion
2nd to 5th digit
MIP extension
2nd to 5th digit
DIP flexion
2nd to 5th digit
PIP flexion
Toe abduction PIP
Toe adduction PIP

Extensor hallucis longus
Flexor hallucis longus
Flexor hallucis brevis
Extensor digitorum longus
Flexor digitorum longus
Flexor digitorum brevis
Dorsal interossei
Plantar interossei

MUSCLES OF THE HEAD, FACE, AND SCALP REGION

Muscle	Function
Auricularis—anterior	Draws the ear forward and downward
Auricularis—posterior	Elevates and retracts the ear
Auricularis—superior	Slightly elevates the ear
Buccinator	Aids in chewing food and compressing the cheeks
Corrugator	Causes the eyebrows to draw medially and downward (eg, causes a frowning expression)
Depressor anguli oris	Depresses the angle of the mouth (eg, causes a grieving expression)
Depressor labii inferioris	Depresses the lower lip
Depressor septi	Causes the nostrils to close inward
Pterygoideus lateralis	Assists in chewing and protrusion
Levator anguli oris	Elevates the corners of the mouth
Levator labii superioris	Elevates the upper lip
Nasalis	Enlarges or compresses the nostrils, causing them to either flare in or flare out
Masseter	Clenches the teeth, elevates the jaw, assists in chewing
Pterygoideus medialis	Elevates and protracts the lower jaw, assists in chewing
Mentalis	Causes the lower lip to protrude and rise (eg, causes an expression of doubtfulness)
Orbicularis oris	Causes the lips to protrude and compress
Occipitofrontalis	Moves the scalp backward and forward (eg, raises eyebrows, causes a surprised expression)
Orbicularis oculi	Assists in closing the eyelids
Procerus	Causes the eyebrows to draw down and in medially
Risorius	Causes the mouth to retract backward (eg, causes a grinning face)
Temporalis	Elevates the jaw and clenches the teeth
Temporoparietalis	Draws back the skin of the temples (eg, tightens the scalp)
Zygomaticus	Causes the mouth's angles to draw upward and backward (eg, causes a laughing face)

CHART OF COMBINED ACTIONS TO BE TESTED WITH MUSCLES

ACTION	MUSCLE
Shoulder shrug, scapular upward rotation	Upper trapezius
Shoulder protraction and scapular upward rotation	Serratus anterior
Scapular elevation and downward rotation	Levator scapula
Scapular adduction, elevation, downward rotation	Rhomboids
Shoulder abduction with lateral rotation	Supraspinatus, infraspinatus
Shoulder adduction with medial rotation	Latissimus dorsi, teres major, and subscapularis
Shoulder abduction, flexion, extension	Deltoid
Hip flexion, abduction, lateral rotation	Sartorius
Hip flexion, abduction, medial rotation	Tensor fascia lata
Hip extension, knee flexion, and leg lateral rotation	Biceps femoris
Hip extension, knee flexion, and leg medial rotation	Semitendinosus, semimembranous

INNERVATION OF MUSCLES

Upper Extremity Muscle	Nerve	Origin
Biceps	Musculocutaneous	C5, C6
Brachialis	Musculocutaneous	C5, C6
Coracobrachialis	Musculocutaneous	C6, C7
Deltoid	Axillary	C5, C6
Infraspinatus	Suprascapular	C4, C5, C6
Latissimus dorsi	Thoracodorsal	C6, C7, C8
Levator scapulae	Cervical 3 and 4, dorsal scapular	C4, C5
Pectoralis major	Lateral and medial pectoral	C5, C6, C7
Pectoralis minor	Medial pectoral	C7, C8, T1
Rhomboid major	Dorsal scapular	C4, C5
Rhomboid minor	Dorsal scapular	C4, C5
Serratus anterior	Long thoracic	C5, C6, C7, C8
Sternocleidomastoid	Cranial nerve XI	C1, C2, C3, C4
Subclavius	Subclavian	C5, C6
Subscapularis	Upper/lower subscapular	C5, C6, C7
Supraspinatus	Suprascapular	C4, C5, C6
Teres major	Lower subscapular	C5, C6, C7
Teres minor	Axillary	C5, C6
Trapezius	Cranial nerve XI, ventral ramus	C2, C3, C4

CHART OF THE THREE PRIMARY HAND/FOREARM NERVES

Radial Nerve (C5, C6, C7, C8)	Medial Nerve (C6, C7, C8, T1)	Ulnar Nerve (C7, C8, T1)
Abductor pollicis longus	Flexor pollicis longus	Opponens digiti minimi
Anconeus	Palmaris longus	Palmar brevis
Brachialis	Lumbricales 1 & 2	Lumbricales 3 & 4
Brachioradialis	Flexor digitorum superficialis	Flexor carpi ulnaris
Extensor carpi		
Radialis longus	Pronator quadratus	Flexor digiti minimi
Extensor carpi ulnaris		
Extensor digitorum longus		Abductor digiti minimi
Extensor digitorum minimi		
Extensor indicis proprius	Opponens pollicis	
Extensor pollicis brevis	Abductor pollicis brevis	
Extensor pollicis	Flexor carpi radialis	Adductor pollicis longus
Supinator	Pronator teres	Interossei
Triceps	Flexor digitorum profundus 2 & 3	Flexor digitorum profundus 4 & 5

Radial nerve: the largest branch of the brachial plexus, arising on each side as a continuation of the posterior cord.

Medial nerve: a branch of the brachial plexus that, along with the lateral pectoral nerve, supplies the pectoral muscles.

Ulnar nerve: one of the terminal branches of the brachial plexus that arises on each side from the medial cord of the plexus.

Trunk

Muscle group	Innervation Level
Rectus abdominis	T7 to 12
Internal oblique	T7 to L1
External oblique	T5 to 11

Lower Extremity

Muscle Group	Innervation Level
Sartorius	L1 to 3
Adductors	L2 to 4
External rotators	L3 to S2
Tensor fasciae latae	L4 to S1
Hamstrings	L4 to S3
Quadriceps	L2 to 4
Anterior tibialis	L4 to 5
Gastrocnemius	L5 to S1
Flexor hallucis longus	S1 to 2
Extensor digitorum brevis	S2 to 3

LOWER EXTREMITY INNERVATION

Tibial Nerve (L4, L5, S1, S2, S3)

Plantaris
Gastrocnemius
Popliteus
Soleus
Posterior tibialis
Flexor digitorum longus
Flexor hallucis longus

The Tibial Nerve Divides Into:

Lateral Plantar Nerve
Dorsal interossei
Plantar interossei
Abductor digiti minimi
Flexor digiti minimi
Opponens digiti minimi
Quadratus plantae
Lumbricales 2, 3, and 4
Adductor hallucis

Medial Plantar Nerve
Flexor digitorum brevis
Flexor hallucis brevis
Abductor hallucis
Lumbricales 1

The Common Peroneal Nerve (L4, L5, S1, S2)

Superficial Peroneal Nerve
Peroneus longus
Peroneus brevis

Deep Peroneal Nerve
Tibialis anterior
Peroneus tertius
Extensor hallucis longus
Extensor digitorum longus
Extensor digitorum brevis

Femoral Nerve (L2, L3, L4)
Iliacus
Pectineus

Sciatic Nerve (L4, L5, S1, S2, S3)
Biceps femoris
Semitendinosus

Sartorius
Rectus femoris
Vastus medialis
Vastus lateralis
Vastus intermedius

Semimembranosus
Adductor magnus

Superior Gluteal (L4, L5, S1)
Gluteus medius
Gluteus minimus
Tensor fasciae latae

Inferior Gluteal (L5, S1, S2)
Gluteus maximus

Obturator Nerve (L2, L3, L4)
Obturator—external
Adductor brevis
Adductor longus
Adductor magnus
Gracilis

Lumbar Plexus (L1, L2, L3, L4)
Psoas major
Psoas minor

Sacral Plexus (L4, L5, S1, S2, S3)
Piriformis
Obturator—internal
Quadratus femoris
Gemelli—superior and inferior

MUSCLES WITH DUAL INNERVATION

Muscle	Nerves
Flexor digitorum profundus	Median nerve—digits 1 and 2
	Ulnar nerve—digits 3 and 4
Flexor pollicis brevis	Median nerve
	Ulnar nerve—deep head of muscle
Adductor magnus	Sciatic nerve
	Obturator nerve
Lumbricales—hand	Median nerve—digits 1 and 2
	Ulnar nerve—digits 3 and 4

COMMON MUSCLE ATTACHMENTS

Upper Extremity

Greater Tuberosity of Humerus
Supraspinatus
Infraspinatus
Teres minor

Lesser Tuberosity of Humerus
Subscapularis

Medial Epicondyle of Humerus
Common flexor tendon's origin
Common injury is golf elbow

Lateral Epicondyle of Humerus
Common extensor tendon's origin
Common injury is tennis elbow

Lower Extremity

ASIS—Anterior Superior Iliac Spine
Sartorius

Anterior Inferior Iliac Spine

Rectus femoris

Greater Trochanter
Gluteus minimus
Gluteus medius
Piriformis
Obturator—internal
Gemelli—inferior and superior

Lesser Trochanter
Psoas major

Ischial Tuberosity
Semitendinosus
Semimembranosus
Biceps femoris
Adductor magnus

Iliac Crest
Tensor fasciae latae

Pubic Ramus
Pectineus
Adductor magnus
Gracilis
Adductor brevis

Medial Femoral Condyle
Gastrocnemius

Lateral Femoral Condyle
Popliteus

Navicular Tubercle
Tibialis posterior

JOINT INTEGRITY

Shoulder Joint

Ball and socket joint/enarthrodial joint
1. Coracoclavicular ligament: connects the clavicle and coracoid process of the scapula.
    a. Trapezoid ligament
    b. Conoid ligament
2. Acromioclavicular ligament: located at the outer end of the clavicle and connects to the acromion process of the scapula.
    a. Inferior ligament
    b. Superior ligament
3. Coracohumeral ligament: from the coracoid process, it connects to the greater tuberosity of the humerus.

Elbow Joint

Hinge joint/ginglymus joint
1. Orbicular ligament: surrounds the head of the radius.
2. Radial collateral: restricts lateral displacement of the elbow joint.
3. Ulnar collateral: restricts medial displacement of the elbow joint.

Hip Joint

Ball and socket joint/enarthrodial joint
1. Iliofemoral ligament: y-shaped ligament that limits extension of the hip.
2. Pubofemoral ligament: limits extension of the hip.
3. Ischiofemoral ligament: limits anterior displacement of the hip.

Knee Joint

Hinge joint/ginglymus joint
1. Anterior cruciate: prevents anterior displacement of the tibia on the femur.

2. Posterior cruciate: prevents posterior displacement of the tibia on the femur.
3. Medial collateral ligament: stabilizes the medial aspect of the knee joint (tibiofemoral joint).
4. Lateral collateral ligament: stabilizes the lateral aspect of the knee joint.
5. Popliteal: provides lateral and posterior support to the knee joint.

Ankle Joint

Hinge joint/ginglymus
1. Deltoid ligament: lateral stability between medial malleolus, navicular bone, talus, and calcaneus.
2. Lateral ligaments: lateral ligament support; injury results in inversion sprain.
   a. Anterior talofibular: secures fibula to talus.
   b. Calcaneofibular: secures fibula to calcaneus.
   c. Posterior talofibular: secures fibula to talus.

Foot

1. Plantar calcaneonavicular ligament (spring ligament): supports the medial aspect of the longitudinal arch.
2. Long plantar ligament: supports the lateral aspect of the longitudinal arch.

BONY LANDMARKS WITH THEIR CORRESPONDING VERTEBRAL LEVEL

BONY LANDMARK	VERTEBRAL LEVEL
Sacroiliac (SI) joint/ posterior superior iliac spine	S2
Sacral promontory	L5, S1
Crest of ilium	L4, L5
Spinal cord ends	L2
Navel, umbilicus	T10
Inferior angle of scapula	7th rib level, T7
Superior angle of scapula	2nd rib level, T7
Bifurcations of the trachea	T4
Spine of scapula	T3

CHAPTER 2

Physiology

FUELS FOR EXERCISE

1. Three primary food sources are carbohydrates, proteins, and fats. Each food source converts adenosine triphosphate (ATP) energy to exercise.
2. Carbohydrates are the major fuel, utilized first during prolonged, low-intensity and short, high-intensity exercises. Glucose is the end product of CH_2O digestion. Glucose that is not readily needed for energy is stored in muscle cells in the form of glycogen.
3. The basic form of fat used for fuel is called free fatty acid. This is stored in adipose tissue as a triglyceride. This fuel source is utilized after carbohydrates during prolonged, moderate exercises.
4. Proteins are very rarely utilized as a fuel source for exercise.
5. Definition of calorie: the amount of heat it takes to raise the temperature of one kilogram of water 1°C.
6. The amount of calories required in the conversion process to energy is different for protein, carbohydrates, and fats. One gram of CH_2O yields 4 calories. One gram of fat yields 9 calories. One gram of protein yields 4 calories.

ENERGY SYSTEMS

AEROBIC SYSTEM	VERSUS	ANAEROBIC SYSTEM
Oxygen system		Lactic acid
Slow process		Rapid process
Fuel source = fats		Fuel source = Glycogen
Unlimited ATP production		Limited ATP
Low fatigue		Easily fatigued
Long-duration activities, long distance		1- to 3-minute activities
		Sprint or high power, short duration
		Byproduct causes fatigue (lactic acid)

MUSCLE FIBERS

SLOW TWITCH	VERSUS	FAST TWITCH
High aerobic capacity		Low aerobic capacity
Low anaerobic capacity		High anaerobic capacity
High capillary density		Low capillary density
Slow contraction		Fast contraction
Slow fatigue		Fast fatigue
Long-distance activity		Short-distance activity
Example: Marathon		*Example: Sprinting*

MUSCLE CONTRACTION

Concentric Contraction

1. Isotonic or dynamic are other names for this contraction.
2. The muscle shortens as it develops tension.

Eccentric Contraction

1. The muscle lengthens as it develops tension.
2. Example: lowering a weight during a hard press is considered a negative repetition or eccentric contraction.

Isotonic Contraction

Speed is variable; the muscle will shorten and develop tension.

Isometric Contraction

No change in muscle length, but muscle will develop tension.

Isokinetic Contraction

Speed is constant; muscle will shorten in length and maintain maximum tension throughout range of motion.

THEORY OF SPECIFICITY OF TRAINING

- Specific training patterns will cause specific physiological responses.
- The effects of training are specific to the sport/activity.
- Specific physiological training applies to each sport because each needs different capacities.

OXYGEN TRANSPORT SYSTEM

The oxygen transport system is important during endurance exercise. For a successful performance, one must be able to efficiently transport oxygen to the working muscles.

Definition of Terms

- VO_2 = oxygen transported
- SV = stroke volume—amount of blood the heart pumps per beat
- HR = heart rate—beats per minute

Formulas

1. AVO$_2$ Diff Arterial Mixed Venous O$_2$ Difference = oxygen—the muscle extracts from arterial blood; the more extracted, the less venous blood.
2. MAX VO = SV x HR x AVO$_2$ Diff

MUSCLE SORENESS THEORY

(The following are only theories as to why muscle soreness may occur)
1. Tearing of muscle fibers, which results in tissue damage.
2. Muscle spasms, which reduce blood flow to muscle.
3. Retention of water/inflammation in tissue.
4. Overstretching of connective tissue (epimysium), which surrounds muscle.

STRENGTH DURATION CURVE

Strength duration curve is a graphic showing the relationship between the intensity (Y axis) and various durations (X axis) of the threshold electric stimulus for a muscle, with the stimulating cathode positioned over the motor point. The strength duration curve may be utilized to determine if a muscle is innervated, partially innervated, or denervated.

DEFINITIONS

Action Potential

A brief regenerative electrical potential that propagates along a single axon or muscle fiber membrane. The action potential is an all-or- none response to a stimulus. When the stimulus is at or above the threshold, the action potential generated has a constant size and configuration.

Chronaxie

The time required for an electrical current twice the rheobase to elicit the first visible muscle twitch.

Epimysium

The connective tissue that surrounds the entire muscle. It provides muscular strength and integrity to the muscle.

Excitability

The capacity to be activated by or react to a stimulus.

Golgi Tendon Organ

Located in the tendons and responds to stretch. The golgi tendon organ complements the muscle spindle, and acts as a safeguard against injury. The golgi tendon tells the muscle to relax if the contraction is too strong and would cause injury.

Latency

Interval between the onset of the stimulus and the response. Peak latency is the interval between the onset of the stimulus and a specified peak of the evoked potential.

Motor Point

The point over a muscle when a muscle contraction may be elicited by a minimal-intensity, short-duration electrical stimulus.

Motor Unit

The motor unit consists of the anterior horn cells, its axon, neuromuscular junctions, and all of the muscle fibers innervated by the axon. A motor unit or fibers can manifest a fast and slow twitch. It is described as the functional unit of skeletal muscle.

Motor Unit Action Potential

Action potential showing the electrical activity of a single motor unit.

Muscle Spindle

Located in the muscle fibers, a sensory nerve is located in the center portion of the spindle. When a spindle is stretched, the following will occur: the nerve impulse will begin, the rate of the stretch is given, and the magnitude of the stretch is given.

Muscle Stretch Reflex

Activation of a muscle following a stretch of the muscle.

Myofibril

Component of a muscle cell composed of contractible filaments. Contains two basic proteins that give the striated pattern:
1. Actin—thin filaments, attached to the Z line
2) Myosin—thin filaments, called the I band.
   Sarcomere: smallest functional unit of a myofibril. It is the distance between two Z lines.

Rheobase

The intensity of an electrical current necessary to produce a minimal visible twitch of a muscle when applied to the motor parts.

Resting Membrane Potential

The voltage across the membrane of an excitable cell at rest.

Sliding Filament Theory

A theory of muscular contraction that states when a muscle performs an isotonic contraction action, filaments will slide over myosin filaments toward the sarcomere, creating cross-bridges, overlapping thick and thin filaments with great force.

Smooth Muscle Tissue

Found in vessel and artery walls, various tissues of the vascular system, lungs, and intestinal and reproductive systems. Differs from skeletal muscle, secondary to lack of a cross-striated pattern. It is under involuntary control.

Stimulus

An external stimulus (eg, electrical stimulation) that influences the activity of a cell, tissue, or organism. A threshold stimulus is a stimulus that produces a detectable response.

Striated Muscle

Called striated muscle secondary to arrangement of contractible proteins in the muscle that gives a cross-striation pattern. Under voluntary control and innervated by the somatic nervous system.

CHAPTER 3

Neuroanatomy & Physiology

CRANIAL NERVES

NERVE #	NAME	ACTION
1	Olfactory	Smells
2	Optic	Sees
3	Oculomotor	Moves the eyes
4	Trochlear	Moves the eyes and controls the contralateral superior oblique
5	Trigeminal	Chews/sensory to face
6	Abducens	Accommodates, moves eyes
7	Facial	Moves the face—taste/salivates/cries
8	Vestibulocochlear	Hears/regulates balance
9	Glossopharyngeal	Tastes/swallows, monitors carotid, body, and sinuses
10	Vagus	Tastes/swallows
11	Accessory	Turns the head, and lifts the shoulders
12	Hypoglossal	Moves the tongue

Sensory nerves = 1, 2, 8
Motor nerves = 3, 4, 6, 11, 12
Mixed nerves/motor and sensory = 5, 7, 9, 10

DERMATOME DISTRIBUTION

Sensory distribution of the cutaneous nerves

Upper Extremity

C1   Top of head
C2   Temple, forehead, occiput
C3   Neck, posterior cheek
C4   Superior part of chest above axilla (clavicle area)
C5   Lateral aspect of the arm, deltoid muscle region
C6   Anterior arm, lateral side of hand to thumb and index finger
C7   Lateral arm and forearm to index, long, and ring fingers
C8   Middle arm and forearm to long, ring, and little fingers

Trunk

    T1   Medial side of forearm to base of little finger
    T2   Axillary region
    T4   Nipple level
    T6   Xiphoid process level
    T10 Umbilicus level
    T12 Anterior superior iliac crest level

Lower Extremity

    L1   Lower abdomen and groin region
    L2   Anterolateral thigh (back and front of thigh to knee)
    L3   Anteromedial thigh, leg, upper buttock
    L4   Medial buttock, lateral thigh, medial leg, dorsum of foot, large toe
    L5   Posterior lateral thigh, lateral leg, dorsum of foot, medial half of sole, first to third toes
    S1   Lateral plantar surface of foot, posterior thigh and leg
    S2   Posterior thigh and leg
    S3   Groin, medial thigh to knee
    S4-5 Perineum, genitals, lower sacrum

LEVELS OF COGNITIVE FUNCTIONING (RANCHO LOS AMIGOS SCALE)

Level

1   No response: patient is unresponsive to any stimuli and appears to be in a deep sleep.
2   Generalized response: patient occasionally reacts to stimuli but not in a purposeful pattern. Responses are limited and inconsistent.
3   Localized response: patient reacts to stimuli but continues to be inconsistent. May follow simple commands in a delayed manner.
4   Confused/agitated: patient responds to stimuli but he or she is unable to process information purposefully. Patient is in a heightened state of activity and behavior is bizarre.

SPINAL SEGMENT WITH MOVEMENTS TO TEST

SPINAL SEGMENT	MOVEMENTS TO TEST
Upper Extremity	
C4	Shoulder shrug
C5	Shoulder abduction, external rotation
C6	Wrist extension, elbow flexion
C7	Wrist flexion, elbow extension
C8	Wrist ulnar deviation
Trunk	
T1	Abduction/adduction of fingers
Lower Extremity	
L2	Hip flexion
L3	Hip flexion, knee extension
L4	Knee extension, ankle dorsiflexion
L5	Ankle dorsiflexion
S1	Ankle plantar flexion and eversion
S2	Knee flexion, ankle plantar flexion

5   Confused/inappropriate/nonagitated: patient is alert and able to follow very simple commands. However, consistency fluctuates.

6   Confused/appropriate: patient can follow directions but only with direct assistance from another individual.

7   Automatic appropriate: patient goes through daily routine automatically but robot-like with shallow recall of activities.

8   Purposeful/appropriate: patient shows carryover for new learning and needs no supervision once activities are learned. Patient is able to recall and is aware of and responsive to environment.

CENTRAL NERVOUS SYSTEM (CNS)

Consists of the brain and spinal cord, both of which are protected by bone. The brain lies within the cranial vault and the spinal cord is protected by the vertebral canal. The brain joins the spinal canal at the foramen magnum.

Covering of the Central Nervous System

Underneath the bony covering is an inner covering of membranes called meninges. The meninges consist of three layers:
1. Dura mater
   - Thick, fibrous connective tissue
   - Outermost meningeal layer
   - Surrounds the meningeal arteries and veins
   - Adheres to the skull
2. Arachnoid
   - Fine, filamentous network
   - Middle meningeal layer
   - Bridge between the dura and inner meningeal layer
   - Cerebrospinal fluid circulated in the space
   - Considered the hydraulic cushion for the CNS
3. Pia mater
   - Single thickness
   - Innermost meningeal layer
   - Adheres to the surface of the CNS

Ventricles

There are four ventricles or cavities that are filled with cerebrospinal fluid. Cerebrospinal fluid provides a support system to cushion the brain. It also aids in the exchange of nutrients and waste.
1. Lateral ventricles (2): large irregular-shaped ventricles with anterior, posterior, and inferior horns. They communicate with the third ventricle through the foramen of Monro.
2. Third ventricle: located posterior and deep between the two thalami and communicates with the fourth ventricle through the cerebral aqueduct.
3. Fourth ventricle: located in front of the cerebellum and behind the pons and upper part of the medulla oblongata. They are pyramid shaped. The openings (foramina) of Luschka and Magendie create communication between the fourth ventricle and subarachnoid space.

Divided into Six Parts

1.   **Cerebrum:** the cerebrum is also called the telencephalon. The telencephalon and diencephalon together constitute the prosencephalon or forebrain. It consists of grayish matter composed of crests (*gyri*) and fissures (*sulci*). The islands of gray matter within each cerebral hemisphere are called basal ganglia. These form an associated motor system in the subthalamus and midbrain. The central sulcus separates the frontal lobe from the parietal lobe. The lateral central fissure, also called the *fissure of Sylvius,* separates the temporal, frontal, and parietal lobes of the brain. The longitudinal cerebral fissure separates the two hemispheres. The parietal hemisphere consists of six lobes on each side:
     1. The frontal lobe, which controls the motor aspects of speech, emotions, judgments, and primary motor cortex for voluntary muscle activation.

2. The parietal lobe, which controls integration of sensations, touch, pain, temperature, and proprioception.
3. The temporal lobe, which controls auditory stimuli and language comprehension.
4. The occipital lobe, which controls the visual stimuli.
5. The insula, which assist with visceral function.
6. The limbic system, which controls feeding, aggression, sexual response, and emotions.

2. **Diencephalon:** consists of the thalamus, subthalamus, hypothalamus, and epithalamus. The thalamus contains sensory nuclei and motor nuclei. The subthalamus is involved in the control of pathways for motor, sensory, and reticular functions. The hypothalamus controls and integrates the peripheral autonomic nervous system, endocrine processes, and many somatic functions, such as body temperature, sleep, and appetite. The epithalamus secrets hormones that control the pituitary gland.

3. **Midbrain:** the midbrain is also called the mesencephalon. It is one of the three parts of the brainstem lying just below the cerebrum and just above the pons. It connects the pons to the cerebrum and the midbrain to the cerebellum. It assists with motor control, muscle tone, suppression of pain, vision, hearing, and certain auditory and visual reflexes.

4. **Pons:** connects the medulla oblongata to the midbrain, allowing the ascending and descending tracts to pass information. The pons consists of white matter and a few nuclei and is divided into a ventral and dorsal portion. It assists in modulation of pain and controlling arousal.

5. **Medulla oblongata:** the most vital part of the brain, continuing as the bulbous portion of the spinal cord just above the foramen magnum and separated from the pons by a horizontal groove. It assists in control of head movements, vestibulo-ocular reflexes, voluntary motor control, center for vital functions, such as cardiac, respiratory, and vasomotor.

6. **Cerebellum:** linked to the brainstem by three pairs of peduncles—superior, middle, and inferior. It is located behind the dorsal pons and medulla in the posterior fossa. It assists in controlling equilibrium and regulation of muscle tone, posture, and coordination of voluntary muscular activity.
   - The cerebellum, pons, and medulla all lie in the posterior fossa and together are known as the hindbrain or rhombencephalon.

PERIPHERAL NERVOUS SYSTEM (PNS)

The PNS consists of nerves referred to as lower motor neurons and ganglia outside the vertebral canal. Forty-three pairs of nerves originate from the CNS and make up the peripheral nervous system. Twelve pairs are cranial nerves, which originate from the brain. Thirty-one pairs are spinal nerves, which originate from the spinal cord. The spinal nerves are divided into the following groups: eight cervical, twelve thoracic, five sacral, five lumbar, and one coccygeal. These spinal nerves correspond to a particular vertebral segment and consist of a ventral and dorsal root, except for C1, which has no dorsal root. The ventral root is an efferent fiber to voluntary muscle, viscera, smooth muscle, and glands. The dorsal root is an afferent fiber that provides sensory receptors from skin, joints, and muscles.

Arteries

1. **Internal carotid:** arteries that arise off of the common carotids and branch to form anterior middle cerebral arteries. Each of two arteries start at the bifurcation of the common carotid arteries, through which blood circulates to many structures and organs in the head.
2. **Vertebral arteries:** arteries branching from the subclavian arteries, arising deep in the neck from the cranial and dorsal subclavian surfaces. They supply the brainstem, cerebellum, occipital lobe, and thalamus.
3. **Circle of Willis:** formed by the interconnection of the internal carotid, anterior cerebral, posterior cerebral, anterior communicating, and posterior communicating arteries.

Covering of Peripheral Nervous System

1. Endoneurium
   - Fine, single layer
   - Covers nerve processes
2. Perineurium
   - Thick membrane
   - Encloses large groups of processes

3. Epineurium
   - Thick, tough layer
   - Surrounds the PNS

PNS has Two Subdivisions

1. Afferent fibers carry sensory impulses to the CNS.
2. Efferent fibers carry motor impulses away from the CNS by cranial or spinal nerves. The efferent division is further divided into two subdivisions based on the type of effector supplied.
   - Somatic nervous system innervates skeletal muscle and is usually under voluntary control.
   - Autonomic nervous system innervates cardiac muscle, smooth muscle, and glands.

MAJOR ASCENDING TRACTS OF THE SPINAL CORD

1. **Dorsal Columns**
   Fasciculus gracilis
   Origin: C1 to T6
   Function: Discrete somatotropic transfer of touch, vibration, and kinesthesia.
   Fasciculus cuneatus
   Origin: T5 to C1
   Function: Discrete somatotropic transfer of touch, vibration, and kinesthesia.
2. **Spinothalamic Tracts**
   Anterior (ventral)
   Origin: Laminae I, IV, V
   Function: Somatotropic transfer of affective light touch, pain, and temperature.
   Lateral
   Origin: Laminae, I, IV, V
   Function: Somatotropic transfer of affective light touch, pain, and temperature.
3. **Spinocerebellar Tracts**
   Ventral (anterior)
   Origin: Dorsal horn
   Function: Somatotropic transfer of proprioception.
   Dorsal
   Origin: L3 to C8
   Function: Somatotropic transfer of spinal interneuron activity.
   Cuneocerebellar
   Origin: C7 to C2
   Function: Somatotropic transfer of spinal interneuron activity.
4. **Spinobrainstem Tracts**
   Spinoreticular
   Origin: Dorsal horn
   Function: Nondiscriminative transfer of touch, proprioception.
   Spinotectal
   Origin: Dorsal horn
   Function: Nondiscriminative transfer of touch, proprioception.
   Spino-olivary
   Origin: Dorsal horn
   Function: Somatotropic transfer of spinal interneuron activity.

MAJOR DESCENDING TRACTS OF THE SPINAL CORD

1. **Corticospinal Tracts**
   Lateral corticospinal
   Origin: Primary motor and sensory cortex
   Function: Controls alpha and gamma motor neurons, modulates 1° afferent.

Anterior corticospinal
Origin: Primary and secondary motor cortex, sensory cortex
Function: Controls alpha and gamma motor neurons, modulates 1° afferent.

2. **Rubrospinal Tract**
Origin: Red nucleus
Function: Controls alpha and gamma motor neurons, modulates 1° afferent.

3. **Tectospinal Tract**
Origin: Superior colliculus
Function: Controls alpha and gamma motor neurons.

4. **Vestibulospinal Tracts**
Lateral vestibulospinal
Origin: Deiters' nucleus
Function: Controls alpha and gamma motor neurons.
Medial longitudinal fasciculus (MLF)
Origin: Vestibular nuclei
Function: Controls alpha and gamma motor neurons.

5. **Reticulospinal Tracts**
Somatomotor
Origin: Reticular formation
Function: Controls alpha and gamma motor neurons.
Autonomic
Origin: Reticular formation
Function: Controls autonomic preganglionic neurons.
Sensory
Origin: Raphe nuclei; reticular formation
Function: Modulates 1° afferent.

AUTONOMIC EFFECTS

Parasympathetic

Craniosacral division. Primarily involves the protection, conservation, and restoration of body resources; slows heart rate, increases intestinal peristalsis and gland activity, and relaxes sphincters.

Sympathetic

Thoracolumbar division. Prepares the body for fight-or-flight responses; accelerates heart rate, constricts blood vessels, and raises blood pressure.

	PARASYMPATHETIC	*SYMPATHETIC*
Bronchi	Constriction	Dilation
Heart	Decreased heart rate	Increased heart rate
Intestines	Increased peristalsis	Decreased peristalsis
Pupils	Constriction	Dilation
Blood pressure	Decreased blood pressure	Increased blood pressure

MOTOR PATHWAYS

Corticospinal Tract

1. Also called pyramidal tract
2. Responsible for:
   - Voluntary movement
   - Grading motor response for fine movements
   - Inhibiting muscle tone

3. Pathway is originated in motor cortex of brain, travels down the corticospinal tract to the brainstem, crosses over the medulla (pyramidal decussation), and travels via the lateral corticospinal tract to the anterior horn cells (ventral gray matter). Approximately 10% of fibers do not cross over in the medulla. They will travel in the anterior corticospinal tracts to assist in voluntary motor control in the cervical and upper thoracic segments.

4. Upper motor neuron disorders

Cerebellar System

1. Responsible for:
   - Equilibrium
   - Posture control
   - Muscular activity
   - Sensory and motor input
2. Pathway varies: cortex or basal ganglia or sensory receptors; anterior horn cells
3. Lower motor neuron disorders

Extrapyramidal System

1. Responsible for:
   - Muscle tone
   - Control of body movements
2. Complex system of pathways between basal ganglia, brainstem, cerebral cortex, spinal cord, and anterior horn cells.

CHAPTER 4

Neurology

DISORDERS

Alzheimer's Disease

- A common degenerative disease that usually begins in later middle life with slight defects in memory and behavior.
- It occurs with equal frequency in men and women.
- The cerebral hemisphere undergoes marked atrophy with a widening of the sulci and lateral ventricles which can be seen on a C-scan.
- The disease is characterized by the patient's forgetfulness, paranoia, hostility, speech disturbances, confusion, and inability to carry out purposeful movements.
- Patient may become bedridden. It has no known cause, prevention, or cure.

Aneurysm

- A ballooning out of an arterial wall.
- It is usually caused by atherosclerosis and hypertension and less frequently by trauma, infection, or a congenital weakness in the vessel wall.
- Aneurysms most often occur in circle of Willis and are called berry aneurysms.

Anterior Cerebral Artery Lesion

- Contralateral hemiplegia
- Incontinence
- Hemiparesis
- Behavioral changes
- If this occurs in the nondominant hemisphere, apraxia would be indicated.
- If it occurs in the dominant hemisphere, aphasia would be indicated.

Anterior Communicating Artery Lesion

- Incontinence
- Impairment of intellect
- Innovative abilities lost
- Paraparesis

Anterior Inferior Cerebellar Artery Lesion

- Ipsilateral ataxia
- Contralateral pain and temperature deficits

- Ipsilateral deafness
- Ipsilateral facial paralysis
- Ipsilateral sensory loss to the face

Basal Ganglia Disorder

- Parkinson's disease: resting tremors, rigidity, shuffling gait, and mask-like face.
- Chorea: sudden uncontrolled movements; very jerky and brisk movements.
- Athetosis: very slow movements.
- Hemiballismus: sudden wild movements that involve only one side of the body.
- Tremor: an involuntary movement, usually with a consistent rhythm and amplitude.

Bell's Palsy

- Paralysis of the facial nerve.
- Typically occurs unilaterally and results in facial paralysis.
- It may be temporary or permanent.
- May result from infections, compression on a nerve by a tumor, or trauma to nerve.

Brown-Séquard's Syndrome

- Hemisection of the spinal cord; may be seen after knife-type injury to the spinal cord.
- Ipsilateral lower motor neuron paralysis at lesion level.
- Ipsilateral upper motor neuron paralysis below lesion.
- Contralateral loss of pain/temperature below lesion.
- Ipsilateral loss of vibration and proprioception below lesion level.
- Ipsilateral loss of kinesthetic sense/muscle tone below lesion level.

Brain Tumors—Neoplasm

- Tumors are space-occupying lesions that produce edema and epileptic-like seizures.
- They may cause increased intracranial pressure, headache, and vomiting.
- Tumors of the cerebellum can cause ataxia and falling.
- Frontal pole tumors can cause personality changes or loss of smell.
- Pituitary edema can cause optical and visual disturbances.

Cerebellar Disorders

- Ataxia: person will have poor coordination, as well as posture and gait difficulties.
- Athetosis: slow, writhing, continuous involuntary movement of the extremities.
- Chores: involuntary muscle twitching.
- Dysmetria: when reaching for an object, the person will overshoot the goal/object.
- Dysdiadochokinesia: person will demonstrate an inability to perform alternating movements.
- Asthenia: person will get tired very easily.
- Tremors: rhythmic, involuntary, nonpurposefully movements.
- Decreased tendon reflexes
- Slurred speech

Cerebral Vascular Accidents

- May be defined as damage to the brain as a result of a pathological condition of the blood vessels.
- Characterized by occlusion by an embolus or cerebrovascular hemorrhage, which results in ischemia of the brain tissues normally perfused by the damaged vessels.

Encephalitis

- An inflammation of the brain.
- May be caused by an infected mosquito bite, poisoning, or hemorrhage.
- Characterized by fevers, headache, nausea, vomiting, and neck pain.
- Patient may demonstrate neurological disturbances, seizures, paralysis, weakness, and irritability.
- Severity of condition depends on many factors, such as age of patient, time of diagnosis, cause and level of inflammation.

Epilepsy

- Repeated seizures due to sudden uncontrolled electric discharge of the nerve cells of the cerebral cortex.
- Symptoms may include altered consciousness, convulsions, stiffness of muscles, movement spasticity of muscles.
- They can be petit mal seizures, which are brief, or grand mal seizures, which last 2 to 5 minutes.

Guillain-Barré Syndrome

- Peripheral polyneuritis (also called infectious polyneuritis).
- Associated with viral infections or immunizations.
- Results in symmetrical wasting away of the extremities.
- Course of disease varies in symptoms (from mild to severe) and length of recovery.

Hydrocephalus

- A blockage in the ventricular system.
- The cerebrospinal fluid is prevented from flowing out and instead accumulates in the ventricles. This increases pressure in the cranial vault and causes a thinning out of the brain and widening of the ventricles.
- Most often occurs in newborns in which cranial bones are not yet fused.
- The fluid separates the bone and the head enlarges.

Internal Carotid Artery Lesion

- Aphasia when in the dominant hemisphere
- Contralateral hemiplegia
- Hemianesthesia
- Hemianopia
- Unilateral loss of vision

Amyotrophic Lateral Sclerosis (Lou Gehrig's Disease)

- Amyotrophic lateral sclerosis
- Upper and lower motor neuron disease
- Sensory losses
- Ataxia
- Decreased muscle tone
- Loss of kinesthetic sense
- Progressive

Middle Cerebral Artery Lesion

A. Involves the **dominant side** main trunk of the middle cerebral artery
- Motor aphasia
- Sensory aphasia
- Contralateral hemianesthesia
- Hemiplegia
- Homonymous hemianopsia

B. Involves the **nondominant side** main trunk of the middle cerebral artery
- Denial of the disease
- Contralateral hemiplegia
- Contralateral hemianesthesia
- Homonymous hemianopia
- Neglect of the left side
- This lesion occurs in the perforating branches of the artery
- Contralateral hemiplegia
- Contralateral rigidity
- Tremor

Multiple Sclerosis

- Progressive disease resulting from demyelination of nerve fibers of the spinal cord or brain.
- It has periods of remission and exacerbation.
- Disease usually shows up in young adults.
- Results in ataxia, abnormal reflexes, paresthesia, muscle weak-ness, vertigo, and vision disturbance.
- Symptoms will vary and there is no known cure.

Myasthenia Gravis

- Result is a fluctuation of muscle strength/weakness, especially muscles of the eyelid, face, jaws, and limbs. As a result, the patient has a drooping jaw, difficulties with swallowing, speech, facial expression, and changing.
- Treatment: muscle strengthening, range of motion.

Parkinson's Disease

- A slow, progressive, degenerative neurologic disorder that usually affects people over 50 years of age.
- The disease is characterized by resting tremors, slow shuffling gait, forward flexion of the trunk, muscle rigidity and weakness, and a masklike face.
- It has no known cause, prevention, or cure.

Polio

- Involves damage to anterior horn cells
- Lower motor neuron involvement
- Weakness
- Atrophy
- Fasciculation
- Hyperflexion

Posterior Cerebral Artery Lesion

- The main trunk
- Contralateral hemiparesis
- Sensory aphasia—dominant side
- Hemianopia
- Loss of superficial touch
- Loss of deep sensation

Posterior Inferior Cerebral Artery Lesion

- Ataxia
- Contralateral hemianalgesia
- Difficulty swallowing
- Intentional tremors
- Ipsilateral weakness of the tongue
- Ipsilateral weakness of the vocal cords
- Nystagmus

Superior Cerebral Artery Lesion

- Contralateral hemianesthesia
- Contralateral hemianalgesia
- Contralateral facial weakness
- Ipsilateral ataxia

Transient Ischemic Attack (TIA)

- Defined as an episode of cerebrovascular insufficiency or occlusion of a small artery.
- This causes the patient to lose consciousness briefly, be confused and disoriented, experience difficulty with speech and tongue movement, but awake with no paralysis.
- The attack is usually brief, lasting a few minutes.

Upper Motor Neuron Lesion

- Spastic paralysis
- No muscle atrophy
- Hyperactive reflexes
- Pathological reflexes, Babinski sign
- Fasciculation/fibrillation not present

Lower Motor Neuron Lesion

- Flaccid paralysis
- Muscle atrophy
- Absent reflexes
- No pathological reflexes
- Fasciculation/fibrillation present

Vertebrobasilar Artery Lesion

- Anesthesia of both sides of the body
- Areflexia
- Coma
- Confusion/loss of memory
- Dizziness
- Headache

REFLEX

An involuntary response to a sensory stimulus.

Cross Extension Reflex

Functions to coordinate reciprocal limb movement as in gait patterns.

Flexor Reflex

Functions as a protective withdrawal reflex to move the body away from a harmful stimulus.

Inverse Stretch Reflex

Functions to provide agonist inhibition and decreases the force of the agonist contraction.

Stretch Reflex

Functions to support agonist muscle contraction and maintenance of muscle tone by providing feedback about muscle length.

Grades of Muscle Stretch Reflexes

0	Areflexia
+	Hyporeflexia
1 to 3	Average
3+ to 4+	Hyperreflexia

MUSCLE STRETCH REFLEXES

SEGMENTAL AND NERVE LEVEL	REFLEX	STIMULUS	RESPONSE
Pons, trigeminal	Jaw maxillary nerve	Tap mandible, half open position	Closure of jaw
C5, C6 musculocutaneous nerve	Biceps	Tap biceps tendon	Contraction of biceps
C5, C6 musculocutaneous nerve	Brachioradialis	At insertion of brachioradialis, styloid process of radius	Flexion of elbow and pronation of forearm
C5 to T1	Scapular, interscapular	Stroking skin between scapulae	Contraction of scapular muscles
C6, C7, C8 radial nerve	Triceps	Tap triceps tendon	Extension of elbow
C7, C8 radial nerve	Wrist extension	Tap wrist extensor tendons	Extension of wrist
C6, C7, C8 median nerve	Wrist flexion	Tap wrist flexor tendons	Flexion of wrist
L4, L5 superior gluteal nerve	Gluteal	Stroking skin of buttocks	Contraction of gluteus
L2, L3, L4 femoral nerve	Patellar	Tap patellar tendon	Extension of leg at knee
S1, S2 tibial nerve	Tendocalcaneus	Stroke Achilles' tendon	Plantar flexion at ankle
S1, S2 tibial nerve	Plantar	Stroke sole of foot	Plantar flexion of toes

PATHOLOGICAL REFLEXES

NAME	STIMULUS	RESPONSE
Asymmetrical tonic reflex	Rotate the head to one side	Flexion of skull limbs and extension of jaw limbs
Babinski's sign	Stroke the outer edge of the sole of the foot	Extension of great toe, flexion of small toes, and spreading of toes
Clonus—upper extremity	Rapid extension of wrist	Rapid reciprocal flexion and extension
Clonus—lower extremity	Rapid dorsiflexion of the ankle	Continued and prolonged reciprocal plantar flexion and dorsi flexion of the ankle
Cross extension	Patient supine, both legs flexed at hip, stimulate the sole of the foot	Extension of contralateral extremity
Extensor thrust	Therapist vigorously dorsiflexes the foot of a leg that has been flexed at hip	Extension of that entire lower extremity
Flexor withdrawal	Lower extremity in extended position stimulates sole of foot	The leg will withdraw from the stimulus; cause an over-response of hip and knee flexion
Forced grasping	Stroke the patient's palm in radial direction	Grasp reaction
Hirschberg's sign	Stroke the medial border of foot	Adduction and inversion of foot
Klippel-Weil thumb sign	Patient's flexed fingers are rapidly extended	Flexion and adduction of the thumb
Marie-Fox	Forcefully flex the patient's toes	Flexion at hip and knee
Negative support reaction	Have patient bounce several times on soles of feet, but do not allow weightbearing	Flexor tone in lower extremities will increase

PATHOLOGICAL REFLEXES, CONTINUED

NAME	STIMULUS	RESPONSE
Positive support reaction	Have patient bounce several times on soles of feet, allowing the lower extremities to bear weight	Extensor tone in the lower extremities will increase
Righting reaction	Push the patient forward/backward and laterally	Head will try to orient itself, maintain midline
Rossolimo's sign	Tap on the balls of patient's foot	Flexion of toes
Strümpell's tibialis anterior sign	Patient flexes the hip	Dorsiflexion and adduction of the foot
Strümpell's pronation sign	Patient flexes the forearm	The hand touches the shoulder
Symmetrical tonic neck reflex	Place the head in flexion or extension	In flexed position, flexion of arms, extension of legs; with head extension, extension of arms, flexion of legs
Tonic labyrinthine	None required. Response depends on patient positioning	Prone: flexor tone increase. Supine: extensor tone increase. Sidelying: extensor tone in side lying limbs will increase; flexor tone in nonweightbearing limbs will increase

SYNERGY PATTERNS

Synergy occurs as a result of the following:
- The muscles work together as one bound unit
- Reflexes occur at the spinal cord level
- The reflexes are primitive or automatic in nature

UPPER EXTREMITY

JOINT	FLEXION	EXTENSION
Shoulder girdle	Elevation, retraction	Depression, protraction
Shoulder	Abduction	*Adduction
	External rotation	Internal rotation
Elbow	*Flexion	Extension
Forearm	Supination	*Pronation
Wrist	Flexion	Extension
Fingers	Flexion	Flexion

Note: Wrist/fingers will vary
*Strong components of the synergism

LOWER EXTREMITY

JOINT	FLEXION	EXTENSION
Hip	*Flexion	Extension
	*Abduction	*Adduction
	*External rotation	Internal rotation
Knee	Flexion	*Extension
Ankle	*Dorsiflexion	*Plantar flexion
Foot	Inversion	*Inversion
Toes	Dorsiflexion	Plantar flexion, great toe may extend

*Strong components of the synergism

THREE STAGES OF RECOVERY IN A CVA

1. **Flaccid Stage**
   - Mobility in turning from supine to sidelying and sitting to supine
   - Preparation for sitting up
   - Preparation for standing up, control of leg
   - Trunk balance
   - Control of upper extremity
   - Stimulation and facilitation to increase tone/voluntary movements

2. **Spasticity Stage**
   - Progression of treatment to work on rehabilitation of patient in the sitting and standing positions as much as possible. Some treatment started in stage 1 will still be performed in the supine position.
   - Inhibition techniques to supine spasticity
   - Weightbearing on extremity
   - Sitting
   - Standing
   - Progression to treatment in prone lying and kneeling
   - Gait training
   - Working for independent control of extremity joints
   - Facilitation for voluntary movement
   - Placing

3. **Stages of Relative Recovery**
   - Treatments to improve patient's gait, balance, and coordination
   - Dissociation of mass patterns of movements
   - Activities of daily living

DIAGONAL PATTERNS

PNF (proprioceptive neuromuscular facilitation) diagonals are named according to the movement that takes place. The pattern starts with the opposite positioning so that the maximal movement can take place. For example, D1 flexion for glenohumeral will start with the patient positioned in internal rotation, extension, and abduction. The finished position is then external rotation, flexion, and adduction.

UPPER EXTREMITY DIAGONALS

JOINT	FLEXION	EXTENSION
Diagonal One (D1)		
Scapula thoracic	Rotation, abduction, anterior elevation	Rotation, adduction, posterior depression
Glenohumeral	External rotation, flexion, adduction	Internal rotation, extension, abduction
Elbow	Flexion	Extension
Radioulnar	Supination	Pronation
Wrist	Flexion, radial deviation	Extension, ulnar deviation
Fingers	Flexion, adduction to radial side	Extension, abduction to ulnar side
Thumb	Flexion, adduction	Extension, abduction
Diagonal Two (D2)		
Scapula thoracic	Rotation, abduction, posterior elevation	Rotation, abduction, anterior depression
Glenohumeral	External rotation, flexion, abduction	Internal rotation, extension, adduction
Elbow	Flexion	Extension
Radioulnar	Supination	Pronation
Wrist	Extension, radial deviation	Flexion, ulnar deviation
Finger	Extension, abduction to the radial side	Flexion, adduction to ulnar side
Thumb	Extension, adduction	Flexion, abduction

LOWER EXTREMITY DIAGONALS

JOINT	FLEXION	EXTENSION
Diagonal One (D1)		
Hip	External rotation, flexion, adduction	Internal rotation, extension, abduction
Knee	Flexion or extension	Extension or flexion
Ankle	Dorsiflexion	Plantar flexion
Subtalar	Inversion	Eversion
Toes	Extension, abduction to tibial side	Flexion, adduction to fibular side
Diagonal Two (D2)		
Hip	Internal rotation, flexion, abduction	External rotation, extension, adduction
Knee	Flexion or extension	Extension or flexion
Ankle	Dorsiflexion	Plantar flexion
Subtalar	Eversion	Inversion
Toes	Extension, abduction to the fibular side	Flexion, adduction to the tibial side

PNF TERMS

Manual contact: firm contact over muscles facilitates the agonist to contract. Light touch may facilitate movement. Maintaining touch may facilitate a holding response. The therapist applies pressure (firm, light, or maintains pressure) for the purpose of stimulating the muscle, tendon, and joint afferent.

Maximal resistance: the therapist applies maximal resistance to stronger muscles in an attempt to create an overflow response to weaker muscles.

Reinforcement: the utilization of major muscle groups or other body parts coordinated to produce a desired movement pattern.

Timing for emphasis: maximum resistance in a sequence of contractions is used to elicit overflow from strong to weaker components. May be used for weakness or incoordination.

Traction: force used to separate a joint surface by manual contact.

PNF TECHNIQUES

Approximation: joint compression to stimulate afferent nerve endings. This is utilized to promote stability and facilitate postural extension.

Contract/relax: the therapist passively moves the body part to its limited point of range of motion. The patient then contracts the muscle against therapist resistance. The therapist resists all motion except for rotation. The patient then relaxes and the therapist moves it passively in the opposite direction caused by the contraction. This technique is used to increase range of motion of the agonist muscle.

Hold/relax: the therapist passively moves the body part to its limited point of range of motion. The patient contracts and the therapist provides resistance, allowing no movement to occur. This is different than contract/relax, in which rotation may occur. Next the patient is asked to relax allowing movement to take place and the therapist passively moves in the newly gained range of motion. Hold/relax is utilized to increase range of motion movement and decrease muscle spasms.

Repeated contractions: isometric contraction followed by repeated isotonic contraction and quick stretches. Can be performed anywhere within the patient's range of motion. Utilized to facilitate the agonist and relax the antagonist. It is performed on patients to increase strength, coordination, and endurance.

Rhythmic initiation: passive motion, then assistive motion, then resistive motion by alternating patterns to promote the ability to initiate movement, promotes relaxation, and decreases rigidity.

Rhythmic stabilization: performed by having the patient alternate isometric contraction of the agonist and antagonist muscles. Utilized to promote stability and to relax the antagonist.

Slow reversal: an alternating pattern of opposing muscle groups to stimulate the agonist through active motion, then relaxation of the antagonist, then coordination between agonist and antagonist. Utilized for a patient who has an inability to reverse direction and muscle imbalance. It will increase muscle strength, improve coordination, and increase endurance.

Slow reversal-hold: an alternating pattern of opposing muscle groups with a pause between reversals to cause relaxation of the antagonist and to stimulate the agonist. Utilized for a patient who has an inability to reverse direction and muscle imbalance. It will increase muscle strength, improve coordination, and increase endurance.

Slow reversal-hold-relax: the patient, through active range of motion, brings the body part to the point of limitation and then reverses direction. The therapist applies resistance to rotation and isometric contraction of the shortened muscle. Next, the patient relaxes and moves the body part in the direction of limitation. This technique is utilized repeatedly to increase range of motion of the agonist.

BERTA BOBATH THEORY OF AUTOMATIC REACTIONS

Berta Bobath, PT, and Karl Bobath, MD, developed this approach. Their treatment was based on the theory of inhibiting abnormal reflex patterns and facilitating righting and equilibrium reaction. The righting and equilibrium reactions are performed in a special sequential order according to development pattern to facilitate movement and control tone.

Three Automatic Reactions

Righting Reactions
- Maintain and restore normal position of the head in space.
- Maintain and restore normal position of the head with regard to trunk alignment.
- Maintain and restore normal position of the head and the four extremities.
- Align the body as necessary for various motor activities.
- Overlap with equilibrium reactions.
- Adjust posture.

Equilibrium Reactions
- Automatic reactions that maintain and restore balance during activities.
- Inhibition of abnormal patterns of posture and movement.

Automatic Adaptation of Muscle Joints to Changes in Posture
- Postural reflex mechanisms
- Postural adaptation to growth
- Assessment
  - Balance
  - Range of motion
  - Postural tone
  - Motor patterns (quality of movement)
  - Sensory deficit—pressure/light touch
  - Proprioception
  - Stereognosis
  - Postural reactions
  - Placing
- Emphasis on the quality of movement available, postural and protective reactions, and postural tone.

SIGNE BRUNNSTROM'S THEORY OF REHABILITATION FOR A CVA

Brunnstrom, unlike Berta Bobath, believed that you should enhance the synergy patterns for treatment. Signe Brunnstrom's theory describes six stages of recovery for the hemiplegic patient. They are:

1. **Initial stage:** no voluntary movement of the affected limb can be initiated; spasticity is absent. Through evaluation, no voluntary movements are present, little or no resistance to passive movements.

2. **Recovery stage:** basic limb synergies are now appearing as weak associated reactions on voluntary attempts to move by the patient. The basic limb synergies in their components now make their appearance as weak associated reactions. This is where you start to see the beginning of flexor synergy patterns of the upper extremity and extensor synergy patterns of the lower extremity. Evaluation of the patient will demonstrate that when movement is attempted there is associated movements through synergy patterns.

3. **Stage three:** the basic limb synergies are performed voluntarily by the patient. In this stage spasticity is also increasing. Upon evaluation, there is full upper extremity synergy patterns along with ankle flexion.

4. **Stage four:** the patient progressed beyond stage three and the spasticity begins to decrease. Here you might observe some initial movement combinations that deviate from the basic limb synergy patterns. The patient may have lateral prehension and semivoluntary finger extension. Upon evaluation, the patient can place his or her hand behind the back, flex the glenohumeral joint with elbow extension, pronate and supinate the forearm with elbow flexion at 90°, sit and dorsiflex the foot while keeping the foot on the floor, sit and slide the foot on the floor by flexing the knee past 90°.

5. **Stage five:** spasticity continues to decrease and the patient increasingly becomes independent from the basic limb synergies. The patient has palmar prehension and voluntary extension of digits. Upon evaluation the patient can perform the test in stage four with greater ease and efficiency. He or she can abduct at the glenohumeral joint with elbow extended, flex the shoulder past 90° with elbow extended, pronate/supinate the forearm with elbow extension and abduction of glenohumeral joint, stand nonweightbearing with affected limb, knee flexed and hip extended, stand with heel forward, knee extended, and dorsiflex the ankle.

6. **Stage six:** patient demonstrates isolated joint movements that are now freely performed. Movements appear to be well coordinated and near normal. The basic limb synergies no longer interfere with the patient's movement. Upon evaluation, the patient can perform the test in stage five with greater ease and efficiency. The patient can stand and abduct the hip, sit and reciprocally contract the medial and lateral hamstring muscles, causing inversion and eversion.

Brunnstrom's Stages of Recovery for the Upper Extremity

1. **Stage one:** initially, the upper extremity is flaccid and no voluntary movement on the affected limb can be initiated.
2. **Stage two:** the beginning of spasticity. Basic limb synergies or some other components are present.
3. **Stage three:** the active initiation of synergies. Spasticity has increased and becomes marked.
4. **Stage four:** patient's movement deviates from the synergies. Example: patient has elevation of the arm to forward horizontal position with the elbow fully extended. Movement deviating from the synergy would be stage four. There are some movement combinations that deviate from the basic limb synergies.
5. **Stage five:** patient performs movement independent of the synergy. Spasticity is decreasing. Example: patient can abduct the arm to the side position with the elbow fully extended and the forearm pronated.
6. **Stage six:** isolated joint movement. Movements are well coordinated and appear normal. Example: patient would have lateral prehension for grasping small objects, such as a card.

Brunnstrom's Stages of Recovery for the Lower Extremity

1. **Stage one:** flaccidity.
2. **Stage two:** minimal voluntary movements of the lower limb.
3. **Stage three:** the ability to perform hip-knee-ankle flexion in sitting.
4. **Stage four:** the ability to perform voluntary dorsiflexion of the ankle in sitting.
5. **Stage five:** the ability to stand isolated, nonweightbearing with knee flexion and hip extended.
6. **Stage six:** the ability to stand and perform outward rotation of the leg at the knee, as well as inversion and eversion of the ankle.

Brunnstrom's Stages of Recovery for the Hand

1. **Stage one:** flaccidity.
2. **Stage two:** no active finger flexion.
3. **Stage three:** mass grasp.
4. **Stage four:** lateral prehension.
5. **Stage five:** palmar prehension.
6. **Stage six:** control of all prehension.

Brunnstrom Evaluates the Quality of Movement as Follows

- Nonfunctional (NF)
- Assistive (A)
- Functional (F)

The therapist is instructed to select a grade (NF, A, or F) for movement of the upper extremity, lower extremity, and trunk.

ROOD SENSORY STIMULATION TECHNIQUES

Theory by Margaret Rood, who was a physical therapist and occupational therapist.

Basic Principles

1. Motor output is dependent upon sensory input. Therefore, you can use sensory stimulus to activate and inhibit a motor response.
2. Motor response follows a normal developmental sequence pattern.
   Stages of muscle development:

- Full range of shortening and lengthening and reciprocal innervation
- Patterns of cocontraction and stability; tonic postural set
- Patterns of heavy weight movement and movement in weightbearing position
- Skilled or coordinated movement; movement in nonweightbearing position with stabilization at proximal joint

3. In early stages, patients who do not demonstrate motor control would benefit from sensory stimulus.
4. Early use of stimulus should be discontinued as soon as patient demonstrates active control. This decreases dependence upon the therapist.
5. Patients who show a low-level response to stimuli may need repeated application of stimulus or a combination of stimulus to produce results.
6. Avoid overloading a patient with too much sensory stimulation and causing an overload effect.

STIMULATION TECHNIQUES

Exteroceptive Stimulation Techniques

- High-frequency vibration (50 to 300 Hz): facilitation of agonist, inhibition of antagonist.
- Low-frequency vibration (5 to 50 Hz): inhibition of agonist.
- Neutral warmth (35° to 37°C): relaxation, inhibition of postural tone, decreased pain, calming effect.
- Pressure on tendons: firm, constant pressure to decreased tone, and generalized inhibition.
- Prolonged icing: inhibition of muscle tone, spasms, and pain.
- Quick icing facilitation of muscles.
- Quick stretch, tapping of muscle belly or tendon: facilitation of agonist.
- Prolonged stretch: inhibition of muscle response or decrease of tone.

Vestibular Stimulation Techniques

- Fast spinning: facilitates postural tone, promotes head righting and increased motor coordination.
- Head down position, prone over a large ball: can activate postural extensors of neck, trunk, and proximal joints. Soothing effect, especially sympathetic responses.
- Slow rocking, rolling on ball: inhibits postural tone; calming effect and relaxation.

Proprioception Stimulation Techniques

- Quick stretch
- Tapping of muscle belly or tendon
- Joint approximation
- Joint traction
- High-frequency vibration
- Low-frequency vibration
- Prolonged slow stretch
- Firm pressure to tendons

LEVELS OF COGNITIVE FUNCTION

Rancho Los Amigos Scale

1. Level one—No response.
   Patient is unresponsive to any stimulus and appears to be in a deep sleep.
2. Level two—Generalized response.
   Patient occasionally reacts to stimuli but not in a purposeful pattern. Response is limited and inconsistent.
3. Level three—Localized response.
   Patient reacts to stimuli but continues to be inconsistent. May follow simple commands in a delayed manner.
4. Level four—Confused/agitated.
   Patient responds to stimuli but is unable to process information purposefully. Patient is in a heightened state of activity and behavior is bizarre. Patient is not able to cooperate with treatment program.

5. Level five—Confused/inappropriate/nonagitated.
   Patient is alert and able to follow very simple commands with fluctuating consistency. If instructions are increasing in complexity, the patient will demonstrate inconsistency.
6. Level six—Confused/appropriate.
   Patient can follow directions but only with direct assistance from another individual. Goal-oriented behavior with directions.
7. Level seven—Automatic/appropriate.
   Patient can go through daily routine automatically but robot-like, with shallow recall of activities.
8. Level eight—Purposeful/appropriate.
   Patient shows carryover for new learning and needs no supervision once activities are learned. Patient is able to recall and is aware of and responsive to environment.

LEVEL OF CONSCIOUSNESS

Glasgow Coma Scale

- This scale is utilized to determine the level of consciousness of the patient.
- The patient is scored according to three categories:
  1. Eye opening
  2. Verbal response
  3. Motor response
- The test is administered and the score added. If the patient has a score of 9 or above, he or she is determined not clinically diagnosed to be in a coma. A score of 7 or less would indicate that the patient is in a coma.

GLASGOW COMA SCALE

EYE OPENING	MOTOR RESPONSE	VERBAL RESPONSE
Spontaneous: 4 points Indicates that brain arousal systems are active.	Obeys commands: 6 points May not have a grasp reflex or a change in posture as a response	Oriented: 5 points Patient will know who, where they are, month, year, and season
To sound: 3 points Eyes will open to sound stimulus	Localized: 5 points Will attempt to respond to stimulus by moving extremity	Confused: 4 points Responds to questions but will have some degree of confusion and disorientation
To pain: 2 points Eyes will open to pain stimulus applied to extremities	Flexor normal: 4 points In response to stimulus, will flex entire shoulder or arm	Inappropriate: 3 points Speech is understandable but patient cannot sustain a conversation
Never: 1 point	Flexion abnormal: 3 points Response to painful stimulus is decorticating rigidity posture	Incomprehensible: 2 points Speech is not understandable but patient can make sounds of moaning and groans
	Extension: 2 points Response is abnormal adduction with internal rotation of the shoulder and pronation of the forearm	None: 1 point
	None: 1 point	

NEUROLOGY DIAGNOSTIC TEST

Cerebral Angiography

An x-ray procedure for visualizing the vascular system of the brain. Radiopaque contrast material is injected into a carotid, subclavian, brachial, or femoral artery with x-rays at specific intervals.

Computed Tomography (CT Scan)

An x-ray technique that produces a film representing a detailed cross-section of tissue structure. CT scan employs a narrowly collimated beam of x-rays that rotates in a continuous 360° motion around the patient. The image is created by computer, using multiple readings of the patient in cross-sectional slices. This is a noninvasive and painless procedure for the patient.

Echoencephalogram

A recording produced by an echoencephalograph, which uses ultrasound to study the intracranial structures of the brain.

Electroencephalography (EEG)

The process of recording brainwave activity. Electrodes are attached to various areas of the patient's head. The patient must refrain from talking or moving and must remain still. The test is used to diagnose seizure and brainstem disorders, focal lesions, and impaired consciousness.

Electromyogram (EMG)

A record of the intrinsic electric activity in a skeletal muscle is obtained by applying surface electrodes or by inserting a needle electrode into the muscle. The physician observes electric activity with an oscilloscope and a loudspeaker. EMGs also measure electric potentials induced by voluntary muscular contraction.

Evoked Potential (EP)

A tracing of a brainwave measured on the surface of the head at various places. The evoked potential is elicited by a specific stimulus that may affect the visual, somatosensory and auditory pathways, producing a characteristic brainwave pattern.

Lumbar Puncture (LP)

The introduction of a hollow needle and stylet into the subarachnoid space of the lumbar portion of the spinal canal at the third and fourth lumbar vertebrae. The patient is placed in a lateral recumbent position, with the back as near the edge of the bed as possible. The legs should be flexed with the thighs flexed on the abdomen. Head and shoulders should be bent down, curving the spine convexly to grant the greatest amount of space between the vertebrae. The test is done to evaluate spinal fluid and measure intracranial pressure. The complications of testing may include headaches, infections, and epidural hematomas.

Magnetic Resonance Imaging (MRI)

Medical imaging that utilizes nuclear magnetic resonance as a source of energy. This procedure is noninvasive and painless for the patient. Allows for three-dimensional viewing and high resolution.

Myelography

A radiographic process by which the spinal cord and spinal subarachnoid space are viewed and photographed. A contrast medium is introduced. This test is used to identify spinal lesions.

Nerve Conduction Velocity (NCV)

Refers to the maximum nerve conduction velocity, which is the speed with which an electrical impulse can be transmitted through excitable tissue.

Position Emission Tomography (PET)

Radioisotopes are injected and emissions are measure by a gamma ray detector system.

This test does provide information on the cerebral blood flow and brain metabolism, however, it is not as detailed as computerized tomography or magnetic resonance imaging.

Ventriculography

An x-ray examination of the head after an injection of air or another contrast medium into the cerebral ventricles, or an x-ray examination of a ventricle of the heart after the injection of a radiopaque contrast medium.

CHAPTER 5

Cardiac Anatomy & Physiology

BLOOD SUPPLY

Arteries

Transport oxygenated blood to the heart through the heart pump to maintain arterial circulation.

Right Coronary Artery

Supplies the right atrium, most of the right ventricle, inferior wall of the left ventricle in most humans; bundle of His, atrioventricular node, and sinoatrial node in approximately 60% of humans.

Left Main Coronary Artery

Supplies most of the left ventricle mass and splits into two branches: the circumflex artery and left anterior descending artery. The circumflex artery supplies the inferior wall of the left ventricle when not supplied by the right coronary artery, left atrium, and sinoatrial node in approximately 40% of humans. The left anterior descending artery supplies the left ventricle, interventricular septum, right ventricle, and inferior areas of the apex and both ventricles.

Coronary Artery Dominance

The right coronary artery is dominant in approximately two-thirds of humans and branches into the posterior descending branches. The right coronary artery will supply part of the left ventricle and ventricular septum. This is called "right dominance." In one-third of humans the branch of the circumflex artery is dominant. Dominance is from branches of both the right coronary artery and the circumflex artery. This is called left dominance.

Capillaries

These are tiny blood vessels that assist in exchange of nutrients and fluids between the blood and tissue. In the heart, they connect the arteries to the veins, creating a large network system.

Veins

These transport unoxygenated blood from the whole body (except the lungs) to the right atrium of the heart. The coronary sinus drains the left atrium and both ventricles and the posterior right atrium and ventricles. The anterior cardiac vein drains the anterior right ventricle. The small cardiac vein (thebesian) drains both atria.

Conduction

Conduction of the heart originates through the sinoatrial node. This sends an impulse to both atria. Next the impulse conducts to the atria ventricle node, which is transmitted to the Purkinje's fibers. This sends an impulse to the ventricles, which contract.

Atrioventricular (AV) node is located in the junction of the right atrium and right ventricle. It merges with the bundle of His. It consists of both parasympathetic and sympathetic innervators.

Sinoatrial (SA) node is located in the junction of the right atrium and superior vena cava. It consists of both parasympathetic and sympathetic innervators and is considered the main pacemaker of the heart.

Purkinje's fiber is located on either side of the intraventricular septum in the right and left branches of the atrioventricular node. It provides special conduction tissue in the ventricles, Purkinje's fibers.

HEART VALVES

Aortic Valve

Composed of three semilunar cusps that are located between the left ventricle and aorta. They prevent blood from flowing back into the left ventricle from the aorta. Area to auscultate is the second right intercostal space at the right sternal border (base of heart).

Atrioventricular Valve

A valve in the heart through which blood flows from the atria to the ventricles. This valve prevents backflow of blood into the atria and closes when the ventricular walls contract. The valve located between the left atrium and left ventricle is the mitral valve. The right atrioventricular valve is the tricuspid valve.

Bicuspid or Mitral Valve

Consists of two cusps (bicuspid) and is located between the left atrium and left ventricle. Allows blood to flow from left atrium to left ventricle but closes to prevent backflow of blood into the atrium. Area to auscultate is the fifth left intercostal space at the midclavicular line (apical area).

Pulmonic Valve

Composed of three semilunar cusps that close during each heartbeat to prevent blood from flowing back into the right ventricle from the pulmonary artery. Area to auscultate is the second left intercostal space at the left sternal border.

Tricuspid Valve or Right Atrioventricular Valve

A valve consisting of three main cusps (ventral, dorsal, and medial cusps) and is located between the right atrium and right ventricle of the heart. The tricuspid allows blood flow into ventricles and closes to prevent backflow into the atria. Area to auscultate is fourth left intercostal space along the lower left sternal border.

HEART TISSUE

Epicardium

The inner layer of one of the pericardium. One of three layers; it is composed of a single sheet of squamous epithelial.

Endocardium

The lining of the heart chamber composed of small blood vessels and smooth muscles.

Myocardium

The middle layer of the heart composed of thick muscle cells, which form a major portion of the heart wall.

Pericardium

A tough white fibrous sac that surrounds the heart and roots of the great vessels. It consists of the serous pericardium and the fibrous pericardium. It protects the heart and the serous membranes.

HEART CHAMBERS

Left Atrium

Receives oxygenated blood from pulmonary veins. Sends blood into the left ventricle from the atria during diastole.

Left Ventricle

High-pressure circulatory that pumps blood through the aorta and systemic arteries, the capillaries, and back through the veins to the right atrium.

Right Atrium

Sends deoxygenated blood from the superior and inferior vena cava and the coronary sinus into the right ventricle.

Right Ventricle

Low-pressure pump that sends blood from the pulmonary artery to the lungs for oxygenation.

HEART RATE

- Normal: 80 to 100 beats per minute
- Bradycardia: heart rate under 60 beats per minute
- Tachycardia: heart rate above 100 beats per minute
- Maximum heart rate: 220 minus age

BLOOD PRESSURE

Systole

The period of cardiac contraction. Correlates with first heart sound when taking blood pressure.

Diastole

The period of cardiac relaxation or filling. Correlates with last heart sound when taking blood pressure.

Normal

Depends on age and will vary.

AGE	SYSTOLIC	DIASTOLIC
1 month	80	45
6 months	90	60
2 years	80 to 90	55 to 65
4 years	100 to 115	55 to 75
6 years	105 to 125	60 to 80
8 years	105 to 125	65 to 80
10 years	110 to 135	65 to 80
12 years	115 to 135	65 to 80
14 years	120 to 140	70 to 85
Adult	110 to 140	60 to 80
Elderly	Slightly higher than adult	Slightly lower than adult

Hypertension

Blood pressure at 140/90 or above must be tested three times to be conclusive.

Hypotension

Abnormally low blood pressure
- Occurs in shock
- Orthostatic hypotension—can occur as a result of patient assuming an upright position; especially common after long periods of bedrest

HEART SOUNDS

Normal Heart Sounds

1. S1 (lub): atrioventricular valves closing. This is the sound heard when the tricuspid and mitral valves are closing inside the heart.
2. S2 (dub): this is the sound heard when the pulmonic and aortic valves are closing inside the heart.

Abnormal Heart Sounds

1. S3 (ventricular gallop): may be audible immediately following the second heart sound. This would indicate decompensated heart functioning or heart failure if heard in an older person or someone with heart disease. When heard in healthy children, young adults, or athletes, it is considered a physiologically normal sound.
2. S4 (atrial gallop): may be heard immediately preceding the first heart sound and is associated with increased resistance to ventricular filling. Sign of ventricle noncompliance. Often heard in persons with hypertensive heart disease, coronary artery disease, and myocardiopathy.
3. Murmur: turbulent blood flow through a valve. Can be stenosis or prolapsed valve.
4. Pericardial friction rub: inflammation of pericardial sac. High-pitched scratching sound.

GRADING SYSTEM

1 Softest audible murmur
2 Medium audible murmur
3 Loud murmur without thrill
4 Murmur with thrill
5 Loudest murmur that cannot be heard with stethoscope off the chest
6 Audible murmur that can be heard with stethoscope off the chest

EKG WAVES

Electrocardiogram (EKG): test that measures the electrical activity of the heart.

Normal

P wave: Atrial depolarization
QRS complex: Ventricular depolarization
ST segment: Pause
T wave: Ventricular repolarization

Abnormal EKG Readings

- Abnormal P wave could result in an atrial or ventricular arrhythmia.
- QRS wave elevation on an EKG is indicative of possible hypertrophy of the myocardium. QRS wave depression is indicative of possible heart failure or chronic obstructive disorder.

- Abnormally elevated ST segment is indicative of an acute heart attack or a myocardial infarction.
- Abnormal Q wave shows a past history of a possible myocardial infarction. Determining when the infarction occurred is beyond the capabilities of an EKG alone. Clinical follow-up should be performed on the patient to determine the age of the infarct.
- An abnormal or inverted T wave could be indicative of ischemia.

CHAPTER 6

Cardiology

TREATMENT OPTIONS

Angioplasty

Also called percutaneous transluminal coronary angioplasty, it is a nonsurgical technique for coronary artery disease (atherosclerosis). A balloon-tipped catheter is inserted and inflated under the radiographic or ultrasonic visual field. The balloon is inflated and deflated until it is confirmed that there is arterial dilation and reduced pressure in the artery. The balloon-tipped catheter is then removed from the patient and the artery is left unoccluded. The angioplasty also helps alleviate anginal pain. This procedure's advantage over bypass surgery is that the patient does not have to undergo open chest surgery, thereby eliminating the risks associated with surgery and having a shorter recovery period.

Coronary Artery Bypass Graft (CABG)

An open-heart surgical technique utilized to bypass clogged, blocked, and narrowing vessels. The saphenous vein, from the patient's leg, is used as a graft to route blood around the blockage to an alternative route to the heart. Another option for the graft is to use the internal mammary artery. It is possible for the patient to have double, triple, and quadruple bypass surgery. This is utilized to relieve anginal pain and improve blood flow to the heart muscle.

Coronary Stents

A coronary stent may be utilized on a severely occluded or blocked coronary artery.

The surgical procedure involves placing a stent in the occluded artery to keep the artery open and maintain a normal blood flow. The stent allows the blood to flow to the heart muscle. A balloon expandable stent is placed in the artery to keep it open; the balloon can be inflated to open the artery up to normal blood flow and is left inside the patient. An advantage to the stent over angioplasty and coronary artery bypass graft is that the stents require less repeat surgeries. Approximately 30% of patients receiving angioplasty and coronary artery bypass grafts have repeated surgery due to renarrowing of the arteries within 3 years.

Transplantation

- Patients are accepted as heart transplantation candidates because they cannot survive without the transplantation.
- Patients may also be considered candidates if they have an ejection fraction of less then 20%.
- Absolute contraindications include uncontrolled malignancy or infections.
- Other possible contraindications are individual and decided by each facility.
- Homologous transplants are from another human.
- Orthotopic homologous transplantation refers to the grafting of the donor heart into the normal heart site.
- Heterotopic homologous transplantation refers to when the patient's heart remains intact and the donor's heart is placed parallel.
- Post-transplantation concerns include infections and rejection.
- Physical therapy starts in the coronary care unit (CCU).

Ventricular Assistive Device

- A mechanical device also called a left ventricular assistive device (LAVD).
- This device is being developed to help patient's stay alive while awaiting heart surgery.
- The device provides circulatory support by pumping blood through the body.

Medication Therapy*

A wide variety of medications may be utilized in treatment of cardiac disease and disorders. Medications may be used to alleviate symptoms (eg, nitroglycerin to decrease angina pain). Listed below are samples of pharmacology agents that are used in cardiac treatments:

1. **Antiarrhythmics**
   - Used to alleviate, prevent, or correct a cardiac arrhythmia
   - Alters conductivity
   - Prolongs the refractory period
   - Improves cardiac output
   - Goal is to have diastolic at 90 or lower
   - Quinidine, disopyramide, and procainamide

2. **Anticoagulants**
   - Used to prevent blood clot formation
   - Coumadin, aspirin, and platelet inhibitors

3. **Antihypertensives**
   - Reduces high blood pressure
   - Reduces myocardial oxygen demands
   - Decreases myocardial force and rate of contraction
   - Diazoxide, guanethidine, and propranolol

4. **Beta Adrenergic Blocking Agents**
   - Reduces blood pressure
   - Decreases rate and force of heart contractions
   - Blocks sympathetic conduction at B-receptors
   - Also utilized for angina, arrhythmias, and hypertension
   - Acebutolol, metoprolol, Lopressor, Inderal, and propranolol

5. **Calcium Channel Blocking Agents**
   - Inhibits the flow of calcium ions across the membranes of smooth muscle cells
   - Lowers heart rate and blood pressure
   - Helps to control chest pain and arrhythmias
   - Relaxes smooth muscle tone
   - Diltiazem (Cardizem), nifedipine (Procardia), and verapamil

6. **Digitalis**
   - Decreases heart rate
   - Increases myocardial contractions
   - Slowing down of A-V nodal conductors
   - More regular apical heart rate
   - Used to inhibit atrial flutter, congestive heart failure, congenital heart block, and myocarditis
   - Dosage must be monitored for toxicity
   - Digoxin is used for congestive heart failure patients

7. **Diuretics**
   - Reduces the volume of extracellular fluid
   - Controls fluid retention
   - Reduces myocardial workload
   - Used for hypertension, congestive heart failure, and edema
   - Most common drug is Lasix; Diuril and Aldactone are also used

8. **Lipid-Lowering Drugs**
   - Decreases serum lipid levels
   - Interferes with metabolism of blood fats
   - Lowers cholesterol

---

*Commonly known drug names are listed in this section. Please note that some are generic or chemical names and some are brand names.

- Used to assist in prevention of atherosclerosis
- Colestrid, Lopid, Mevocor, and Zocor

9. **Nitrates**
    - Dilates coronary arteries
    - Reduces angina pain
    - Improves coronary blood flow
    - Most common is nitroglycerin
    - Isodril, Iso-bid, and isosorbide dinitrate
10. **Vasodilators**
    - Dilates the peripheral blood vessels
    - Used in combination with diuretics
    - Nitroglycerin and isosorbide dinitrate

CARDIAC REHABILITATION

Risk Factors Associated With Heart Disease

- Smoking
- Hypertension
- Elevated cholesterol levels
- Family history
- Sedentary lifestyle
- Diabetes
- Age
- Male gender

Overall Treatment for Cardiac Disease

- Diet
- Medication
- Exercise
- Behavioral changes

Note: *A multiphasic approach to risk factor reduction is key. No single element alone is an effective treatment.*

CARDIAC RESPONSE TO EXERCISE

Normal Response

1. Under normal conditions the cardiac output and heart rate will increase in a linear relationship with the increase in work load and oxygen consumption demand.
2. Maximum heart rate will decrease with age (220 minus age = maximum heart rate).
3. Blood pressure: systolic will rise but diastolic will remain level or slightly increase.

Abnormal Response

1. On EKG, the ST segment will depress or elevate, denoting heart injury.
2. Blood pressure:
    - Systolic: will remain level during exercise or remain high after exercise
    - Diastolic: will increase above 20 mmHg or decrease after exercise
3. Angina symptoms during exercise
4. Abnormal heart rate—bradycardia or tachycardia

Note: **Stop** *exercising the patient if any of the above occur during exercise. Continue to monitor pulse and blood pressure while calling for assistance.*

POSSIBLE BENEFITS OF A CARDIAC REHABILITATION PROGRAM

- Decreases serum lipid level
- Improves maximum oxygen consumption
- Increases HDL levels
- May decrease high blood pressure
- Improves activity/exercise tolerance
- Improves or relieves angina
- Improves aerobic capacity
- Decreases depression following myocardial infarction
- Decreases heart rate at rest
- Improves heart rate recovery after exercise
- Improves respiratory capacity during exercise
- Increases stroke volume
- Assists in weight reduction

ENERGY COSTS OF SELECTED ACTIVITIES—MET LEVELS

METABOLIC EQUIVALENTS (METS) ARE USED TO COMPARE THE ENERGY COSTS OF VARIOUS ACTIVITIES TO REST.

LEVEL	ACTIVITIES
1 ½ to 2 METS	Sitting, self-feeding, reading, active assistive exercise to extremities in supine or sitting, standing, walking (1 mph), desk work
2 to 3 METS	Typing, level walking (2 mph), level bicycling (5 mph), light woodworking, playing an instrument, active exercise standing or light mat activities, light weights (2 to 3 pounds) may be used, lawn mowing with a riding mower
3 to 4 METS	Cleaning windows, walking (3 mph), cycling (6 mph), archery, golf (pulling the golf bag cart), fishing, slow stair-climbing, balance and mat activities with mild resistance
4 to 5 METS	House painting, walking to 3.5 mph, cycling (8 mph), raking leaves, light dancing, resistance exercise sitting to 10 to 15 pounds maximum
5 to 6 METS	Shoveling light soil, walking (4 mph), horseback riding, ice skating, stairs/step aerobics to tolerance, hand lawn mowing
6 to 7 METS	Shoveling 10 pounds, cycling (11 mph), light snow shoveling, light downhill skiing, walking (5 mph)
7 to 10 METS	Jogging to rapid running, basketball, heavy shoveling, vigorous skiing, rapid cycling up and down hills, cycling (13 mph), horseback riding/galloping, walking (5.5 mph)
11 to 12 METS	Backpacking, climbing hills, handball, racquetball, jumping rope 120 to 140 skips/minute, running 5-minute mile
13 to 14 METS	Running 7-minute mile, cross-country skiing vigorously, shoveling wet snow

CARDIAC REHABILITATION PROGRAM

Contraindications for Cardiac Rehabilitation Program Participation

- Unstable angina
- Fever
- Thrombophlebitis
- Uncontrolled diabetes
- Acute illness
- Uncontrolled dysrhythmias
- Uncontrolled tachycardia
- Recent embolism

- Third-degree heart block
- Symptomatic congestive heart failure
- Resting systolic blood pressure over 200 mmHg
- Resting diastolic blood pressure over 100 mmHg

Borg 10-Grade Scale for Perceived Exertion

0	Nothing
0.5	Very, very weak
1.0	Very weak
1.5	Weak (light)
3.0	Moderate
4.0	Somewhat strong
5.0	Strong (heavy)
6.0	
7.0	Very strong
8.0	
9.0	
10.0	Very, very strong (almost maximum)

Exercise Prescription

1. **Intensity**
   - Cardiac patient should have an exercise stress test prior.
   - The cardiac patient should initially start at a low-level intensity.
   - Age adjusted heart rate for maximum is 220 minus the patient's age. This can then be multiplied by 65% to 95% to determine workload level.
   - 50% to 85% of maximum oxygen consumption.
2. **Duration**
   - Fifteen to 60 minutes of scheduled exercise period.
3. **Frequency**
   - Three to 5 days per week with no more than 2 days of rest between sessions.

Phase I—Inpatient Cardiac Rehabilitation

- Phase I is the beginning protocol for the patient's cardiac rehabilitation programs. This begins as an inpatient in the coronary care unit. Phase I is the acute phase.
- It may include some of the following activity levels:
  1. Monitored ambulation, which typically uses Holter monitoring and involves monitoring the patient's heart and blood pressure while the patient is ambulating with the physical therapist or cardiac nurse.
  2. Passive range of motion (ROM), ankle pumps and breathing exercises progressing to active ROM supine, active ROM sitting, walking 50 to 75 feet.
  3. Phase I may also include low-level exercise testing.
  4. ADL training for bathroom procedures is typical.
  5. Ward activities start and progress; bedside commode, feeding, and partial self-care; sitting in chair 15 minutes to 30 minutes; showers; dressing; bathroom privilege; and exercise testing.
  6. Calisthenics progressing from 1.0 to 4.0 METS.
  7. Education on pulse monitoring, activity diary, blood pressure, nutrition, home exercise program, and exercise prescriptions.
- Discharged after a submaximal or low-level treadmill test.

Phase II—Outpatient Cardiac Rehabilitation

- Phase II is considered an outpatient cardiac rehabilitation program. This is conducted after the patient is discharged from phase I and enters outpatient cardiac rehabilitation. Phase II is the subacute phase.
- Phase II program includes an increase in the patient's exercise program, again with continued monitoring. Phase II also includes continued patient education, typically regarding risk factors, diets, stress, and medication.

- Phase II includes more aggressive stress testing for the patient.
- Phase II is typically an 8 to 12 week program. Payers (insurance companies) typically cover 36 sessions, which are usually scheduled three times a week for 12 weeks.
- Duration of exercise is usually 30 to 60 minutes per session.
- It begins with the completion of a low-level treadmill test and ends with the maximal treadmill test. MET functional level at exit is typically 9.
- Phase II may include some of the following activities:
  1. Group support program
  2. Walking
  3. Treadmill
  4. Ergometer
  5. Circuit training
  6. Risk factor modification
  7. Teach energy conservation techniques
  8. Patients should now be independent in self monitoring or vital signs

Phase III—Community Exercise Program

- Phase III is typically referred to as a maintenance program. It is the process of ongoing exercise performed by the patient under supervised conditions of a self-regulated exercise program.
- Phase III is a high-level exercise conditioning phase. Patients exercise at 65% to 85% of their maximum heart rate, which is obtained from their treadmill test.
- Duration is typically 45 to 60 minutes per session.
- Frequency is a minimum of three times a week and may be daily.
- Discharge is typically 6 to 12 months.
- Supervision during the exercise session is still encouraged.
- Insurance does not typically cover the maintenance program and patients may exercise at a community center, private club, or a hospital-based program if available.

Phase IV—Ongoing for Life

Phase IV is promoting a life-long commitment to cardiac care, including exercise, diet, and behavior modification.

GOALS OF THE CARDIAC REHABILITATION PROGRAM

Phase I

Some examples include the following:
- Assessment of the patient's response to activities of daily living and self care.
- Determining the patient's response to monitored ambulation activities.
- Assisting the patient in identifying risk factors and methods to reduce them.
- Educating the family.
- Identifying diet and medication assessment.
- Patient should be able to pass a mild stress test.

All these areas may be assessed during phase I and appropriate goals set up for the patient. For example, one specific goal under education might be for the patient to independently list the risk factors associated with his or her evaluation and identify what steps he or she can take to modify those risks.

Phase II

Some examples of goals include the following:
- Determining the patient's response to exercise in a safe manner.
- Evaluating the home environment for the patient's transition from an inpatient to outpatient basis.
- Assessing whether response to exercise is appropriate.
- Monitoring the patient's social and emotional response to the program.
- Patient should be able to pass a maximal stress test.

Phase III

Some examples of maintenance goals include the following:
- Patient should be able to exercise independently in a safe manner.
- The patient should be educated in independent management of risk factors, medication, diet, and stress.
- Patient should be able to independently perform activities of daily living in a safe manner.

DISORDERS/DISEASES

Aneurysm: a bulging of the wall secondary to weakness of the tissue. Aneurysms are usually located in the aorta but may also occur in the peripheral vessels. The arterial aneurysm is usually caused by atherosclerosis, hypertension, or occasionally by trauma, infection, and congenital weakness in the vessel wall. One sign of an arterial aneurysm is a blowing murmur heard on auscultation.

Angina pectoris: a symptom of myocardial ischemia secondary to coronary artery disease. It may be stable, predictable in appearance, occurs after exercise, eating, and exposure to intense cold or emotional stress. Rest, nitrates, or vasodilators typically alleviate this. It may also be unstable, which can occur with activity or rest. This pain is more intense than stable and may last several hours. The pain is typically substernal, epigastrium, and pericardium, with radiation symptoms in the left arm, jaw, or neck. Levels of angina are:

1+ light or barely noticeable

2+ moderate or bothersome

3+ severe and very uncomfortable

4+ most severe pain ever experienced

Arrhythmia: a disorder of the electrical activity of the heart causing an absence or irregularity of the heart's normal rhythm.

Atherosclerosis: an arterial disorder that results from an accumulation of plaque, lipids, cholesterol, and cellular debris in the inner layers of the walls of the arteries. The inner layers become progressively thickened, calcification of arterial walls, and a loss of elasticity. This decreases or prevents blood flow through the arteries to the organs. Signs and symptoms may include changes in skin color, headaches, dizziness, intermittent claudication, and changes in peripheral pulses. It may cause a thrombosis and is a major cause of myocardial infarct, angina pectoris, and coronary heart disease.

Atrial septal defect: a congenital heart defect of an abnormal opening between the atria. Atrial septal defect causes an increased flow of oxygenated blood into the right side of the heart. This causes the right heart volume to overload and enlargement of the right atria. The defect is corrected by surgical closure depending on the child's age and severity of the enlargement.

Backward heart failure: venous return to the heart is decreased resulting in venous stasis and congestion. Pulmonary edema occurs due to the ventricles not emptying and the blood backing up in the pulmonary veins and lungs.

Cardiac tamponade: accumulation of blood or fluid in the pericardial sac. Signs and symptoms include hypotension, decreased heart sounds, weak or absent peripheral pulses, tachypnea, and pericardial friction rub. It may also be called cardiac compression because of the compression of the heart caused by the accumulation of blood or fluid. Intervention for treatment places the patient on monitored bedrest with aspiration of the blood or fluid. Surgical intervention is necessary to repair the bleeding vessel or vessels.

Congestive heart failure: an impaired cardiac pumping that results in edema and systemic congestion. Left heart failure results from an inability of the left ventricles to pump blood into the systemic circulation. This results in elevated end diastolic left ventricular pressure and pulmonary congestion, fatigue, central cyanosis, cardiac asthma, tachycardia, and pulmonary edema. Hypertension, aortic valve disease, or cardiac failure may cause left heart failure. Right heart failure results in elevated end diastolic right ventricular pressure. This causes systemic congestion, fatigue, cyanosis of the capillary stasis, pleural effusion, enlarged liver, and pitting edema. Mitral stenosis, ineffective endocarditis, and tricuspid valvular disease may cause right heart failure.

Forward heart failure: left ventricle failure results in a greatly reduced cardiac output. This may be caused by loss of contractility of the ventricle or after myocardial infarction.

Heart failure: a condition that results in the heart not being able to pump enough blood to meet the metabolic needs of the body. There are five types of heart failure.

High-output heart failure: cardiac heart failure from an increased amount of circulation. This may be caused by anemia or large arteriovenous fistula.

Low-output heart failure: the heart cannot maintain adequate circulation due to a decreased venous return. This may be caused by a hemorrhage.

Myocardial infarction: also called heart attack; it results in necrosis of a portion of the cardiac muscle. The necrosis or death of the heart muscle tissue is caused by obstruction in the coronary artery. This may be caused by a spasm, thrombus, atherosclerotic heart disease, embolism, and drug overdoses. The myocardial infarction sites may include the right coronary artery, causing an inferior myocardial infarction; circumflex artery, causing a lateral myocardial infarction; and the left descending artery, causing an anterior myocardial infarction. Signs and symptoms include chest pain, sense of heaviness in the chest, nausea, vomiting, sweating, hypotension, weakness, shortness of breath, light-headedness, and chest pain radiating to the left arm and neck. Myocardial enzymes are released into the blood as a result of necrosis. Blood enzyme and an electrocardiograph may be utilized to assist with patient diagnosis.

Patent ductus arteriosus: a congenital heart defect resulting in an abnormal opening between the pulmonary artery and aorta. The patent duct, located between the descending aorta and pulmonary artery, is bifurcate and does not close after birth. This allows left to right blood flow from the aorta to the pulmonary artery, causing increased workload on the left side of the heart. Surgery is utilized to correct the defect if there is no spontaneous closing and the child is old enough to tolerate the procedure.

Tetralogy of Fallot: a congenital heart defect that results in four specific defects causing a mixing of oxygenated and unoxygenated blood. The four defects are as follows: ventricular septal defect, malpositioning of the aorta, pulmonary stenosis, right ventricular hypertrophy. Surgery is utilized to correct the defect, optimally after the child is 1 year old; and supportive measures are utilized early on to assist the child with comfort and function.

Transposition of the great arteries: a congenital heart defect resulting in the great arteries being reversed. The aorta leaves the right ventricle and pulmonary artery leaves the left ventricle. This prevents communication between the systemic and pulmonary circulation. Surgery is utilized to correct the defect, optimally after the child is at least 6 months of age; and supportive measures are utilized early on to assist the child with comfort and function.

Ventricular septal defect: a congenital heart defect resulting in an opening in the ventricular septum. This allows mixing of the left ventricle's oxygenated blood with the right ventricle's unoxygenated blood. The defect is corrected by surgical closure unless it is small and could close spontaneously.

Cardiac Diagnostic Test

Cardiac catheterization: the coronary arteries are injected with a contrast material for visualization through a cinefluoroscopy or x-ray. This is utilized to determine cardiac output, measure pulmonary artery and blood gas pressure, abnormal wall movements, ventricular function, and anatomy of the heart.

Echocardiography: the reflections of ultrasound waves from the cardiac surfaces are analyzed. This is utilized to determine left ventricular systolic functioning, observe chambers, evaluate movement of valves, and evaluate structure and function of cardiac walls. This can assist in identifying tumors or pericardial effusion.

Electrocardiogram: 12 surface electrodes are placed on the patient to record the electrical activity of the patient's heart. The electrodes will provide feedback on cardiac rhythm, rate, conduction, and myocardial infarctions or ischemia.

Exercise stress test: an exercise test performed typically on a stationary bike or treadmill where the physician can monitor the patient's response to a variety of exercise levels. Typically, heart rate, blood pressure, respiratory rate, patient's perceived level of exertion/workload, and electrocardiogram are monitored to provide feedback to how the patient's cardiovascular system responds under stress.

Holter monitoring: electrocardiograph reading with an ambulatory EKG unit to monitor patient for typically 24 hours. This monitors the patient while performing normal activities. Utilized to monitor the effects of medication, activities of daily living, ambulation, pacemaker functions, and evaluation of patient's symptoms with patient's daily activities.

Phonocardiography: an electroacoustic device that will produce and record heart sounds. A microphone is placed over the base of the heart and on the chest over the apex of the heart. This records aortic and pulmonary components of the heart sounds. This information is utilized to confirm auscultatory findings.

Radionuclide angiocardiography: red blood cells marked with radionuclide are injected into the blood. They are then monitored to determine ventricular wall motion, ejection fraction, congenital defects, and abnormal blood flow.

Technetium 99m scanning: the patient's blood is injected with technetium 99m, a radionuclide, which is taken up by the myocardial tissue. This is also called hot spot imaging and is utilized to evaluate and locate myocardial infarctions.

Thallium 201 myocardial perfusion imaging: thallium 201 is injected into the blood at the patient's peak exercise level. This is also called cold spot imaging and is utilized to identify ischemic myocardium, infarcted myocardium, and diagnose coronary artery disease.

CHAPTER 7

Pulmonary Anatomy & Physiology

LUNG STRUCTURE

The lungs are divided into a right lung, which contains three lobes, and a left lung, which contains two lobes. The right lung consists of 10 segments. The left lung consists of eight segments. The pleura is a delicate membrane enclosing the lung. The pleura is divided into the visceral pleura, which covers the lungs, and the parietal pleura, which lines the chest wall and covers the diaphragm. The pleural cavity is the space within the thorax that contains the lungs. The pleural space is the potential space between the visceral and parietal layers of the pleura. It contains a small amount of fluid that acts as a lubricant.

UPPER AND LOWER AIRWAYS

The upper airway entry point into the respiratory system is the nose or mouth. The pharynx serves as a passageway for the respiratory and digestive tracts. The pharynx is composed of muscle, is lined with a mucous membrane, and contains the opening of the larynx. The larynx is the air passage that connects the pharynx with the trachea. The trachea conveys air to the lungs. The trachea starts the lower airways. At the fifth thoracic vertebra, the trachea divides into two bronchi: primary and secondary. The bronchiole extends from the bronchi into the lobes of the lung. The terminal branches allow passively inspired air from the bronchi to the respiratory bronchioles. The respiratory bronchioles allow the exchange of air and waste gases between the alveolar ducts and the terminal bronchioles.

MUSCLES OF INSPIRATION

Inspiratory muscles act to draw air into the lungs to exchange oxygen for carbon dioxide. The major muscle of inspiration is the diaphragm.

Primary

- Diaphragm phrenic innervation (C3, C4, C5)
- Levatores costarum
- External intercostal
- Internal intercostal

Accessory

- Scaleni
- Sternocleidomastoid
- Trapezius
- Serratus anterior—posterior superior
- Pectoralis major

- Pectoralis minor
- Latissimus dorsi
- Thoracic spine extensors
- Subclavius

MUSCLES OF EXPIRATION

Expiration is the moving of air out of the lungs, or exhalation. Expiration is a result of passive relaxation of inspiratory muscles and elastic recoil of lungs.

Primary

- Internal oblique
- External oblique
- Rectus abdominis
- Transverse abdominis
- Internal intercostal—posterior
- Transverse thoracic

Accessory

- Latissimus dorsi
- Serratus anterior—posterior inferior
- Iliocostalis lumborum
- Quadratus lumborum

BREATHING SOUNDS

Normal

- **Bronchial:** inspiration shorter than expiration. Short pause between inspiration and expiration. Loud and high pitched.
- **Bronchovesicular:** inspiration equals expiration in duration, with no pause between. Lower intensity than bronchial. Medium pitched.
- **Tracheal:** inspiration and expiration are equal in duration. Short pause between inspiration and expiration. Loud and high pitched.
- **Vesicular:** longer inspiration and shorter expiration with no pause between. Relatively faint and low pitched.

Abnormal

- **Bronchophony:** an increase in intensity and clarity of vocal resonance. This may result in an increase in lung tissue density (eg, pneumonia).
- **Crackles:** result of secretions, as in pneumonia or early tuberculosis. Characterized by popping or bubbling sounds.
- **Egophony:** a change in voice sound when a patient is asked to make an "e" sound and it sounds like an "a" over the peripheral chest wall. May be caused by pleural effusion.
- **Friction rub:** a dry, grating sound similar to footsteps on packed snow. Caused by rubbing of pleural surfaces against one another.
- **Pectoriloquy:** abnormal transmission of whispered syllables that cannot be heard clearly.
- **Rhonchi:** airways obstructed by thick secretions, muscular spasm, neoplasm, or external pressure causing a continuous rumbling sound.
- **Wheeze:** a high-pitched musical quality, caused by airway obstruction. Airways may be narrowed by inflammation of secretions or bronchospasm.

DIVISION OF LEFT AND RIGHT LUNGS

LEFT LUNG (EIGHT SEGMENTS)

LEFT UPPER LOBE	LEFT LOWER LOBE
ap = apical—posterior	s = superior
an = anterior	ab = anterior medial basal
sl = superior lingula	lb = lateral basal
il = inferior lingula	pb = posterior basal

RIGHT LUNG (10 SEGMENTS)

RIGHT UPPER LOBE	RIGHT MIDDLE LOBE	RIGHT LOWER LOBE
ap = apical	l = lateral	s = superior
an = anterior	m = medial	ab = anterior basal
p = posterior		lb = lateral basal
		pb = posterior basal
		mb = medial basal

EVALUATION OF SPUTUM

Sputum is described in terms of quantity, viscosity, color, and odor. The color will assist in determining the condition that the patient is experiencing.

- Red: blood
- Pink: pulmonary edema
- Yellow: infection starting to clear
- Green: acute infection
- Gray: abscess
- Rust: pneumonia
- White or clear: may equal chronic cough, cystic fibrosis, or chronic bronchitis
- Thick tenacious sputum: asthmatic bronchitis

CHAPTER 8

Pulmonary

PULMONARY FUNCTION TEST

OBSTRUCTIVE VERSUS RESTRICTIVE

TEST	OBSTRUCTIVE	RESTRICTIVE
Total lung capacity	Increases	Decreases
PCO_2	Increases	Decreases
FEV1	Sharply decreases	Normal
Functional residual capacity	Increases	Decreases
Residual volume	Increases	Decreases
Vital capacity	Decreases	Decreases
Vital capacity as a percent of predicted value	Normal > 80% Mild obstructive 80% Mild restrictive 60 to 80% Severe obstructive < 80% Severe restrictive < 50%	
FEV1/FVC ratio	Normal > 75% Mild obstructive 60 to 75% Moderate obstructive 40 to 60% Severe obstructive < 40% Restrictive—normal	

PULMONARY PHARMACOLOGY

Antibiotics

Antimicrobial agents derived from cultures of a microorganism or produced semisynthetically and used to treat infections by destroying or interfering with the development of a living organism.

- Erythromycin
- Penicillin
- Tetracycline

Antihistamines

- Azatadine
- Brompheniramine
- Dimenhydrinate
- Diphenhydramine
- Loratadine
- Phenindamine

Bronchodilators

- Epinephrine
- Isoproterenol
- Metaproterenol
- Terbutaline
- Salbutamol
- Theophylline
- Albuterol
- Procaterol

Corticosteroids

- Glucocorticoids—prednisone
- Mineral corticoids—aldosterones
- Dexamethasone
- Prednisolone
- Triamcinolone

Mucokinetics

- Bland aerosol
- Acetylcysteine—reduces viscosity of secretions

Oxygen: odorless, tasteless, colorless transparent gas that is slightly heavier than air.
1. Low-flow oxygen therapy: provides only part of the patient's required minute volume.
2. High-flow oxygen therapy: provides all of the gas the patient needs.

LUNG VOLUMES

- **Dead air space:** area in which no gas exchange takes place.
- **Residual volume (RV):** amount of gas left over after maximum expiration, which helps prevent the lungs from collapsing.
- **Tidal volume (TV):** amount of gas inspired and expired at rest.
- **Forced expiratory volume (FEV):** amount of air that can be forcibly expelled after maximum inspiration.
- **Total lung capacity (TLC):** amount of gas in the respiratory system after a maximal inspiration.
- **Vital capacity (VC):** maximum volume of air forcibly expired after a maximal inspiration.
- **Inspiratory capacity (IC):** maximum volume of air inspired from resting level of expiratory air.
- **Functional residual capacity (FRC):** volume of gas in lungs after normal expiration.
- **Inspiratory reserve volume (IRV):** maximum volume inspired after normal inspiration.
- **Expiratory reserve volume (ERV):** maximum volume expired after normal expiration.

PULMONARY CLASSES OF IMPAIRMENT

Class 1—0% Impairment

1. Roentgenographic appearance is usually normal but may show healed or inactive disease
2. Dyspnea may occur but is consistent with the activity

3. FEV and FVC (forced vital capacity) tests are not less then 85% of predicted value
4. Arterial oxygen saturation is not applicable

Class 2—20 to 30% Impairment

1. Roentgenographic appearance may be either normal or abnormal
2. Dyspnea does not occur at rest and during the performance of usual activities of daily living. Patients comparable to person of same age and body build on level surfaces but not unleveled
3. FEV and FVC tests are 70 to 85% predicted value
4. Arterial saturation is not applicable

Class 3—40 to 50% Impairment

1. Roentgenographic appearance may be normal but is typically not
2. Dyspnea does not occur at rest but may occur during the normal activities of daily living. The patient cannot keep pace with other persons of the same age and built
3. FEV and FVC tests are 55 to 70% predicted value
4. Arterial saturation is usually 88% or greater at rest and after exercise

Class 4—60 to 90% Impairment

1. Roentgenographic appearance is usually abnormal
2. Dyspnea occurs during activities (eg, climbing one flight of stairs or walking 100 yards level surface); it may even occur at rest
3. FEV and FVC tests are less then 55% of predicted value
4. Arterial saturation is usually less than 88% at rest and after exercise

PULMONARY SURGERY

1. **Lobectomy:** removal of a lobe of lung
2. **Pneumonectomy:** removal of portion of a lung
3. **Pleurectomy:** removal of the pleural sac
4. **Decortication:** removal of any restrictive membrane that limits pulmonary function from the surface of the lung
5. **Segmental resection:** excision of a segment of the lobe
6. **Wedge resection:** excision of a portion of a segment of the lobe

PULMONARY TERMS

Apnea: absence of ventilation
Atelectasis: incomplete expansion of lung secondary to collapse of alveoli
Barrel chest: increased anterior-posterior diameter of the thorax
Bradypnea: slow respiratory rates, shallow abnormal depth; this is normal during sleep
Cyanosis: caused by low oxygen saturation; the skin has a bluish tint
Dyspnea: rapid rate, shallow depth (accessory muscle activity)
Flail chest: when two or more ribs are broken, the chest will move paradoxically during breathing
Hemothorax: blood in the pleural space
Hypercapnia: blood, CO_2 in arterial blood
Hyperpnea: rapid rate, increased depth
Hyperventilation: fast rate, increased depth
Hypoxia: fluid CO_2 in the blood, diminished availability of oxygen to the body tissue.
Orthopnea: difficulty breathing when in a position other than erect
Pes carinatum: the sternum protrudes forward and is abnormally prominent
Pectus excavatum: the sternum is abnormally depressed
Tachypnea: abnormally fast rate of breathing

PULMONARY DISEASES/DISORDERS

Asthma

- Increased sensitivity of trachea and bronchi to irritants
- Spasms of smooth bronchi muscle
- Narrowing of airway
- Inflammation and production of mucus
- Increased respiratory rate
- Chest wall movements normal or symmetrically decreased
- Dry, irritating, or wheezing cough
- Symptoms may include anxiety, bronchial spasm

Adult Respiratory Distress Syndrome

- Respiratory syndrome characterized by hypoxemia and respiratory deficiency
- May be caused by aspiration of a foreign object, oxygen toxicity, trauma, pneumonia, respiratory infections, and multiple blood transfusions
- Patient may demonstrate tachypnea, hypoxemia, breathlessness, and decreased lung compliance
- Other names for this include acute respiratory distress syndrome, shock lung, wet lung, pump lung, and congestive atelectasis

Atelectasis

- Collapsed or airless alveolar unit
- Prevents the respiratory exchange of oxygen and carbon dioxide
- May be caused by internal bronchial obstruction, postoperative pain, external bronchial compression, narcotic overdose, rib fracture, and neurological trauma
- Patient may demonstrate decreased breathing sounds, tachycardia, increased temperature, and dyspnea

Bronchiectasis

- Abnormal condition of the bronchial tree
- Chest wall movement may be reduced over affected side
- Increased vocal sounds
- Sputum, possibly foul smelling, and hemoptysis may occur
- Characterized by irreversible dilatation and destruction of the bronchial walls
- Symptoms include a constant cough with sputum, chronic sinusitis, clubbing of fingers
- Treatment includes postural drainage, antibiotics

Bronchogenic Carcinoma

- A malignant lung tumor that originates in the bronchi
- May cause coughing, fatigue, chest tightness, aching joints
- Surgery is the most effective treatment; however, approximately 50% of cases are advanced and inoperable
- Treatment can include radiotherapy and chemotherapy

Bronchopulmonary Dysplasia

- Obstructive pulmonary disease
- The lungs have abnormal development and pulmonary immaturity
- Seen in premature infants
- Symptoms may include decreased breath sounds, increased bronchial secretions, crackles/wheezing, and hyperinflation

Chronic Bronchitis

- Distinguished by excessive secretion of mucus in the bronchi, including a productive cough for at least 3 consecutive months

- Other symptoms may include chest infections, cyanosis, hypoxemia and hypercapnia, wheezing and rhonchi
- Chest wall movement normal or symmetrically decreased
- Normal vocal sounds
- Productive cough with sputum with infection
- Treatment includes cessation of cigarette smoking, postural drain

Cystic Fibrosis

- Genetically determined systemic disease of the exocrine glands
- Increased secretions with rales and wheezing
- Overproduction of mucus
- Congenital disease
- Chest walls movement normal or reduced
- Vocal sounds may have egophony
- Cough is productive and sputum may have hemoptysis

Emphysema

- Lung tissue loses its elasticity
- Lungs remain overinflated; diaphragm flattens and is then less effective
- Destruction of alveolar walls allows airways to collapse
- Barrel chest
- Pink puffers
- Chest wall movement normal or symmetrically reduced
- Vesicular breath sounds
- Patient's cough and sputum variable

Hemothorax

- Blood and fluid in the pleural cavity between the parietal and visceral pleura
- Usually a result of trauma
- Emergency care necessary, as shock may occur from hemorrhage, pain, and respiratory failure
- Symptoms may include chest pain, respiratory distress, signs of blood loss, and decreased breath sounds

Hyaline Membrane Disease

- Respiratory distress syndrome of the newborn (RDS)—acute lung disease
- Characterized by airless alveoli, inelastic lungs, more than 60 respirations per minute, nasal flaring, intercostal and subcostal retractions, grunting on expiration and peripheral edema
- Most often in premature babies
- Treatment includes measures to correct shock, acidosis, and hypoxemia and use of continuous positive airway pressure especially developed for infants

Lung Contusion

- Blood and edema within the alveoli and interstitial space
- The injury does not break the skin
- Caused by trauma or a blow to the lung area
- Symptoms may include swelling, pain, decreased breath sounds, and cyanosis

Peripheral Airway Disease

- Inflammation of distal conducting airways
- Associated with smokers and obesity
- Decrease in forced expiratory flow (FEF) 25 to 75%

Pneumonia

- Chest wall movement reduced on affected side

- Breath sounds are vesicular or bronchial
- Vocal sounds are egophony, or whispering pectoriloquy
  - **Aspiration pneumonia** is an inflammatory condition of the lungs and bronchi. It is caused by inhalation of foreign matter or vomitus containing acid gastric contents.
  - **Bacterial pneumonia** is a bacteria infection in the interalveolar. The most common type is streptococcal. Symptoms may include fever, cough, shaking, chills, crackle sound, and decreased breath sounds.
  - **Viral pneumonia** is a pulmonary infection caused by a virus.

Pneumothorax

- A collection of air or gas in the pleural space, which causes the lung to collapse
- May be the result of an open chest wound that permits entrance of air
- Onset is a sudden, sharp chest pain followed by difficult rapid breaths
- Cessation of normal chest wall movements on affected side
- Vocal sounds decreased
- A dry cough
- Symptoms may include local or referred pain, chest pain, cyanosis
- Treatment includes being placed in bed in Fowler's position, oxygen unless contraindicated, and air aspirated from the pleural space. Intermittent positive pressure breathing may be administered. Educate the patient on passive exercise, how to turn, cough, and breathe deeply

Pulmonary Edema

- Excessive fluid from the pulmonary vascular system into the interstitial space
- Chest wall movement is normal or symmetrically reduced
- Vocal sounds are normal
- Cough may include frothy white or pink sputum
- Symptoms may include rales, crackles, dyspnea, and tachypnea

Pulmonary Effusion

- Excessive fluid between the visceral and parietal pleura
- Reduced or absent chest wall movement on the affected side
- Breath sounds are decreased or absent; high-pitched bronchial may be present
- Vocal sounds are reduced or absent
- May have pleural rub
- Cough is absent or nonproductive
- Symptoms may include pain and/or fever

Pulmonary Embolism

- A thrombus that becomes embolic and is lodged in the pulmonary circulation
- Chest wall movement is reduced on the affected side
- Breath sounds may be reduced
- Vocal sounds are normal
- Symptoms may include wheezing, pleural friction rub, rales, dry hacking cough with hemoptysis, and possible pleuritic pain

Rib Fracture

- A break in the bone of thoracic skeleton
- May be caused by a blow, crushing injury, or violent coughing
- Most common rib fracture occurs at the fourth to eighth ribs
- Breathing is rapid and shallow
- Site of break is tender to the touch
- Symptoms may include decreased or absent breath sounds, rales and rhonchi, crackling of bone fragments rubbing together
- Confirmation by chest x-ray

Tuberculosis (TB)

- Chronic granulomatous infection caused by an acid-fast bacillus
- Transmitted by inhalation or ingestion of infected droplets
- Listlessness, vague chest pain, pleurisy, fever, and weight loss
- Hospitalization for the first weeks of treatment with a combination of drugs, rest and good nutrition

RESPIRATORY DISEASES

OBSTRUCTIVE	VERSUS	RESTRICTIVE
Something interferes with the normal airflow		Reduction of actual lung volume
Increased secretions		Structural deformity
Spasms		Chest wall stiffness
Inflammation		Loss of lung tissue
May be reversible		Difficult to treat
Examples: asthma, cystic fibrosis, emphysema, bronchitis, pulmonary edema		Examples: scoliosis, pectus excavatum, burns, pneumothorax, collagen diseases, neuromuscular diseases

CLINICAL PRESENTATION IN COPD (CHRONIC BRONCHITIS AND EMPHYSEMA)

BLUE BLOATER	VERSUS	PINK PUFFER
Chronic productive cough		Little sputum, shortness of breath
Obese, edematous		Thin, nonedematous, pink
Cyanotic, right side congestive heart failure		Typically no congestive heart failure
Inflammatory cells in submucosa, edema		Destruction of airways
Hypertrophy of bronchial, smooth muscles		

POSTURAL DRAINAGE CONTRAINDICATIONS (POSITION HEAD DOWN)

1. Shunt
2. Head trauma
3. Cerebral hemorrhage
4. Cardiac condition in which increased venous return increases patient's chance of cardiac failure
5. Hypertension

PERCUSSION CONTRAINDICATIONS

1. Angina
2. Skin breakdown, wounds
3. Pneumothorax
4. Osteoporosis
5. Pulmonary emboli
6. Tumor

CHEST PHYSICAL THERAPY

INDICATIONS	VERSUS	CONTRAINDICATIONS
Airway resistance		Cerebral edema
Poor ventilation		Aneurysm
Poor oxygenation		Severe hypertension
Fluid/mucus in airways		Cardiac complications
Poor chest mobility		Pulmonary edema
Dyspnea		Gastric regurgitation
Poor mucocilliary movements		Recent hemoptysis
Aspirations		Fractured rib
Pulmonary secretions		Pneumothorax
Atelectasis		Pulmonary embolus
		Open thoracic wounds
		Immediately after chest tube removal
		Osteoporosis

PATIENT POSITIONS

Upper Lobes

1. Apical
   - Sitting upright
   - Percussion: between clavicle and scapula
2. Anterior
   - Supine, knees in a slightly flexed position, pillows underneath knees
   - Percussion: between clavicle and nipple
3. Posterior
   - Sitting in chair, patient leaning forward approximately 20° to 30°, resting on pillows
   - Percussion: top of shoulder blade
4. Left lingular
   - Right sidelying position, rotated backward one-quarter of a turn, foot of bed elevated 14 to 18 inches
   - Percussion: left side at nipple level

Middle Lobe

1. Right middle lobe
   - Left sidelying position, rotated backward half a turn, foot of bed elevated 14 inches, pillows under right hip
   - Percussion: right side at nipple level

Lower Lobes

1. Apical
   - Prone, pillows under stomach
   - Percussion: middle of back at inferior angle of scapula
2. Anterior
   - Supine, pillows under knees, foot of bed elevated 18 inches, chest tilted 20°
   - Percussion: anterior lower ribs
3. Posterior
   - Prone, pillows under the hips, foot of bed elevated 18 inches, chest tilted 20°
   - Percussion: posterior ribs, level should be close to the spine area

4. Lateral basal
   - Prone position, turned a half turn upward, foot of bed elevated 18 inches, chest tilted 20°
   - Percussion: lateral lower ribs

PULMONARY THERAPY

Treatment Components

1. Airway Clearance Techniques
   - Cough: the patient is instructed to cough to assist in clearing secretions. The patient will perform coughing in the sitting position if possible.
   - Assisted cough: the therapist utilizes his or her hand/hands to assist the patient with coughing. The therapist will push inward and upward, forcing coughing and assisting the rapid exhalation of air.
   - Huff: the patient will deeply inhale and forcibly expel the air while saying "Ha, ha." This is affected in patients who have collapsed airways and cannot tolerate high intrathoracic pressure.
   - Forced expiratory technique: the therapist uses this technique with the patient to assist in the removal of peripheral secretions. The patient starts with diaphragmatic breathing, performs thoracic expansion exercises, controlled diaphragmatic breathing, inhales resting tidal volume, lastly contracts the abdominal muscles to produce forced expiratory huffs.
   - Tracheal stimulation: this technique is used for patients who cannot cough when asked. The therapist places his or her finger or thumb above the suprasternal notch. Then the therapist applies quick inward and downward pressure on the trachea to elicit the cough reflex.
2. Bagging
   - Purpose: to provide artificial ventilation, restore oxygen, and re-expand the lungs.
   - Technique: to coordinate with the patient's breathing pattern. Attach manual resuscitator bag to the oxygen source and then connect it to the tracheal tube. Squeeze bag rhythmically to deliver volume of air to patient. Patient expires passively.
   - Indications: before and after suctioning a patient who is not mechanically ventilated.
3. Breathing Exercises
   - Purpose: to assist with the removal of secretions, relaxation, and increase thoracic cage mobility, tidal volume, increase ventilation, and improve gas exchange.
   - Technique: teach patient to produce a full inspiration followed by a controlled expiration. Use hand placement for sensory feedback and lateral and diaphragmatic costal excursion. Use gentle pressure through exhalation breathing activity.
   - Indications: utilize with spontaneously breathing patients.

Breathing Exercises

1. Diaphragmatic Breathing
   - Purpose: to increase ventilation, improve gas exchange, improve chest wall mobility, and prevent pulmonary compromise.
   - Technique: position the patient semireclined. The therapist will place his or her hand over the subcostal angle of the patient's thorax, then apply gentle pressure when the patient exhales and increasing to firm pressure at the end of exhalation. The patient will then inhale and the therapist will instruct the patient to resist the therapist's hand on inhalation. The therapist will then release pressure so the patient can fully inhale.
   - Indications: post-trauma patients. Postoperative patients, obstructive lung disease, and restrictive lung disease.
2. Pursed Lip Breathing
   - Purpose: increase tidal volume, reduce the respiratory rate, reduce dyspnea, and facilitate relaxation.
   - Technique: patient will slowly inhale through nose or mouth and passively exhale through pursed lips.
   - Indications: obstructive disease and to get the patient who has an unproductive breathing pattern to relax.
3. Segmental Breathing
   - Purpose: to prevent pulmonary compromise, improve chest wall mobility, increase ventilation to hyperventilated lungs, and redistribute gas.
   - Technique: position patient in a specific segment for postural drainage (eg, upright sitting). The therapist will

apply gentle pressure over the thorax of the patient during exhalation. The pressure will increase to firm just prior to inspiration. The patient will breathe in against the therapist's resistance. The therapist will lastly release pressure, allowing the patient to take a full inspiration.

- Indications: post-trauma, incisional, pleuritic pain with decreased movement in the thorax.

4. Sustained Maximal Inspiration
   - Purpose: to increase inhaled volume, improve alveolar inflation, and restore functional residual capacity.
   - Technique: have the patient inspire slowly through the nose or pursed lips to maximal inspiration, hold for 3 seconds, and passively exhale the volume.
   - Indications: acute lobar collapse, acute post-trauma pain, and acute postoperative pain.

5. Coughing
   - Purpose: to remove secretions from the larger airways.
   - Technique: inspiration gasp followed by closing of the glottis. Contraction of expiration muscles followed by opening of the glottis.
   - Indications: utilize with spontaneously breathing patients.

6. Patient Mobilization
   - Purpose: to prevent injurious sequelae from bedrest and immobility and to reduce the rehabilitation time.
   - Technique: turn and passively position the patient, passive and active range of motion, exercises, sitting, standing, and ambulation.
   - Indications: use with all patients according to their diagnosis and tolerance.

7. Percussion
   - Purpose: utilized in addition to postural drainage to mobilize secretions.
   - Technique: during inspiration and expiration, rhythmically clap cupped hands over bare skin or thin material covering the area of involved lung.
   - Indications: when secretions are not adequately cleared from coughing, suctioning, or from breathing exercises and mobilization of the patient.

8. Postural Drainage
   - Purpose: through the assistance of gravity, the patient's retained secretions are mobilized.
   - Technique: position patient so the involved segmental bronchus is uppermost.
   - Indications: when secretions are not adequately cleared from coughing, suctioning, or from breathing exercises and mobilization of the patient.

9. Suctioning
   - Purpose: to remove secretions from the larger airways.
   - Technique: utilizing an aseptic technique, furnish supplemental oxygen. Gently insert a suction catheter, then apply suction while withdrawing catheter. Re-expand the lung with a mechanical ventilator or manually with a resuscitator bag attached to a tracheal tube.
   - Indications: tracheal suctioning is for use only with those patients who have an artificial airway.

10. Vibration
    - Purpose: utilized in addition to postural drainage to mobilize secretions.
    - Technique: only perform during expiration, intermittent chest wall compression over the area of the involved lung.
    - Indications: when secretions are not adequately cleared from coughing, suctioning, or from breathing exercises and mobilization of the patient.

CHAPTER 9

Clinical Disorders

ACQUIRED IMMUNODEFICIENCY SYNDROME (AIDS)

- An immunodeficiency disease characterized by progressive destruction of T-cells and lymphocytes.
- The disease leaves patients highly susceptible to infections.
- HIV (human immunodeficiency virus) is a retrovirus that is unique because some of the cells will escape from the body's immune system.
- Some patients who have HIV may never develop AIDS. Patients who have the disease have different rates of progression.
- **Treatment:** no known cure; different treatment combinations work differently in each patient and may slow progression of the disease or the disease may go into remission. Secondary infections are the leading cause of death. Special implications for physical therapy are the use of universal precautions for health care workers. Exercises for pain relief and prevention of muscle atrophy/strength/endurance are beneficial to patients. Breathing exercises, posture instructions, balance activities, and activities of daily living assessment are also potential physical therapy treatment areas.

BUERGER'S DISEASE

- Also called thromboangiitis obliterans.
- Results in inflammatory changes in arteries and veins.
- Diagnostic test in physical therapy is to place toes/foot in dependent position—will see rubor color; then place toes/foot above heart level—will see pallor color.
- **Treatment:** must stop smoking, avoid extreme temperatures, and avoid wearing tight clothing. Buerger's exercise protocol.

CUSHING'S DISEASE

- Metabolic disorder characterized by abnormally increased secretion of adrenocortical steroids. Caused by increased amounts of adrenocorticotrophic hormone (ACTH), secreted by the anterior lobe of the pituitary gland.
- Results in accumulation of fat and edema on the chest, upper back and face.
- Also called hyperadrenocorticism.
- **Treatment:** removal or destruction of adrenocortical steroid-secreting tissue, usually by surgical or radiologic procedures.

DEEP VENOUS THROMBOSIS

- The formation of an abnormal blood clot in a deep vein.
- The danger is in the clot breaking free, resulting in a pulmonary embolus.

- Symptoms may vary; skin may appear cyanotic, warm, cold, or normal temperature.
- Pain, tenderness, and edema may be present.
- Superficial thrombophlebitis is not an emergency and does not require hospitalization.
- **Treatment:** typically consists of warm compresses over the involved veins and anti-inflammatory drugs. Deep venous thrombosis treatment includes hospitalization, bed rest with elevated lower extremities, and anticoagulants.

DIABETES INSIPIDUS

- Disease involving the imbalance of water secondary to an antidiuretic hormone (ADH) secreted by the posterior lobe of the pituitary gland.
- This disease can be caused by injury or lack of functioning to the following: hypothalamus, posterior pituitary gland, and the neurohypophyseal track.
- This water imbalance results in excessive excretion of diluted urine.
- **Treatment:** no specific physical therapy intervention. Treatment is usually replacement of antidiuretic hormone with synthetic derivatives. Caution is for physical therapist to monitor patient's condition during treatment for high blood pressure, water intoxication, and seizures.

DIABETES MELLITUS

- Results in carbohydrate intolerance.
- Patient is unable to produce a sufficient amount of insulin or, more commonly, develops peripheral resistance to a normal or increased amount of secreted insulin.
- Type I diabetes is considered insulin-dependent to prevent ketosis. This was previously called juvenile-onset diabetes.
- Type II diabetes is considered noninsulin-dependent. Typically, this is adult-onset diabetes.
- Hypoglycemia symptoms include sweating, pallor skin color, headaches, dizziness, irritable and nervous mood, and patient is hungry and shaky.
- Hyperglycemia symptoms include flushed skin, dehydration, thirst, weakness, nausea, vomiting, and lethargic mood.
- **Treatment:** diet adjustment or insulin depending upon the severity of the disease. The goal of treatment is to maintain normal blood glucose levels. Special implications for the physical therapist include knowing the signs and symptoms of a patient going into a diabetic coma, hypoglycemia, or hyperglycemia. A therapist should be aware of how exercises affect a patient with diabetes mellitus. Physical therapist may also be involved with wound care in diabetics.

HEMOPHILIA

- Hereditary disorder resulting in deficiency in the clotting factor. The results are a bleeding disorder that can result in small or large blood losses.
- Hemophilia type A is caused by a deficiency or absence of antihemophilia factor VIII.
- Hemophilia type B is caused by a deficiency of plasma thromboplastin.
- Hemarthrosis and muscle bleeds are of particular concern in physical therapy.
- **Treatment:** splinting, ice, rests, and elevation is needed in the acute stage. In chronic situations, joint protection, maintaining joint function, daily exercise for ROM, strength and endurance, ADL training, and use of appropriate splints and assistive devices.

HEPATITIS

- Acute or chronic inflammation of the liver.
- May be caused by alcohol abuse, drug reactions, chemical reaction, or a virus.
- Hepatitis A is an acute infection acquired through contaminated water/food, or spread by saliva and feces. It does not lead to chronic hepatitis.
- Hepatitis B is the second major cause of cirrhosis in the United States. It is acquired through exposure to blood and infected body fluids.

- Hepatitis C is typically acquired through blood transfusion and 50% of cases progress to chronic hepatitis. It may also be acquired with needlesticks and intravenous drug usage.
- Hepatitis D is uncommon in the United States and is typically associated with drug addicts, sexually active teenagers, and patients receiving several transfusions. This type of hepatitis results in progression to chronic active hepatitis and death.
- Hepatitis E is rare in the United States and typically found in developing countries. Patients at risk are typically travelers. It does not progress to chronic hepatitis. Transmitted through contamination of water.
- **Treatment:** medical management depends on the type of hepatitis found and the extent of the liver damage.

HERNIA

- A protrusion of an organ through an abnormal opening in the wall.
- Most common types are direct and indirect inguinal, femoral, incisional, and umbilical.
- The main reason for occurrence is a weakness in the abdominal muscles.
- Inguinal hernia is the most common type, involving 75% of all hernias.
- **Treatment:** supports and trusses can contain the hernia. Surgical intervention is necessary for correction.

HODGKIN'S DISEASE

- A malignant disorder that results in progressive enlargement in lymph tissue.
- Symptoms include weight loss, low grade fever, anemia, night sweats, and leukocytosis.
- Common areas affected are the spleen, liver, and bone marrow.
- May be fatal, but typically 50% of patients have long-term remission.
- **Treatment:** radiotherapy and/or chemotherapy.

HUNTINGTON'S CHOREA

- Hereditary disease.
- Results in progressive mental deterioration.
- Characterized by irregular movements and tremors.
- Disease typically occurs during the fourth decade of life.
- Average survival rate is 15 years after diagnosis.
- **Treatment:** no specific physical therapy treatment, but symptoms may be alleviated or decreased through medication therapy.

LEUKEMIA

- An abnormal form and amount of immature white blood cells in the bone marrow. The normal cells are replaced with malignant neoplasm, resulting in bone marrow failure.
- The cells are malignant and can overflow from the bone marrow into the peripheral circulation and progress to the lymph nodes, liver, and spleen.
- The three main symptoms are anemia, infection, and bleeding.
- Leukemia can be acute with a sudden onset and rapid progression of the disease.
- Leukemia may also be chronic with a slowly developing onset and progression.
- **Treatment:** chemotherapy, blood transfusion, antibiotics, bone marrow transplants, and supportive measures for pain and infections. Special considerations for physical therapy include awareness that patient is susceptible to infections and bleeding. Physical therapy treatments may include safety instructions because of patient weakness, education on pressure points and prevention of sores, and general range of motion and gentle stretching exercises depending on blood tests.

MARFAN'S SYNDROME

- Hereditary resulting in elongation of the bones.
- Typical appearance is tall, lean person. The extremities are very long and feet and hands are greatly extended. Patient is usually over 6 feet tall.

- Disease will affect muscle, bone, ligaments, and skeletal structures.
- Problems include ligament laxity, lateral curvature of the spine, joint hypermobility, muscular underdevelopment, pes valgus, and genu recurvatum.
- **Treatment:** no specific physical therapy treatment. Orthosis may be utilized to assist with deformities.

PANCREATITIS

- Serious inflammation of the pancreas; may be acute or chronic.
- It can result in the pancreas being digested by its own enzymes.
- Acute pancreatitis may be caused by alcoholism, medications, hereditary, trauma, peptic ulcers, viral infections, and post-surgical inflammation.
- Chronic pancreatitis is caused by structural or functional impairment of the pancreas.
- **Treatment:** medical management of acute pancreatitis consists of management of symptoms, as it typically subsides in several days. Chronic pancreatitis treatment is focused on prevention of further damage to the pancreas.

PSORIASIS

- A chronic, inherited, reoccurring skin disease.
- Characterized by erythematous plaque covered with silvery scales on the skin.
- Fifteen to twenty percent of patients may develop psoriasis arthritis.
- **Treatment:** no known cure; physical therapy intervention is treatment with ultraviolet light.

RAYNAUD'S SYNDROME

- Caused by spasm in small blood vessels.
- Intermittent attacks of ischemia in the extremities.
- Common in the hands; may also be in the toes, ears, and nose.
- Results in intermittent attacks of blanching, cyanosis, and redness.
- The attacks may cause pain, numbness, burning, and tingling sensations.
- **Treatment:** vasodilators; avoid exposure to excessive temperatures, caffeine, and smoking. Education on protecting body from the elements and sometimes biofeedback.

REFLEX SYMPATHETIC DYSTROPHY

- Typically follows an injury (eg, a sprain or fracture).
- Injury results in damage to afferent pathways of sensory processing.
- Characterized by persistent pain above the normally accepted pain level.
- Initially injury will show swelling and increased tissue temperature.
- Later the skin will appear dry, shiny, and leathery.
- **Treatment:** contrast baths, electrical stimulation, range of motion.

RHEUMATIC HEART DISEASE

- Caused by rheumatic fever.
- Result is serious heart defects (valvular) and damage to the heart muscle.
- Heart murmurs present.
- Damage may result in permanent heart deformities.
- **Treatment:** no specific physical therapy. Medical management depends on significance of heart damage.

SCLERODERMA

- Result is a thickening of skin and subcutaneous tissues caused by new collagen formation.
- Most common in middle-age women.
- Serious if it affects the organs.

- Frequently it is accompanied by Raynaud's syndrome.
- **Treatment:** maintain range of motion, prevent contractures, and muscle strengthening.

Systemic Lupus Erythematosus

- Collagen vascular disorder.
- Primarily affects the connective tissue in the skin, joints, blood vessels, and internal organs.
- Inflammatory response seen.
- Characteristics are fever, butterfly rash, polyarthritis, vasculitis, pericarditis, and renal involvement.
- Women are more commonly affected—two to three times more than men.
- **Treatment:** medications, joint conservation techniques. Ultraviolet treatment is contraindicated.

Thrombus

- Formation of a clot from accumulation of fibrin, platelets, cellular elements of blood, and clotting factors.
- May be either blood or fat clot.
- Typically, the clot is attached to the interior wall of a vein or artery.
- **Treatment:** anticoagulant drug therapy.

Ulcer (Peptic) Disease

- A break in the protective mucus lining resulting in gastric acid going into the submucosal areas.
- Peptic ulcers involve proteolytic enzymes, which are the main components in the digestion process.
- Gastric ulcers are a type of peptic ulcer that affects the lining of the stomach.
- Duodenum ulcers are a type of peptic ulcer that occurs in the duodenum.
- Stress may also cause ulcers in varying degrees.
- **Treatment:** medical management utilizing drug therapy to promote healing, pain relief, and prevention of complications. Prevention of future ulcers may be helped through education on stress reduction. Surgical intervention is necessary in severe cases where there is perforation.

CHAPTER 10

Kinesiology & Physics

PLANE CLASSIFICATION

- Frontal plane (coronal or XY plane): divides the body into front and back parts
- Sagittal plane (YZ plane): divides the body into right and left sides
- Horizontal plane (transverse or XZ plane): divides the body into upper and lower parts

LEVER CLASSIFICATION

1. **First-class lever:** the fulcrum is located between the weight and the force. Favors force or speed/distance.
   Example: seesaw utilizes a force arm and weight arm to gain force or distance
   Example: the atlantooccipital joint (axis) head (weight)
2. **Second-class lever:** the weight lies between the fulcrum and the force. Favors force with little range of motion (ROM).
   Example: crowbar utilizes a force advantage where small force can move large weight
   Example: brachioradialis and wrist extensors on elbow flexion
3. **Third-class lever:** the force is applied between the fulcrum and the weight. Produces ROM and speed at the expense of force. The weight arm is longer than the force arm, designed for producing speed, or for moving a small weight over a long distance. This is the most common lever in the body.
   Example: elbow flexion

LEVER TERMS

Force arm: the distance of the lever between the fulcrum (joint) and the effort force (muscle attachment).
Fulcrum: point of rotation.
Mechanical advantage: the ratio of the force arm over the resistance arm.
Resistance arm: (also known as weight arm) the distance of the lever between the fulcrum and the weight.

DEGREES OF FREEDOM CLASSIFICATION

Joints are classified according to the number of axes or planes in which they move. Maximum number that a single joint can possess is three.
   1. **One degree of freedom:** one axis of movement
      Example: elbow joint
   2. **Two degrees of freedom:** two axes of movement
      Example: metacarpophalangeal joints in the hand
   3. **Three degrees of freedom:** three axes of movement
      Example: shoulder joint

TERMS

Accessory movement: small translating motion; a few millimeters of passive ROM. Example: lateral glide at the elbow joint

Closed kinematic chain: distal segment of the chain is fixed in space. Example: exercising on a stair machine, foot fixed on step during exercise.

Electrogoniometry: technique for electrically recording movement.

Goniometry: the measurement of range of motion in a joint; degrees of movement available in each plane of movement for a joint.

Kinematic chain: several joints in successive segments.

Kinematics: describes the positions and motions of the body in space.

Kinesiology: the study of muscular activity and of the anatomy, physiology, and mechanics of the movement of body parts.

Open kinematic chain: distal segment of the chain terminates free in space. Example: short arc quads, foot not connected during exercise

TYPES OF SYNOVIAL JOINTS

There are typically six types of synovial joints in the body. These joints are classified according to the shape of the articulating surface, as well as the type of movement that is permitted by the joint.

Ball and Socket

These are highly moveable joints. They allow flexion, extension, abduction, adduction, medial and lateral rotation, and circumduction. Example: hip or shoulder joint

Condyloid Joints

These joints allow movement in three directions, either flexion and extension, abduction and adduction, or circumdu Example: metacarpophalangeal joint

Hinge Joint

The hinge joint permits movement in one axis. It may also be referred to as a ginglymus joint. A hinge joint only permits flexion and extension. Example: elbow joint

Plane Joint

A plane joint allows movement typically in only one axis, generally in a gliding or sliding movement. Example: acromioclavicular joint

Pivot Joint

The pivot joint allows rotation around an axis. Example: atlantoaxial joint

Saddle Joint

A saddle joint allows a concave/convex relationship. Example: carpometacarpal joint of the thumb

PHYSICS

Methods of Heat Transfer

Conduction: heat is transferred from one part of a body to another through molecular collision. Example: hot packs, paraffin

Convection: heat is transferred by the combined mechanisms of fluid mixing and conduction. Example: whirlpool, paraffin

Radiation: heat is transferred in the form of electromagnetic waves without heating the intervening medium. Example: warming by the sun

PHYSICAL LAWS

Cosine Law

The cosine law states that the intensity of radiation to a surface is altered by the cosine of the incident angle formed between the source and the patient. Clinically this means the source (eg, ultrasound) should be perpendicular to the patient for best results.

Inverse Square Law

The inverse square law states that the intensity of radiation from a light source varies inversely to the square of the distance from the source. Clinical application means the further (eg, the infrared light) is moving from the patient, the greater the decrease in intensity will be.

Joule's Law

Joule's law states that the amount of heat produced is proportional to the square of the current, the resistance, and the time that the current flows.

Ohm's Law (V = IR)

V = (volt) – electromotive force
I = current
R = resistance

Ohm's law states that the strength of an electrical current in a circuit is directly proportional to the applied electromotive force and inversely proportional to the resistance of the current.

WAVEFORMS/CURRENT

Alternating Current (AC)

AC, sinusoidal pattern of any frequency, current flow where the direction reverses at regular intervals.

Asymmetrical Biphasic Pulsatile

Uneven ion distribution with ion flow in both directions.

Faradic

Low amplitude, long duration, one direction.

Galvanic

Direct current (DC), steady and uninterrupted direct current, unidirectional.

Modulation

Three clinical waveforms to choose from in set-ups of most units:
1. Continuous
2. Interrupted
3. Surge

Monophasic Pulsatile

Ion flow in one direction.

Pulsatile

A rectangular-patterned waveform (common clinical rate: 1 to 100 pulses per second)

Symmetrical Biphasic Pulsatile

Ions flow equally in both directions.

COMMON TERMS

AC: alternating current; an electric current that may reverse directions

Amplitude: magnitude

Anode: positive electrode

Cathode: negative electrode

Chronaxie: minimal time that a stimulus of twice rheobase stimulates a tissue (strength-duration curve)

Circuit: pathway along which an electrical current will flow

Current: a flow of electrons along a conductor in a closed circuit or an electrical current; the current may be directed or alternating

DC: direct current; an electrical current that flows in only one direction and is basically constant in value

Frequency: rate of oscillation

Impedance: resistance in an electrical system

Microamp: 1/1,000,000 of an amp

Milliamp: 1/1000 of an amp

Ohm: the basic unit of resistance

Pulse width: duration of a pulse

Rheobase: minimum intensity of an electrical stimulus to elicit a minimal contraction

Waveform: shape of electron flow in an electrical current

Voltage: the potential energy difference between two entities

FORMULAS

Joule's Law (Q = 1 RT)

Q = Joule's law =   1 = current
                     R = resistance
                     T = time

Power = volts x amps

(watts) = (force) x (current)

Temperature Conversions

Celsius = (temperature in Fahrenheit − 32) x 5/9

Fahrenheit = (temperature in Celsius x 9/5) + 32

Work = E x C

Joule's law = (volts) x (coulombs)

CHAPTER 11

Arthritis

GOUT

- Disturbance in the uric acid metabolism, resulting in increased serum urate levels.
- Diagnosis is through urate crystals in the synovial fluid, connective tissue, and/or articular cartilage.
- Usually affects one or two joints.
- Site of initial attacks may include the metatarsophalangeal joint, ankle, instep, knee, elbow, and fingers.
- Symptoms include redness, swelling, fever, and severe pain over the affected joint.
- Affects males more than females.
- **Treatment:** medication (salicylates); have patient avoid extreme temperatures, alcohol, fatigue, or exhaustion.

MARIE-STRÜMPELL DISEASE

- Another name is ankylosing spondylitis.
- Disease is a bony ankylosis of all the vertebral joints. Characterized by recurrent back pain (especially the sacroiliac joint), which may progress up to the thoracic spine, resulting in kyphosis.
- Varies between periods of exacerbation and remission.
- "Bamboo spines" in the vertebral column.
- Most common in males.
- Fever, anorexia, eye problems, other systems and joints may be affected.
- **Treatment:** maintain joint mobility through exercise and stretching, heat, and postural instructions. Strengthening of the trunk extensor and preventing muscle imbalance are important. During acute exacerbation, aggressive stretching and exercises must be avoided.

OSTEOARTHRITIS (DEGENERATIVE JOINT DISEASE)

- Most common type of arthritis.
- Also called degenerative joint disease because it is a slow progressive degeneration of the joint structure.
- Associated with aging and referred to as wear-and-tear arthritis.
- May affect only one joint.
- Most common joints involved include lumbar spine, cervical spine, hip, knee, and first metatarsophalangeal and carpometacarpal joint.
- Begins in the articular cartilage rather than the synovial membrane.
- Diagnosis is usually made based on radiographic examination, patient history, and physical examination.
- **Treatment:** there is no cure; symptoms can be minimized with proper exercise, medication and rest. Joint conservation techniques to prevent excess force to the joint. Postural instructions to decrease wear and tear from abnormal alignment stress. Prevention and treatment of muscle imbalance and home education program.

PSORIATIC ARTHRITIS

- A seronegative inflammatory joint disease.
- This affects a small percentage (5% to 7%) of patients who have psoriasis.
- Psoriatic arthritis results in inflammation in the synovitis.
- The synovium inflammation can progress to the joint space filling with dense fibrous tissue.
- Joints typically affected include the distal interphalangeal, digits, and sacroiliac.
- **Treatment:** no known cure; medications are utilized to assist with pain and inflammation. Typically the disease is mild and not destructive.

RHEUMATOID ARTHRITIS

- Chronic systemic connective tissue disease with many characteristics.
- Joints are usually symmetrically involved. The synovium is inflamed and edematous.
- Female gender and age (typically third or fourth decade) are the two primary risk factors associated with rheumatoid arthritis.
- A proliferation of granulation tissue, known as pannus, occurs. Pannus eventually will destroy the joint cartilage, bone, and other periarticular tissues.
- The end results are destroyed joint cartilage, ankylosis, joint instability, and joint deformity.
- Morning stiffness is common.
- **Treatment:** heat, aquatic therapy, gentle exercise, and stretching exercises to maintain range of motion. Treatment goals to reduce pain, minimize stiffness, decrease edema, maintain joint mobility, and education.

STILL'S DISEASE

- Another name for juvenile arthritis.
- Can range from mild to severe, resulting in permanent disabilities.
- Severe pain in inflamed joints.
- Systemic effect more severe in children.
- A fever and rash mark the disease.
- The rash typically appears on the trunk and extremities.
- May even destroy growth plate in children.
- Twenty percent have disabilities when they reach adulthood.
- **Treatment:** aspirin in high doses, depending on the size of the child. Physical therapy utilized for pain and maintaining mobility.

TYPICAL JOINT PROBLEMS WITH RHEUMATOID ARTHRITIS

JOINT	PROBLEM
Cervical	Decreased rotation, especially C1 to C2
Temporomandibular (TMJ)	Decreased mouth opening
Shoulder	Loss of range of motion
Elbow	Instability and flexion contractures
Metacarpophalangeal (MCP)	Ulnar drift
Proximal interphalangeal (PIP)	Swan neck or boutonniere deformities
Distal interphalangeal (DIP)	Rarely affected
Hip	Not commonly affected
Knee	Flexion contractures
Ankle/foot	Hallux valgus (bunion), hammer, and claw toe deformities

OSTEOARTHRITIS VERSUS RHEUMATOID

OSTEOARTHRITIS	RHEUMATOID
Nonsystemic disease	Systemic disease
Cartilage thinning	Bony erosion
Affects weightbearing joints	Single joint affected first
Heberden's nodes	Ulnar deviation
No clinical or lab findings	Aspirate synovial fluid
Bony spurs form	Pannus formation
Narrowing of joint space	Fibrous adhesions
Osteophytes	Painful joint
Surface becomes rough	Inflammatory reaction
Stiffness/pain	Swelling/redness/heat, tender joint
Treatment: rest, support, heat, and regular exercise	Treatment: rest, heat, joint conservation techniques

CHAPTER 12

Oncology

TERMS

Benign Tumors

A tumor that is localized, slow growing, and does not invade other tissue or metastasize in other body sites. It may grow in size to become harmful if it impairs functions of the body.

Cancer Staging

A system for describing the extent of a malignant tumor and its metastases. It is utilized to plan a treatment program and predict a prognosis. The American Joint Committee on Cancer recommends staging cancer as follows: stage one is the primary tumor, stage two involves the primary tumor and lymph nodes, and stages three involves the primary tumor, lymph nodes, and metastases in other areas.

Cancerous Malignancies

A neoplasm characterized by uncontrolled growth of neoplastic cells. The cells tend to invade surrounding tissue and metastasize to other body sites. Malignant cells are present.

Carcinoma

A malignant epithelial neoplasm that invades surrounding tissue and metastasizes to other body sites. Most commonly in the skin, large intestine, lungs, stomach, prostate, cervix, or breast. Tumor is firm, irregular, and nodular.

Lymphoma

A disorder of a tumor or neoplasm in the lymphoid tissue. Examples include Hodgkin's disease, lymphatic leukemia, adenolymphoma, and Burkitt's lymphoma. Usually malignant but may be benign in rare cases. Characterized by enlarged lymph node(s).

Malignant Tumors

A tumor whose growth may cause death and tends to become worse over time. The tumor will invade surrounding tissue and metastasize to distant sites.

Neoplasm

Any abnormal growth of new tissue; it may be benign or malignant. The new tissue serves no purpose and may cause harm by competing for blood supply.

Oncology

The branch of medicine that studies tumors and cancerous malignancies.

Sarcoma

A malignant neoplasm of soft tissue; presents as painless swelling. The tumors are vascular and usually highly invasive. Tumors occur 40% in lower extremities, 20% in upper extremities, 20% in the trunk, and 20% in the head, neck, or retroperineuma.

Tumors

Characterized by progressive, uncontrolled proliferation of cells. A tumor may be localized, invasive, benign, or malignant. A tumor may be named by the location, the person who first identified this type of tumor, and/or cellular makeup.

TREATMENT OPTIONS

Surgery

- Surgical removal or resection of tissue as allowed by the growth and metastases in other areas.
- Tumor may be completely or partially removed or the entire area may be resected.
- For example, a radical mastectomy to treat breast cancer is the surgical removal of the entire breast. A dissection is the removal of tissue in an area surrounding the operative site.
- Symptoms may include weakness after surgery, soreness, limited range of motion, and edema.

Radiation Therapy

- Utilizing radioactive substances in the treatment of the disease.
- May be utilized prior to surgery to attempt to decrease the tumor size as an option to surgery or postoperatively.
- A radiation oncologist is a physician who specializes in the treatment of cancer through radiation.
- Radiation therapy may cause sickness. Volume of radiation and length of exposure and treatment area determine the severity of sickness.
- Symptoms may include headaches, nausea, vomiting, diarrhea, and anorexia.

Chemotherapy

- Treatment with chemical agents to destroy the cancer cells.
- The chemical agents function to decrease the cell's ability to replicate and destroy cancer cells.
- There are many different chemical agents available, and the physician determines the most appropriate. This could be based on the latest research, if a patient is in a clinical study, location and type of cancer, stage of cancer, and side effects to patient. Side effects vary with type of agents utilized.
- Drugs may be prescribed in conjunction with chemotherapy to prevent side effects, and reduce or assist with symptoms after chemotherapy.

EVALUATION, TREATMENT, AND PRECAUTIONS

Initial Evaluation

Depends on the type, location, and staging of cancer. The evaluation could include muscle weakness, endurance level, range of motion, ability to perform activities of daily living (ADLs), gait evaluation, sensation, and safety of patient.

Treatment Options

Vary with the type, location, and treatment of cancer. Some examples include:
- Education of the patient and family to treatment protocols and procedures, and disease effects on the patient from a physical therapy perspective.
- Development of treatment plans: long- and short-term goals with patient/family.
- Patient and family should be aware of the risk of falling secondary to weakness. Provide home safety assessment.
- Development and increased ability to perform ADLs and functional abilities.

- Referral to support groups and other health care team members.
- Increased activity to tolerance, conditioning, and muscle strengthening.
- Teaching gait and ADLs techniques to patient and family to increase safety.
- Patient position during and after treatment to prevent pressure sores or contractures.
- Modalities as appropriate (eg, long course of treatment in a hospital bed may cause neck and back pain).
- Therapeutic exercises as tolerated, depending on condition. For example, the same patient above may benefit from the Williams/McKenzie exercise for back and neck pain.
- Home program education with family/patient to continue therapy at home.

Precautions

- Tumors in certain locations (eg, bone tumors may cause weakness to bone area, or lower or upper extremities).
- Cancer treatments may affect cardiac and respiratory systems, causing side effects; therefore, cardiac/respiratory systems should be monitored in physical therapy.
- Exercise levels may be decreased and fatigue may occur.
- Infection levels for the patient may be sensitive, watch for any open wounds, and use sterile precautions. Wear a mask when treating a patient if you have a cold or infection.
- Safety of patients, as they may have decreased balance, numbness, and/or neuropathy in extremities.

CHAPTER 13
Obstetrics & Gynecology

PHYSIOLOGICAL CHANGES DURING PREGNANCY

- Most uterine weight gain is during week 20. The average weight gain is typically 20 to 30 pounds.
- No specific neurological disorders result solely from pregnancy.
- The renal system must expand and a common complaint in early stages of pregnancy is the need to go to the bathroom very frequently. Weakness in the pelvic floor walls might result in stress incontinence.
- Respiratory changes result in widening of the thoracic cage, progressive elevation of the diaphragm, and the center part of the diaphragm becomes flat. Breathing patterns become more costal than abdominal because of the elevation of the diaphragm. Hyperventilation and dyspnea may occur during exercise.
- Cardiovascular system changes result in increased blood volume, increased heart rate and cardiac output, decreased arterial blood pressure at the end of the first trimester and throughout pregnancy.
- Gastrointestinal functions change because of hormones and structural changes. Changes may include vomiting or nausea, heartburn, minor abdominal pains, and lactose intolerance.
- Metabolic changes in carbohydrates may result in gestational diabetes.
- Musculoskeletal changes:
  1. Postural changes may result in cervical and/or lumbar lordosis, forward head, and kyphosis.
  2. Hormone release of relaxin results in ligament laxity. This most commonly involves the sacroiliac joint and hypermobility.
  3. Abnormal wall and pelvic floor muscular weakness. Diastasis recti abdominis may occur, resulting in lateral separation of the rectus abdominis.
  4. Back pain occurs as a result of the ligament laxity and weakness of abdominal muscles.
- Balance changes from the pregnancy result in the center of gravity being shifted forward.
- Varicose veins may be a result of pregnancy, causing pain in the lower extremities.
- Gait pattern typically reveals a waddling gait.

TREATMENT OPTIONS

1. First the physical therapist needs to be aware of precautions in treatment program planning.
   - Avoid exercises that strain the pelvic floor muscles.
   - Avoid exercises that strain the abdominal muscles.
   - Avoid deep heating modalities and agents.
   - Have the patient avoid holding her breath during exercises so as not to increase interthoracic pressure.
   - Avoid positions that place the buttocks higher than the chest.
   - Avoid exercises that result in abdominal compression.
   - Avoid stretching that involves the hip flexors and areas of ligament laxity.
2. Transcutaneous electrical nerve stimulation (TENS) may be utilized to assist with pain.
3. A sacroiliac support belt and/or an orthosis may assist in support and help with back pain.

4. Superficial heat and moist hot packs may be utilized to assist with muscle relaxation and pain.
5. Gait instructions to walk avoiding an abducted gait, decreasing the waddling gait pattern.
6. Stretching exercise for postural correction and muscular relaxation. Exercises are modified (eg, single knee to chest stretching, patient should be supported with pillows or towel rolls and sidelying).
7. Modified curl-ups for abdominal wall strengthening.
8. Teach proper body mechanics.
9. Pelvic floor exercises and pelvic stabilization exercises.
10. Postural exercises for stretching and strengthening.
11. Teach the patient to monitor her own vital signs during exercise and activities of daily living.
12. Teach ankle pumps and elevated support positions of lower extremities to assist with edema and varicose veins.
13. Utilize elastic stockings for assistance with varicose veins.
14. Relaxation techniques, breathing exercise, meditation, and yoga.

CHAPTER 14

Wheelchairs

If long-term use of a wheelchair is expected, a physical therapist may prescribe certain personalized requirements, such as size, left or right-hand propulsion, type of brakes, height of armrests, special seat pads, special tires, and weight of the wheelchair.

MEASUREMENTS

There are six key measurements needed to fit someone for a wheelchair. In clinical practice, some of these measurements may be altered by the height and compressibility of the patient's cushion, so ideally you would measure with the patient sitting on the cushion that he or she will be utilizing. These are optimal measurements, but be sure they are functional for the patient's use based on any additional disabilities the patient may present.

1. **Seat width**
   - Measure on the patient: width of hips at the widest part
   - Chair measure: add 2 inches to the patient measure
2. **Seat depth**
   - Measure on the patient: back of buttocks to back of knee
   - Chair measure: subtract 2 to 3 inches from the patient measure
3. **Leg length/foot rest length**
   - Measure on the patient: from bottom of the shoe to just under the thigh
4. **Seat height**
   - Measure on the patient: the leg from the bottom of the foot to the thigh
   - Chair measure: add 2 inches to the leg length measure
5. **Arm rest height**
   - Measure on the patient: from the seat platform to just under the elbow (which is held at 90° with relaxed shoulders)
   - Chair measure: add 1 inch to the patient measure
6. **Back rest height**
   - Measure on the patient: from the seat platform to the axilla (shoulder flexed to 90°)
   - Chair measure: add 4 inches from the patient measurements above

STANDARD DIMENSIONS (IN INCHES)

CHAIR STYLE	WIDTH	DEPTH	SEAT HEIGHT	ARM HEIGHT	BACK HEIGHT
Adult	18	16	20	10	20
Narrow adult	16	16	20	10	20
Tall adult	18	17	20	10	18
Tall narrow adult	16	17	20	10	18
Low seat (propel with feet)	18	16	17	10	16
Junior (9 to 12 yrs)	16	13	18.5	8.5	16
Child's chair	14	11.5	18.75	8.5	16.5
Tiny tot (high)	12	11.5	19.5	6	17.5
Tiny tot (low)	12	11.5	17	6	17.5
Pediatric (2 to 4 yrs)	10	8	19.5	5	15

SPECIALIZED WHEELCHAIRS

Amputee's Chair

Modified by placing drive wheels posterior to back support to increase stability. Recommended for bilateral lower extremity amputees.

Hemi Chair

Low to the ground wheelchair so the patient can use uninvolved lower and upper extremities for propulsion.

One Arm Drive

Patient can propel the lever with one hand.

Powered Wheelchair

Utilizes a power source to move the chair for a patient with decreased exercise tolerance.

Reclining Back Wheelchair

Back may be extended for pressure relief and trunk support.

Sports Wheelchair

Lightweight wheelchair customized for greater maneuverability to utilize for participation in wheelchair sports.

Tilt Wheelchair

Entire seat and back may be tilted backward for pressure relief or so the patient is not thrown out of wheelchair.

CHAPTER 15

Geriatrics

CHANGES IN AGING

Cardiovascular System

- Loss of arterial elasticity
- Increase in peripheral resistance
- Systolic blood pressure increases with age secondary to decreased compliance of the blood vessels
- Decline in cardiac output
- The capacity of circulation to adapt to changes in body positioning decreases
- Decreased myocardial contractility and heart valves may stiffen
- Decreased cardiac output, 40% decline of overall resting cardiac output between third and seventh decade of life
- Decreased stroke volume
- Difficulty in meeting demands for increased cardiac output secondary to maximum heart rate decreasing
- Diminished supply of oxygenated blood, causing fatigue
- Decreased nourishment to vital organs, edema, and impaired waste removal
- After exertion, more time is needed to return to normal cardiac functioning.
- Some elderly people experience increased arrhythmia as conduction through nodal tissues slows
- Pacemaker's cells of the ventricle decline
- Automatic function of Purkinje network slows

Pulmonary System

- Decrease in vital capacity and forced expiratory volume (FEV); FEV can decline 20 to 40 ml per year
- Decreased strength of respiratory muscles
- Stiffening of chest wall
- Loss of bone matrix in the thoracic cage
- More vulnerable to respiratory illnesses
- Decreased elastic recoil of the lungs
- Decreased elasticity of the bronchial walls
- Decrease in rate of oxygen consumed and decreased oxygen delivery, reducing capacity to consume oxygen
- Increased ventilation
- Perfusion mismatch in the exchange of oxygen and carbon dioxide between the lungs
- Reduced ability to cough and breathe deeply
- Increased thinning of alveolar walls
- Decreased inspiratory muscle strength
- Increased mucus layer thickening
- Greater susceptibility to respiratory disease

Skeletal System

- Vertebral column becomes more compressed, shorter, disc atrophy, and less flexibility
- Increased calcification and ossification of ligaments and elastic fibers in cartilage
- Bone mass decreases
- Bone loses resilience and becomes lighter
- Increased sensitivity to bone fractures
- Increased susceptibility to osteoporosis
- Increased anterior/posterior diameter of the thoracic spine
- Increased susceptibility to hip and knee degeneration
- Stiffness of joints as a result of the degenerative process in the synovium
- Stiffness when going from sit to stand or in weightbearing positions
- Skeletal changes in the temporal mandibular joints; loss of teeth can decrease the ability to eat and can affect speech

Muscular System

- Decreased muscle mass
- Decreased endurance and increased muscle fatigue
- Increase in interstitial fluid, collagen, and intracellular fat
- Loss of muscle elasticity
- Articular cartilage tissue water content decreases
- Stiffening of capsules and ligaments
- Increased formation of collagen fibers and loss of elastic fibers
- Prolongation of contraction tone, latency period, and relaxation time
- Enzymes that repair damage are unable to be replaced and repaired effectively
- Decreased endurance, the ability and amount of the enzymes involved in energy metabolism become degraded

Nervous System

- Brain weight decreases during the aging process
- Increased lipofuscin pigment in neurons
- Nerve conduction velocity decreases
- Sleep patterns change, duration of deep sleep levels decreases, and number of arousals from sleep increases
- Central temperature regulation functions become impaired, causing the elderly to be more susceptible to hyperthermia and hypothermia
- Degeneration of the integumentary system
- Decrease in Purkinje cells of the cerebellum
- Atrophy of the medullary olives
- Trunk instability
- Losses in the vestibular, proprioceptive, kinesthetic, and visual mechanisms
- Postural instability
- Memory loss as a result of impaired neuronal function, debranching, shortening within the cortex, marked changes in prefrontal, temporal, and hippocampus

Endocrine and Metabolic Systems

- Adrenal cell degeneration, which can result in elevated blood sugar levels and increased glucose intolerance
- Thyroid activity decreases
- Metabolic energy decreases
- Liver tends to get smaller in measurement in advanced aging
- Body burns fewer calories
- Lower immunity; hormones with the immune system decline

Senses

- Kinesthesia—the ability to perceive changes in body orientation and position in space declines with aging
- Vestibular senses decrease, which can result in accidental falls

- Vibration sensitivity declines
- Temperature sensations decline as well as the ability to maintain constant body temperature
- Visual field may decline, causing difficulty with perception and slower responses to tasks involving spatial ability; acuity and accommodation slow with steady decline
- Hearing loss may occur, which may be dangerous (eg, inability to hear approaching automobile)

ASSESSMENT/SCREENING

1. Home safety
2. Exercise level/current activity level
3. Nutritional problems
4. Observations
   - Does patient appear dehydrated?
   - Difficulty breathing?
   - Skin color
   - Weight/height
5. Overall health/history
6. Medications
7. Vital signs
   - Blood pressure
   - Respiratory rate
   - Pulses
   - Heart rate
8. Musculoskeletal
   - Motor planning/mobility
   - Balance/dynamic and static
   - Range of motion/goniometry
   - Flexibility
   - Muscular endurance
   - Muscular strength/manual muscle testing
9. Cognitive functioning
10. Coordination
    - Equilibrium
    - Nonequilibrium
11. Vascular testing
    - Girth measurements
    - Homan's sign
    - Reactive hyperemia
    - Ischemia and rubor test
12. Skin integrity
13. Sensory abilities
    - Protective sensation
    - Discriminatory sensations
14. Posture
    - Posterior view
    - Lateral views
    - Anterior view
15. Gait
    - Cadence
    - Width of base of support
    - Length of step
    - Center of gravity
    - Arm swing
    - Observation of gait deviations
    - Amount of assistance necessary

16. Family status/support system
17. Sample treatment programs
    - **Cardiovascular:** aerobic exercises to increase oxygen uptake from blood
      Examples: walking, biking, dancing, and swimming
    - **Muscular:** increase muscular endurance
      Examples: walking, swimming, and water aerobics for elderly
    - **Flexibility:** maintain or increase joint flexibility
      Examples: slow stretching exercises; have patient hold stretch 20 seconds and release, then rehold 20 seconds, attempting to reach a little farther
    - **Posture:** emphasize potential problem areas—forward head, rounded shoulders, and tight hip flexor muscles
      Examples: teach chin tucks, pectoral stretch, and hip extension stretch
    - **Balance coordination:** improve balance and coordination to assist with safety
      Examples: yoga exercises, balance exercises such as standing on one foot, walking a line, and moving objects from one place to another
    - **Gait:** teach gait with an assistive device
      Examples: teaching patient the correct side to hold a cane and which lower extremity to advance first
    - **Home safety:** teach patient how to perform a safety home assessment
      Examples: provide patient with a safety checklist form to take home and inventory list for safety issues (sample question: are there any throw rugs on the floor?)
18. Education of patient/family and support system
    - Increase ability to perform activities of daily living
    - Home education
    - Patient education brochures and videos
    - Safety education
    - Nutrition counseling
    - Referral to other services as necessary

CHAPTER 16

Psychology

COMMON DISORDERS

Affective Psychosis

- Psychotic reaction
- Mental disorder of organic or emotional origin
- Characterized by extreme derangement or disorganization of personality
- Accompanied by severe depression, agitation, regressive behavior, illusions, delusions, and hallucinations
- Usually requires hospitalization because the patient is incapable of functioning in society

Alzheimer's Disease

- Chronic, progressive, widespread deterioration of the cerebrum
- Intellectual decline, loss of memory, confusion, anxiety, depression, loss of reasoning
- As disease progresses, there may be some motor impairment, gait problems, or contractures
- Consistency of treatment and redirection to another task if the patient becomes frustrated are considerations during treatment

Conversion Disorder

- May also be known as hysteria
- A response to severe emotional stress, resulting in loss or impairment of some motor or sensory function
- Often connected with the nervous system, resulting in problems with vision, sensation, hearing, or motor disturbances like hemiplegia, paraplegia, quadriplegia, tics, or tremors
- There is no known organic cause for this

Depression

- A feeling of sadness or helplessness
- Patient typically has little drive for activity or achievement. Patient may cry easily and there may be an eating disorder
- May be altered with the assistance of medication. The therapist needs to take a positive attitude, build in successful treatment experiences for the patient, and involve the patient in making choices about the types of treatments available

Hypochondria

- An overconcern with physical health
- Extreme anxiety about health
- May have no physiological basis for health problems

Mania

- Type of psychosis
- State of mental disorder
- Person exhibits a behavior of euphoria

Manic-Depressive Psychosis

- Wide swings in behavior between periods of euphoria and extreme depression
- Patient may be suicidal
- Bipolar disorder

Neurosis

- Inefficient way of coping with anxiety
- Involves the use of the unconscious defense mechanism
- An emotional disturbance

Obsessive-Compulsive Neurosis

- Neurotic condition
- Characterized by the inability to resist the intrusion of persistent, irrational thoughts, ideas, or fears

Obsessive-Compulsive Personality

- Type of personality disorder
- Characterized by an uncontrollable need to perform certain acts or rituals
- When the acts become irrational, they interfere with acts of living in society

Paranoia

- A psychotic state or disorder
- Patient has delusions of persecution or grandiosity
- Patient is typically suspicious in all situations with all people

Psychopathy

- Patient may also be called a sociopath
- An antisocial personality disorder
- Characterized by behavior patterns that lack moral and ethical standards

Psychosis

- Mental disorder of organic or emotional origin
- Characterized by an extreme derangement or disorganization of personality
- Accompanied by depression, agitation, and hallucinations
- Person often requires hospitalization and cannot function in society

Schizophrenia

- Recognized through odd and bizarre behaviors
- Thoughts are distorted
- Very suspicious of others
- Withdrawal into fantasy life
- Patient may be destructive or impulsive

Suicide

- Occurs as a result of feeling hopeless or helpless
- Patient experiences a sense of rejection
- May be prevented. Encourage patient to discuss feelings and refer to appropriate services

Common Terms

Behavior Modification

- Attempt to change the patient's attitude toward pain, grooming or appearance, and willingness to participate in therapy
- Reinforce or reward healthy, positive, and socially appropriate behavior

Defense Mechanism

- An unconscious response by which the ego is protected from anxiety, guilt, or shame.
  - Denial: refusal to recognize external reality
  - Repression: inability to recall past events
  - Displacement: transferring an emotion to a substitute emotion
  - Reaction formation: behavior that is exactly opposite of what is expected
  - Projection: attributing your own unwanted trait to another

Empathy

- Capacity to understand what your patient is experiencing from his or her perspective
- Empathy helps you to better understand the meaning of the illness or disability, thereby strengthening your working relationship as you treat the patient

Grief Process

- Patients who lose body parts, functions, or clarity of mental processing may go through some, or all, of the following stages of grieving:
  - Denial
  - Anger
  - Bargaining
  - Depression
  - Acceptance
  - Perseveration
  - Patient continues to repeat a movement, word, or expression
  - Often accompanies a head injury or brain damage from stroke

Placebo

- Inactive treatment given for potential research benefit
- Used in experimental drug studies to compare the effects of the inactive substance with those of the experimental drug

CHAPTER 17

Therapeutic Modalities

AQUATIC POOL THERAPY

A form of hydrotherapy for patient use to allow exercises in the water. The pool allows greater freedom of movement than traditional whirlpools to allow for therapeutic exercise. The pool provides buoyancy to assist patients with reducing stress on joints while exercising or ambulating, often allowing them to perform activities in the pool that they could not do on land. Exercises in the pool also provide resistant therapy for strengthening.

Precautions

- Pool chemical levels must be tested daily and adjusted accordingly
- Pool cleaning and filters must be regularly maintained
- Patients' fear of the water

Indications

- Increase range of motion
- Provide gait training with less stress on joints
- Improve balance
- Increase endurance/aerobic capacity
- Increase strength
- Improve circulation
- Promote patient relaxation

Contraindications

- Open wounds
- Incontinence
- Urinary infection
- Unstable blood pressure
- Uncontrolled epilepsy
- Upper respiratory infection
- Heat intolerance
- Severe mental disorders
- Uncontrolled diabetes
- Severe respiratory disorders
- Serious cardiac disorders
- Patients who fear water

Application

1. Explain procedures to the patient. The type of ambulation, active exercises, active-assistive exercises, and resistance exercises should be prescribed and monitored by the staff. There are many variations depending on the patient's diagnosis and treatment plan.
2. The patient should be instructed to bring a swimsuit or trunks and a towel.
3. The patient should bathe or shower prior to entering and after leaving the pool. Shoulder length or longer hair should be tied back or in a bathing cap.
4. The patient should have exercise sheets available and staff to monitor the program.
5. The program should be recorded in the clinical record, noting response to treatment.
6. Recommend treatment temperatures remain at 92° to 98°F. Treatment time is 15 to 60 minutes depending on the patient's program and tolerance.

CONTINUOUS PASSIVE MOTION

The passive movement of an extremity through a predetermined range of motion by the use of a mechanical device.

Precautions

- A physician typically predetermines range of motion degrees
- For the safety of the patient, be sure to remove all linen and clothing away from roller tracks

Indications

- Total joint surgery, especially total hip or knee replacement surgery
- Tendon or ligament repair
- Post-immobilization fracture

Contraindications

- Nonstable fracture sites
- Increase in pain to intolerable levels
- Increase in edema

Application

1. Explain the procedure to the patient.
2. Place clean sheepskin on patient's treatment area. Make sure wound areas are covered with a dressing to maintain sterile conditions.
3. Adjust the unit under the patient with the anatomical joint aligning with the mechanical hinge joint on the machine.
4. Place joint in machine and secure safety straps.
5. Set the beginning and end range of motion degrees on the continuous passive motion (CPM) machine.
6. Turn the unit on and monitor for security of treatment area, joint placement, and patient complaints.
7. Provide the patient with an emergency shut-off switch.
8. If the patient can tolerate the initial beginning and end range of motion then gradually increase 5° to 10° every 24 hours based on tolerance.
9. Treatment time is 1 hour to continuous 24 hours or determined by the treatment team and patient tolerance. Duration of treatment-CPM continues until the patient achieves goals for range of motion with CPM. For maximum benefit, the affected limb should be in the CPM machine 20 hours out of every 24 hours.

CONTRAST BATH

The alteration and quick immersion of an extremity into hot and then cold water. The containers are filled with hot water (100° to 110°F) and cold water (55° to 65°F).

Precautions

- Check water temperature prior to treatment
- Wipe floor for any spilled water
- Caution should be used with peripheral vascular disease patients if water temperature is above 40ºC.

Indications

- Sprains, initial 48 hours
- Strains, initial 48 hours
- Arthritis
- Reflex sympathetic dystrophy
- Peripheral vascular disease
- Edema

Contraindications

- Malignancies
- Hemorrhage
- Diabetes
- Sensory loss
- Cardiac problems
- Buerger's disease

Application

1. Explain the procedure to the patient
2. Drape the patient, then expose the area to be treated
3. Place the patient in a comfortable position
4. Begin alternating between the hot and the cold water for a period of 20 minutes
5. Begin by placing the extremity in hot water for 4 to 6 minutes
6. Remove from hot water and then place extremity into cold water for 1 minute
7. The treatment typically ends in the warm water unless treating for edema, which you would end in cold water
8. Remove extremity from the bath and dry off
9. Inspect the skin of the extremity treated

CRYOTHERAPY

There are several types of cryotherapy available including cold packs, ice massage, ice packs, ice-soaked towels, vapocoolant sprays, and cold-compression units. Cold packs are available as canvas or plastic-covered silica gel. Ice packs contain crushed ice in a plastic bag or a towel. Ice massage uses a plastic or insulated cup of frozen water with a wooden tongue depressor in the middle. Ice-soaked towels are typically terrycloth towels put in a slush mixture and then wrung out. Fluori-Methane spray is one type of a vapocoolant spray utilized in the clinic. The bottle emits a fine spray on the patient when inverted. Cold-compression units contain cooled water that is circulated through a sleeve that is applied over extremity.

Precautions

- Frostbite
- Systemic chilling
- Excess pressure may cause blisters
- Protect bony prominences
- Check patient's hypersensitivity to cold and skin sensation
- Hypertensive patients
- Vapocoolant sprays may be an environmental concern

Indications

- Inflammatory conditions
- Edema
- Muscle spasms
- Alleviate pain
- After therapeutic exercise to prevent edema/inflammation
- Spasticity
- Facilitate a muscle contraction
- Postorthopedic surgical swelling and pain
- Myofascial pain syndrome—trigger points

Contraindications

- Ischemia tissue
- Hypersensitivity to cold
- Impaired circulation
- Peripheral vascular disease
- Impaired sensation
- Raynaud's phenomenon

Application

Cold Pack or Ice Pack

1. Explain the procedure to the patient: why ice is being used and the type of sensations that will be experienced, such as cold, burning, and/or numbness.
2. Drape the patient and expose the area to be treated.
3. Apply a wet towel to the skin surface to be treated to insulate for cold packs and ice packs. The damp towel may be covered with a dry towel when less cold application is desired.
4. Patient is positioned so the treatment area is supported.
5. Secure the cold pack or ice pack to the area being treated.
6. Give the patient a signal device in case of any difficulties.
7. Allow 10 to 15 minutes treatment time.
8. Upon completion of treatment, dry and inspect area.

Ice Massage

1. Explain the procedure to the patient and why ice is being used.
2. Describe the sensations the patient should expect to feel. The patient should report to the therapist when she or he feels each of the sensations.
3. Drape the patient and expose the area to be treated.
4. A towel should be utilized to absorb water seepage from the melting ice.
5. Remove the ice from a paper cup or tear cup back to expose the ice. Warn the patient before applying ice.
6. Apply ice to the treatment area in small overlapping circles.
7. Treatment time: 5 to 10 minutes.
8. After drying, inspect the skin.

Ice Towels

1. Explain the procedure to the patient.
2. Drape the patient and exposed area to be treated.
3. Place a towel in the slush mixture.
4. Wring out the towel and place it on the patient.
5. The towel can be on the patient 4 to 5 minutes, then it will need to be changed.
6. After treatment, dry and inspect area.

Vapocoolant Spray

1. Explain the procedure to the patient.
2. Drape the patient and expose the area to be treated.
3. Hold spray 18 to 24 inches from the area to be treated. Invert the spray nozzle can downward.
4. Sweep spray over the treatment area every 4 to 5 seconds at a 30° to 45° angle.
5. The muscle group in the area of treatment should be passively stretched before and during application.
6. Spray the entire treatment area, including the area of referred pain.
7. Moist hot packs may be applied during treatment for 5 to 10 minutes to increase stretching.
8. Total treatment time: 15 to 20 minutes.
9. After drying, inspect the skin.

Cold-Compression Units

1. Explain the procedure to the patient.
2. Clean the area and place elastic stockinet over area to be treated.
3. Place the extremity in the sleeve of the unit.
4. Set temperature on the unit, approximately 10°C to 25°C.
5. Treatment time of 15 to 30 minutes depending on area treated and tolerance.
6. Remove the extremity from sleeve, dry off, and inspect.

ELECTRICAL STIMULATION

Electrical stimulation is the use of electricity to artificially stimulate nerves and muscles. This may be used to accomplish a variety of therapeutic purposes, such as the effects on a denervated muscle are to decrease atrophy and increase the circulation of the muscle. Effects on an innervated muscle are to produce muscle relaxation, decrease spasms, prevent atrophy, decrease spasticity, re-educate muscles, and reduce pain and edema.

Precautions

- Equipment should have an annual biomechanical check-up and be in good condition
- Equipment should be properly grounded
- Use the correct type of current for denervated and innervated muscle
- Use care over areas of impaired sensation
- Make sure intensity of electrical stimulation machine is turned to zero prior to turning on machine

Indications

- Muscle spasms
- Edema
- Spasticity
- Denervated muscle
- Pain
- Muscle re-education
- Impaired range of motion
- Disuse atrophy
- Wound healing

Contraindications

- Pacemaker
- Cardiac problems
- Malignancy
- Hemorrhage
- Directly over uterus
- Directly over an area of infection or inflammation
- Metal implants
- Directly over or near pharyngeal or laryngeal muscles
- Deep vein thrombosis

Application

1. Explain the procedure to the patient.
2. Expose then inspect the area to be treated and drape properly.
3. Position the patient for comfort.
4. Determine which electrodes to use.
    - Soak electrode pads in water and squeeze out excess. Cover with a wet gauze, or
    - Use disposable electrodes or carbonized rubber electrodes and place a small amount of gel on electrode surface.
5. Connect the wires from the machine to the electrodes.
6. Place the dispersive electrode on an antagonistic muscle surface or adjacent area. Place active electrode over area being treated.
7. Secure electrodes with straps.
8. Set intensity at zero prior to turning on and set the timer for a treatment of 10 to 30 minutes.
9. Increase intensity to the patient's tolerance. Utilize the desired wave form.
10. Adjust intensity to achieve the optimal treatment effect within the patient's tolerance. At the first sign of muscle fatigue, switch to another area.
11. Have an emergency shut-off switch or a signaling device of some sort available to the patient.
12. When treatment is completed, turn the intensity to zero, turn off the power, and remove the electrodes.
13. Inspect the patient's skin.

FLUIDOTHERAPY

Fluidotherapy is the circulation of heated silicon or cellulase particles in a dry heat environment; energy is transferred by convection. Primarily used to treat hands, wrists, and forearms. Provides a whirlpool effect in a unit of circulated dry heat.

Precautions

- Check for diminished or absent sensation prior to treatment
- Inspect area for open wounds, scars, or sutures
- Vary or control level of agitation to patients who are beginning desensitization

Indications

- Joint stiffness
- Arthritis
- Increased tissue elasticity prior to stretching to prepare for additional treatment
- Alleviate pain
- Chronic inflammatory conditions
- Post fracture—stable

Contraindications

- Fresh sutures or wounds
- Acute inflammatory conditions
- Infections
- Edema
- Decreased circulation
- Decreased sensation

Application

1. Explain the procedure to the patient.
2. Test area for sensation.
3. Remove jewelry or wrap in gauze and tape prior to treatment.
4. Wash area to be treated.

5. Place extremity in treatment sleeve with protective sleeve or stockinet over the treatment area.
6. Temperature: 102° to 118°F.
7. Treatment time: 15 to 20 minutes.
8. Remove protective sleeve after treatment; dry and inspect the area.

FUNCTIONAL ELECTRICAL STIMULATION

Functional electrical stimulation (FES) is typically a hand-held unit that encompasses a wide variety of stimulator units which are available in the marketplace. The therapist utilizes the units because it allows a wide variety of protocols for specific treatments. FES is also called neuromuscular electrical stimulation (NMES).

Precautions

- Irritation under electrode placement
- Turn intensity to zero prior to turning on the unit

Indications

- Disuse atrophy
- Impaired range of motion
- Gait training
- Muscle re-education
- Spasticity

Contraindications

- Pacemaker
- Cardiac problems
- Malignancy
- Hemorrhage
- Directly over uterus
- Directly over an area of infection or inflammation
- Metal implants
- Directly over or near pharyngeal or laryngeal muscles
- Deep vein thrombosis

Application

1. Explain the procedure to the patient.
2. Drape the patient, expose the area to be treated, and place the patient in a comfortable position.
3. While the machine is off, turn the intensity to zero, and place the electrodes. Arrange disposable electrodes in proper position depending on condition being treated, then secure the electrodes.
4. Intensity, amplitude, pulse rate, pulse duration, and treatment is determined by protocols.
5. Complete treatment, return intensity to zero, turn off power, remove electrodes, and inspect the treated area.

Example

Gait training treatment for dorsiflexion and functional electrical stimulation (FES) to control drop foot and facilitate dorsiflexors and evertors during swing phase of gait.

- Wave form: asymmetric biphasic square
- Pulse duration: 20 to 250 μsec.
- Modulation: utilization of foot switch-heel switch stops stimulation during stance phase and activates stimulation in swing phase.
- Amplitude: tetanic muscle contraction
- Pulse rate: 30 to 300 pps
- Electrode placement: bipolar on anterior tibialis muscle or peroneal nerve near head of fibula.

GAIT TRAINING AND AMBULATORY AIDS

Gait training is the analysis of a patient's gait and the determination if intervention is necessary to correct gait deficiencies and monitor patient safety. Ambulatory aids may be utilized for assistance and safety.

Precautions

- Patient's weightbearing status
  - Nonweightbearing—no bearing of weight is permitted.
  - Partial weightbearing—toes or ball of foot of involved lower extremity may contact floor.
  - Full weightbearing—full weight is permitted on the involved lower extremity.
- Decreased strength and endurance will affect performance of the patient.
- Evaluate the patient's home and/or work site for obstacles to gait training or the use of ambulatory aids. For example, inquire if there are stairs inside or outside or both, verify if the door entrance is 36 inches or wider, and establish if the patient will be walking on carpet, tile or wood floors, cement, or on area rugs.

Indications

- Pre or post surgery for correct weightbearing status on the affected extremity
- Unsafe gait pattern
- Poor balance
- Increase independence
- Impaired ambulation skills

Contraindications

- Excessive edema of foot
- Severe contractures prohibiting safe movement
- Poor cognitive functioning causing unsafe gait patterns
- Bilateral nonweightbearing status
- Injury, infection, and/or open wounds on feet

Application

Canes

When a wider base of support is needed for stability.
1. Explain procedure to patient.
2. Measure cane to allow 20° to 30° elbow flexion. Adjust to proper height (wood or aluminum cane).
3. Utilize single-point cane or quad cane (four contact points), depending on support needed.
4. Cane is placed in the hand of the opposite side of involved extremity.
5. Cane and the involved extremity are advanced together. The cane should be kept flat on the floor.
6. The uninvolved extremity then follows the involved extremity. Steps should be equal.

Crutches

Aid to relieve weightbearing on the lower extremities and to increase the base of support.
1. Measuring crutches' axillary (wood or aluminum crutches).
   - 20° to 30° of elbow flexion
   - Two-finger width between axilla and crutch
2. Determine gait pattern with weightbearing status: nonweightbearing, partial weightbearing, or full weightbearing.
   - Two-point gait procedure:
     - One crutch and opposite extremity move together, then opposite crutch and extremity, two movements for each completed step.
   - Three-point gait:
     - Both crutches and the involved leg move together, then the uninvolved extremity.
   - Four-point gait:
     - One crutch advances forward then the opposite extremity, followed by the remaining crutch and extremity. It will take four movements to complete one step.

- Swing-through gait:
  - Both crutches are advanced forward together. This movement follows with swinging both legs forward in front of crutches.
- Swing-to gait:
  - Both crutches are advanced forward; the patient then shifts weight onto hands and then both legs swing forward to meet crutches.
- Stairs:
  - Ascending stairs: uninvolved extremity goes up, followed by crutches and involved extremity together.
  - Descending stairs: the crutches and involved extremity go down the steps, followed by the uninvolved extremity.

Walker

When a wider base of support is needed to provide anterior and lateral stability.

1. Measure walker.
   - 20° to 30° of elbow flexion
   - Adjust to proper height
2. The walker should be kept flat on the floor when the patient takes a step.
3. Choose the type of walker:
   - Folding walker for ease in traveling—folds up and compact. To increase stability, pick up the walker and move the involved extremity forward, then the uninvolved extremity.
   - Rolling walker (wheels are attached to the walker—either two wheels on the front legs or a total of four wheels). A hand brake may be applied to assist with stopping. Appropriate when therapist wants to facilitate continuous movement of the patient. The patient slowly rolls the walker ahead while taking even-sized steps.
   - Reciprocal walker is a hinged walker that allows advancement of one side of the walker at a time (four-point gait).
   - Hemiwalker is a walker that is modified to use with one hand. The handgrip is located in the center front of the walker.

HIGH-VOLT PULSED CURRENT

High-voltage pulsed current, which provides unidirectional short duration, and twin peak pulses. Modulation may be continuous, surged, or interrupted.

Precautions

- Areas of decreased sensation, skin irritation, and burns may occur under electrodes.
- Intensity of machine at zero prior to turning on.
- Equipment is in good condition and grounded.

Indications

- Pain control
- Decreased edema
- Muscle spasms
- Muscle re-education
- Decreased range of motion in contracted joint
- Decreased atrophy
- Muscle strengthening

Contraindications

- Pacemaker
- Coronary problems
- Pregnant
- Near laryngeal and pharyngeal muscles
- Malignancies

- Infection
- Hemorrhage
- Deep vein thrombosis

Application

1. Explain the procedure to the patient.
2. The patient is positioned comfortably. Only the area to be treated is exposed so the patient is draped to protect his or her privacy.
3. Determine which electrodes to use.
   - Soak electrode pads in water and squeeze out excess. Cover with wet gauze, or
   - Use disposable electrodes or carbonized rubber electrodes and place a small amount of gel on the electrode surface.
4. Connect wires from the machine to the electrodes.
5. A hand-held probe may be utilized instead of electrodes for stimulation of specific motor points or trigger points. If using a probe only, a probe and dispersive pad are needed.
6. Connect the wires from the machine to the electrodes.
7. Place the dispersive electrode on an antagonistic muscle surface or adjacent area. Place active electrode over area being treated.
8. Secure electrodes with straps.
9. Select polarity to use and set the dial.
10. Select pulses per second rate and set the dial.
11. Set pad function switch to reciprocal rate, continuous, or hand-held probe.
12. Set machine intensity to zero, set treatment time, and turn on machine.
13. Slowly turn up intensity to the selected level.
14. Adjust pad balance switch if necessary and intensity switch to patient tolerance.
15. Give the patient the emergency shut-off switch or signaling device.
16. Turn the intensity down to zero before turning the machine off and ending treatment and prior to removal of the electrodes.
17. Inspect the skin of the area that was treated.

MOIST HOT PACKS

Hot packs are a conductive type of superficial moist heat. The outer cover is a cotton fabric and inside is a silicon gel that retains water well. The packs are available in various sizes and are preheated in a hydrocullator unit. The temperature of the water in the hydrocullator should be maintained at 150° to 190°F.

Precautions

- Extra toweling must be utilized so heat is not transferred too quickly and results in a burn.
- Once a hot pack is applied, the treatment area may not be observed.
- Some patients may not be able to tolerate the weight of the hot pack.
- The number of covers/towels used varies with the patient's tolerance to heat, so it may be difficult to determine how many it takes to prevent a burn.
- Patients with circulatory impairments should be treated with caution.

Indications

- Alleviate pain
- Muscle spasms
- Joint stiffness
- Chronic inflammatory condition
- Increase in circulation
- Increase in tissue elasticity
- Improve tissue healing

Contraindications

- Scars
- Burns
- Hemorrhage
- Infection
- Over open wounds or open skin
- Sensory loss
- Acute inflammatory condition
- Circulatory disorders
- Patient's with long-term steroid use if capillary fragility is present
- Malignant tumors
- Deep vein thrombophlebitis
- Edema
- Post-acute trauma with bleeding
- Hemophilia
- Impaired cognitive status

Application

1. Explain procedure to the patient.
2. Drape the patient, expose the area to be treated, and place the patient in a comfortable position.
3. Place the hot pack inside a terrycloth cover upon removing from the hydrocullator.
4. Seal the cover by pressing the velcro parts together.
5. Wrap additional towels around the hot pack and cover depending on the patient's tolerance to heat, typically six to eight covers. For instance, the patient lying on top of the hot pack will require extra protection as the increase in body weight increases the output of heat.
6. Place a towel between the patient's skin or treatment area and the hot pack cover(s).
7. Place the covers and toweling on the area to be treated with the side of the pack with moist towels next to the patient's skin.
8. Cover the opposite pack with folded towels to prevent heat loss.
9. Give the patient a signaling device to locate assistance if necessary.
10. Periodically check on the patient and increase or decrease towel as needed.
11. Secure the pack to the patient.
12. Treatment time: 20 to 30 minutes.
13. Periodically inspect the area being treated.
14. Remove hot packs at the end of treatment and dry the area.
15. Inspect the area and note tolerance to treatment in chart.

INFRARED LAMP

Heat transmission through radiant energy for therapeutic application of infrared lamps. There are two types of lamps: luminous (penetrates dermis and subcutaneous tissue 5 to 10 mm), and nonluminous (penetrates the epidermis 2 mm).

Precautions

- Treatment temperature is not precisely controlled, so careful instruction to the patient on how to discern the difference between a therapeutic response and becoming uncomfortable is important
- Check the area to be treated for sensation prior to treatment
- Check the lamp for lint build-up and to verify that the lamp is in operating order
- Nipples, genitalia, and eyes should be covered

Indications

- Joint stiffness
- Pain
- Muscle spasms

- Preparation for other therapeutic treatment
- Arthritis

Contraindications

- Open wounds
- Scars
- Sutures
- Infections
- Decreased circulation
- Decreased sensation
- Malignant tumors

Application

1. Explain the procedure to the patient.
2. Drape patient, expose area to be treated, and place patient in a comfortable position.
3. Remove all jewelry and metal objects.
4. Turn on lamp for 5 to 10 minutes to allow the lamp to warm up.
5. Place the reflector at a right angle to the surface being treated.
6. The output of the lamp is determined by the wattage.
7. Center lamp 30 to 36 inches over the treatment area if using a nonluminous lamp. Center the lamp 18 to 24 inches over the treatment area if using the luminous lamp. Intensity of treatment can vary depending on the distance of the lamp to the patient.
8. Give the patient a signaling device and advise of the treatment time of 15 to 20 minutes.
9. Inspect the area closely during and after the treatment. Keep the patient 10 to 15 minutes after the end of treatment to recheck the area and to allow the patient to cool down.

INTERMITTENT COMPRESSION PUMP

A pump that applies external pressure to the extremity through an inflatable sleeve. The pump is attached to the sleeve through rubber tubing. Some units have the ability to also produce a coolant effect through the inflatable sleeve.

Precautions

- Check the patient's blood pressure prior to treatment
- Open wounds
- History of cardiac problems

Indications

- Chronic edema
- Traumatic edema
- Post mastectomy
- Injury edema
- Stasis ulcer
- Amputation

Contraindications

- Obstructed lymphatic channel
- Infection
- Thrombophlebitis/deep vein thrombus
- Acute inflammation/infection
- Cancer
- Kidney insufficiency
- Hypertension
- Cardiac insufficiency
- Arterial insufficiency

Application

1. Check the patient's blood pressure.
2. Explain procedure to patient.
3. Measure the extremity and record in the clinical record.
4. Drape the patient, expose the area to be treated, and place the patient in a comfortable position.
5. The extremity should be elevated approximately 40° to 50° and abducted 20° to 70°.
6. Place stockinet over the extremity.
7. Put the compression sleeve over the extremity, being careful to avoid wrinkles on the stockinet.
8. Attach the sleeve to the rubber tubing and pump.
9. Set the inflation rate for approximately 45 to 90 seconds and the deflation rate for approximately 15 to 20 seconds for a 3:1 treatment cycle.
10. Set pressure and slowly increase it to the desired level over two to three cycles.
11. Give the patient a signaling device.
12. Treatment time varies from 20 minutes to 6 to 8 hours, depending on the condition.
13. Turn the machine off after treatment and remove the extremity from the sleeve. Check the extremity for any pressure points.
14. Measure the extremity after treatment and record.
15. If appropriate, reapply the compression stocking after treatment to assist in preventing fluid/edema from returning.

IONTOPHORESIS

The application of a continuous direct current to transfer medical agents through penetration of the skin for therapeutic treatment.

Precautions

- Allergy or sensitivity by the patient to therapeutic agents
- Electrochemical burns may occur
- Anesthetic effect occurs under the electrodes
- Direct current will lower skin resistance

Indications

- Edema reduction
- Inflammation
- Muscle spasms
- Bursitis
- Tendonitis
- Sprain/strain
- Epicondylitis
- Myositis
- Temporomandibular joint (TMJ)
- Carpal tunnel syndrome

Contraindications

- Allergy of patient to ion
- Areas of recent scarring
- Metal near the treatment area
- Pacemaker
- Impaired skin sensation
- Over open wounds, cuts, and bruises
- Pregnant
- Malignancies
- Pharyngeal or laryngeal muscles

Application

1. Explain the procedure to the patient.
2. Drape the patient, expose the area to be treated, and place the patient in a comfortable position.
3. Place the active electrode over the treatment area. The active electrode should have the same polarity as the ion.
4. Place the dispersive electrode at a distant site.
5. Secure both electrodes in place.
6. Determine dosage, current intensity, and time of treatment.
7. Turn on machine and turn intensity up slowly.
8. Check on the patient every 5 minutes and leave the signaling device readily available.
9. Once the treatment is complete, turn off the machine, inspect the skin, and cleanse the treatment site.

MASSAGE

Massage is the manipulation of body tissue and soft tissue by the therapist's hands. There are many therapeutic massage techniques, including effleurage, kneading, friction, tapping, and vibration for the therapist to choose from.

Precautions

- Areas of skin irritations, open wounds, and blisters.
- Tolerance of patient to the pressure of massage.

Indications

- Muscle spasms
- Pain
- Edema
- Scar management
- Contractures (soft tissue restriction)
- Trigger points
- Bursitis
- Tendonitis

Contraindications

- Acute inflammation
- Infection
- Phlebitis
- Hemorrhage
- Venous insufficiency
- Malignancy
- Edema secondary to kidney dysfunction
- Edema secondary to heart failure

Application

1. Explain the procedure to the patient.
2. Drape the patient, expose the area to be treated, and place the patient in a comfortable position.
3. Inspect the massage area and observe any broken skin, the color of skin, and swelling.
4. Explain the procedure or type of massage and benefits to the patient.
5. Select an appropriate skin lubricant (eg, lotion, oil, or cocoa butter).
6. Select one massage technique or a combination of techniques. The types of massage techniques include:
   - Effleurage
   - Friction
   - Kneading
   - Percussion
   - Tapping

- Acupressure massage
- Stroking
- Vibration
- Clapping
7. Determine treatment time (will vary with the patient's tolerance and diagnosis).
8. Upon completion of the massage, wipe the area clean and reinspect.

PARAFFIN BATH

Paraffin bath is the utilization of paraffin wax and mineral oil (melted at a temperature of 125° to 127°F), the wax is melted and contained in a temperature-controlled stainless steel tank. The application of hot wax through dipping or brushing is typically applied to a patient's distal extremities.

Precautions

- Paraffin can easily fall to the floor during treatment/removal, making the floor slippery
- Paraffin wax is flammable
- Body parts should be cleaned prior to treatment
- The patient should be cautioned not to change position after the first dip into the wax, as cracks will allow hot wax to enter and create hot spots
- Do not dip any deeper then the first dip
- Check temperature prior to treatment

Indications

- Rheumatoid arthritis
- Contractures
- Joint stiffness
- Pain
- Increased range of motion to be followed by exercise

Contraindications

- Open wounds
- Infections
- Skin rashes
- Scars
- Burns
- Hemorrhage
- Sutures

Application

Paraffin Dipping
1. Remove jewelry. If the jewelry cannot be removed, cover with gauze and secure with tape.
2. Clean and wash the area to be treated. Explain the procedure to patient.
3. Protect the patient's clothing from the paraffin.
4. Apply wax to the treatment area, then dip the part into the paraffin six to 12 times. Instruct the patient to dip the part into paraffin and do not move the part after the first layer of paraffin is applied.
5. Hold the part over the bath, allowing the excess paraffin to drip off.
6. Allow the paraffin to solidify, then place plastic wrap or wax paper around the final layer, covering all of the paraffin.
7. Place a towel around the plastic wrap or wax paper to retain the heat.
8. Treatment time: 20 minutes.
9. Remove the wrapping and peel off the paraffin.
10. Check the patient's skin and dry off the area.

Paraffin Painting

1. Remove jewelry. If the jewelry cannot be removed, cover with gauze and secure with tape.
2. Clean and wash the area to be treated. Explain the procedure to patient.
3. Protect the patient's clothing from paraffin.
4. Protect the floor from paraffin drippings.
5. Use a paintbrush, dip into the paraffin and brush the paraffin onto the treatment area.
6. Allow the first layer to solidify before continuing.
7. Apply paraffin using the technique of brushing 10 to 12 times to the area being treated.
8. Place plastic wrap or wax paper around the area after the last layer has solidified.
9. Cover the plastic wrap or wax paper with a towel to retain the heat.
10. Treatment time: 20 minutes.
11. Remove the wrapping and peel off the paraffin.
12. Check the patient's skin and dry off the area.

PHONOPHORESIS

Phonophoresis is the use of ultrasound coupled with an anti-inflammatory agent. Ultrasound energy is utilized to penetrate the skin into the deeper tissues by the use of an anti-inflammatory agent. Anti-inflammatory agents include dexamethasone, salicylates, lidocaine, or local analgesics.

Precautions

- Check the patient for sensitivity or allergies to the agents used.
- Keep the sound head moving continuously on the skin throughout the treatment or burning may occur through overheating of tissue.
- Maintain uniform contact between the ultrasound head and the area being treated or burns may occur.
- When the unit is on, do not hold the sound head in the air or break treatment contact, as this could damage the sound head crystal.
- A complaint of sharp pain by the patient indicates the intensity needs to be reduced, more coupling medium needs to be added, and/or move the sound head a little faster.
- Do not treat over bony prominences to eliminate the possibility of concentrated energy causing localized heating.
- Do not treat over or near the heart.

Indications

- Bursitis
- Tendonitis
- Sprains and strains
- Pain
- Inflammatory conditions

Contraindications

- Pacemaker or any external or implanted electrical device
- Malignancy
- Fracture site
- Epiphyseal plate in children
- Acute infections
- Pregnancy
- Metal implants
- Over spinal cord area
- Thrombophlebitis
- Impaired sensation

Application

1. Explain the procedure to the patient.
2. Drape the patient, expose the area to be treated, and place the patient in a comfortable position.
3. Acquire the physician-prescribed agent to be utilized with the ultrasound from the pharmacy.
4. Utilize the medicinal agent to cover the treatment area; additional coupling agent may be used on the sound head.
5. Set the unit for continuous ultrasound mode.
6. Make sure the intensity control is at zero before turning on the unit.
7. Set the unit's automatic timer to the desired treatment time, which is usually 5 to 10 minutes.
8. Apply the sound head to the skin being treated at a right angle and start to move continuously in small circular motions. The small circular motions should overlap circles of approximately 50% of the previous circle. It is essential to keep the sound head in firm, uniform contact with the skin. The right angle must be maintained throughout the treatment.
9. Turn up the intensity of the unit. The dosage varies depending on the treatment area.
10. When the treatment time returns to zero, the machine will shut off.
11. Turn the intensity control to zero.
12. Wipe off the medicinal agent from the sound head.
13. Cleanse the skin while thoroughly inspecting for any reaction.

SHORT-WAVE DIATHERMY

High-frequency current to produce deep heat within body tissues for therapeutic purposes. Produces heat below the skin surfaces through conversion heat transmission.

Precautions

- Patients with pacemakers should not be in the treatment area
- Patients should not move during treatment or touch cables or the machine
- Due to electromagnetic radiation, all watches, jewelry, and hearing aids must be removed
- Overheating is a danger; burns should be avoided by insulating with towels over bony prominences

Indications

- Muscle spasms
- Pain
- Joint contractures
- Degenerative joint disease
- Sacroiliac strains
- Ankylosing spondylitis
- Bursitis

Contraindications

- Malignancy
- Pacemaker
- Acute inflammation
- Diminished sensations
- Metal implants
- Pregnancy
- Hemorrhage
- Thrombophlebitis
- Impaired vascular status
- Space occupying lesions
- Impaired cognitive function

Application

1. Explain the procedure to the patient.

2. Drape the patient, expose the area to be treated, and place patient in a comfortable position. Choose a treatment table without metal contact. Inspect the area to be treated.
3. Place one layer of toweling over the treatment area.
4. Position the treatment area midway between the two electrodes. The electrode/metal plates should be 1 to 3 inches away from the treating surfaces.
5. Allow the machine to warm up, making sure all dials are turned down to low intensity for warm-up.
6. Turn up the intensity until the patient feels a warm sensation (it should not feel hot or burning).
7. Check the patient initially and every 5 minutes to determine if the intensity for heating is correct.
8. Give the patient the emergency shut off or signaling device.
9. Treatment time: 20 minutes.
10. Turn the machine off after treatment time, remove the towel, and dry and inspect area.

THERAPEUTIC EXERCISES

There are many types of therapeutic exercise programs. The general guidelines for exercise applications are as follows:

1. A therapeutic exercise program for a patient may be implemented after an initial evaluation by a qualified therapist and a treatment program design based on the patient's problem.
2. Only a qualified therapist, or an assistant or staff member supervised by a therapist, may perform the application of therapeutic exercise to the patient.
3. The type of exercises to be performed, the purpose, goals, and outcomes should be discussed between the patient and the staff member.
4. The treatment area should be inspected prior to and after each treatment. Record all observations in the patient's chart.
5. The type of procedure/exercise performed, repetitions, amount of weight, number of sets, and the time will be recorded in the clinical record.
6. Home exercise programs will be given to the patient and documented in the clinical record.

Types of Therapeutic Exercises

- Passive exercises
- Active exercises
- Progressive resistance exercises
- Muscle re-education
- Stretching
- Range of motion
- Coordination exercises
- Posture exercises
- Active assistive exercises
- Neuromuscular facilitation
- Mobilization
- Home exercise program
- Prenatal/postpartum exercise
- Isokinetic exercise

Indications

- Increase strength
- Increase range of motion (ROM)
- Prevent atrophy
- Restore posture
- Improve functional ability
- Increase ability to perform activities of daily living (ADLs) independently
- Improve ability to return to work, sports, or play
- Increase coordination
- Increase endurance/conditioning
- Increase circulation
- Assist in pain management

Contraindications

(as determined by the attending physician or therapist after evaluation)
Examples
- Recent surgery restrictions
- Unstable fracture site
- Malignancy
- Tumors
- Pregnancy
- Osteoporosis
- Cardiac pathology
- Pulmonary pathology
- Neurological condition
- Cognitive functioning
- Weightbearing status
- Infection

Application

1. Explain the exercise program to the patient along with the desired outcomes, purposes of exercise, and goals.
2. Observe and examine the injured area before and after exercise.
3. Drape the patient appropriately during exercise and have the patient wear comfortable clothing that won't restrict movement.
4. Record in the clinical record the following information:
   - Exercise program
   - Types of exercises
   - Weight and repetitions
   - Time of exercise
   - Amount of exercise
   - Amount of resistance
5. When possible, give the patient written exercise instructions during the session in the facility to facilitate understanding and compliance.
6. Progress the patient's exercise program as tolerated following the physician's instructions and the patient's limitation.
7. Set the patient up with a home exercise program and written instructions.

TRACTION

Mechanical traction utilizes a mechanical device that can apply a distraction force to the spine to attempt to separate vertebral bodies and elongate spinal structures. Traction can be applied continuously or intermittently. Cervical traction is for the cervical spine. Pelvic traction is for the lumbar spine.

Precautions

- Osteoporosis
- Joint instability
- Claustrophobic patients who cannot relax with traction
- Acute sprains or strains that could be aggravated by traction

Indications

- Disc protrusion
- Herniated nucleus pulposus
- Degenerative disc disease
- Joint hypomobility
- Joint stiffness
- Pain—subacute or chronic

- Nerve root impingement
- Discogenic pain

Contraindications

- Fractures or unstable spinal column
- Pregnancy—lumbar
- Bone tumor
- TMJ—cervical (unless the patient can tolerate a special cervical device such as Saunder's).
- Acute herniated disc
- Spinal infection
- Spinal tumors
- Osteoporosis
- Spinal fusion, 1 year postoperative

Application

Pelvic Traction

1. Explain the procedure to the patient.
2. Place a pelvic belt and thoracic restraint on the table. Utilize a split table if available to decrease friction.
3. Patient is positioned supine on the table with belts underneath.
4. Place a small bench, flexion stool, or pillows beneath the patient's knee.
5. Hook the pelvic belt around the patient so the top edge is around the iliac crest and is secure.
6. Hook the thoracic belt around the patient so the inferior margin is slightly below the lower ribs and is secure.
7. Retighten the straps and double check to make sure the belts are secure. Make sure the thoracic restraint is attached to the end of the table.
8. Hook the "S" hooks on the pelvic belt to the traction machine spreader bar.
9. Adjust the traction machine height for correct pull alignment.
10. Determine treatment mode (intermittent or static).
11. Determine treatment force, poundage (typically low force to start—25 to 65 lbs depending on weight of the patient), adjusting to the patient's tolerance throughout treatments.
12. Remove all slack in the pelvic belt to the machine. Release the split table if in use.
13. Turn on the machine, starting with low poundage. Determine if the angle of pull is correct.
14. Treatment time: 10 to 30 minutes and cycle on/off depending on condition.
15. Have an emergency shut-off device available to the patient.
16. When treatment time is over, unhook the belt from the machine and release the restraints. Remove the belts, and lock the split table, if used.

Cervical Traction

1. Explain the procedure to the patient.
2. Determine whether the patient is supine or seated for treatment. Supine is usually preferred for the patient's comfort.
   - Supine: the patient is lying on his or her back with the machine positioned to pull at 25° to 30° angle. Place a pillow under the patient's knees for comfort.
   - Sitting: the patient sits in a chair with the head under the traction machine. The patient may rest arms on pillows or at the side. The knees should be flexed with feet flat on the floor. The traction machine should pull 25° to 30° of cervical flexion.
3. Choose a cervical halter or, if available, a cervical sliding device, which is the preferred method.
   - The cervical halter is placed on the back of the skull and under the mandible of the patient (use tissue on the harness for sanitary purposes). Secure the halter straps and adjust so that the force is in the occipital area and not on the chin. Attach the cervical halter to the spreader bar and remove the slack.
   - Cervical sliding device: place the patient's head against the padded headrest with 20° to 30° of cervical flexion. A head strap is secured across the forehead and an adjustable yoke below the mastoid process. The device is attached to the spreader bar. All slack is removed.
4. The spreader bar is attached to the "S" hook on the machine.

5. Determine the treatment poundage (initially start with a low force of 10 to 15 lbs and gradually increase tolerance to 20 to 35 lbs).
6. Treatment time: 10 to 20 minutes and cycle depending on condition.
7. Turn on the machine and check with the patient to determine the angle of pull.
8. Provide an emergency shut-off switch and signaling device.
9. At the end of the treatment, release the patient from the sliding device or harness and inspect the area.

Transcutaneous Electrical Nerve Stimulation (TENS)

The application of electrical current through the skin. It is designed to provide afferent stimulation for pain management.

Precautions

- Skin irritation at the electrode site
- Patient accidentally increasing intensity when unit is clipped onto clothing

Indications

- Acute pain
- Chronic pain
- Headaches
- Post-surgery

Contraindications

- Cardiac pacemaker
- Do not place electrodes across the throat or over the eyes, or laryngeal or pharyngeal muscles
- Do not place electrodes over the head or neck of a patient following a cerebral vascular accident
- Do not place electrodes over the head or neck of a patient following an epileptic seizure
- Do not use during pregnancy
- Do not apply electrodes over mucous membranes

Application

1. Explain the procedure to the patient.
2. Drape the patient, expose the area to be treated, and place in a comfortable position.
3. Choose a site for electrode placement depending on the patient's complaint.
   - Acupuncture point
   - Area around incision
   - Trigger point
   - Determine distribution of the involved nerve
   - Around the area of pain or proximal/distal to the pain site
   - Segmental-related myotomes
4. Choose the method of application.
   - Conventional TENS
   - Acupuncture TENS
   - Burst mode
   - Brief intense TENS
   - Modulated mode TENS
   - Point stimulation, hyperstimulation TENS
   - Treatment time varies from 20 minutes to 24 hours
5. After TENS is removed, inspect the area and cleanse and dry the skin well.

Ultrasound

High-frequency sound waves that produce temperature elevation to the deeper structures without causing excessive heating of the superficial layers through the use of a coupling agent.

Precautions

- Keep the sound head moving continuously on the skin throughout the treatment or burning may occur through overheating of tissue.
- Maintain uniform contact between the ultrasound head and the area being treated or burns may occur.
- When the unit is on, do not hold the sound head in the air or break treatment contact, as this could damage the sound head crystal.
- A complaint of sharp pain by the patient indicates the intensity needs to be reduced, more coupling medium needs to be added, and/or move the sound head a little faster.
- Do not treat over bony prominences to eliminate the possibility of concentrated energy causing localized heating.
- Do not treat over or near the heart.
- Check the patient for areas of sensitivity.

Indications

- Bursitis
- Tendonitis
- Joint contractures
- Muscle spasms
- Pain management
- Calcium deposits
- Sprains and strains

Contraindications

- Pacemaker or any external or implanted electrical device
- Malignancy
- Fracture site
- Epiphyseal plate in children
- Acute infections
- Pregnancy
- Metal implants
- Over spinal cord area
- Thrombophlebitis
- Impaired sensation

Application

Direct Contact

1. Explain the procedure to the patient.
2. Drape the patient, expose the area to be treated, and place the patient in a comfortable position.
3. Apply a generous amount of coupling agent. Spread the gel evenly over the transducer.
4. Select continuous or pulsed method.
   - Continuous ultrasound for a heating effect.
   - Pulsed ultrasound for a mechanical effect.
5. Make sure the intensity control is at zero before turning on the unit.
6. Set the unit's automatic timer to the desired treatment time, which is usually 5 to 10 minutes.
7. Apply the sound head to the skin being treated at a right angle and start to move continuously in small circular motions. The small circular motions should overlap circles of approximately 50% of the previous circle. It is essential to keep the sound head in firm, uniform contact with the skin. The right angle must be maintained throughout the treatment.
8. Turn up the intensity of the unit. The dosage varies depending on the treatment area.
9. When the treatment time returns to zero, the machine will shut off.
10. Turn the intensity control to zero.
11. Wipe off the coupling agent from the sound head.
12. Cleanse the skin while thoroughly inspecting for any reaction.

Underwater Application

This technique is used when the surface is uneven, such as the hand, elbow, knee, ankle, or where ever good contact by the sound head is not possible.

1. Explain the procedure to the patient.
2. Fill a container with water high enough to adequately cover treatment areas. A plastic container is preferred to metal.
3. Immerse the part to be treated into the container of water.
4. Immerse the sound head into the water at a right angle to the part being treated. The head of the transducer must be completely covered with water throughout the treatment.
5. Keep the sound head .5 to 1 inch away from the skin while the intensity is up from zero.
6. Turn on the timer for 5 to 10 minutes.
7. Move the sound head while turning up the intensity to the desired level. Move the sound head slowly and continuously.
8. If air bubbles appear on the transducer or the skin, they should be wiped away immediately.
9. When the timer turns off, remove the part treated, and dry and inspect the area.

Ultrasound with Electrical Stimulation

1. Explain the procedure to the patient.
2. Check the area to be treated.
3. A dispersive electrode is to be placed in firm contact and secure to the patient at a point away from the area being treated. The electrode is soaked in warm water and covered with wet gauze.
4. Apply a generous amount of coupling agent to the transducer, which is the active electrode.
5. Place the sound head at a right angle to the area being treated and move constantly in small, slow overlapping circles, maintaining firm contact with the treatment area.
6. Set the treatment timer for 5 to 10 minutes.
7. Turn up the ultrasound intensity to the desired level.
8. Turn up the electrical stimulation intensity to the desired level.
9. A few seconds before the timer shuts off the unit, slowly reduce the intensity to zero and then the ultrasound intensity to zero.
10. Remove dispersive electrodes. Wipe off the coupling agent from transducer and the patient.
11. Thoroughly check the patient's skin.

ULTRAVIOLET RADIATION

Ultraviolet radiation is the application of radiant energy from the ultraviolet portion of the electromagnetic spectrum. There are two types of lamps to provide treatment: hot quartz mercury vapor lamp (luminous) and a cold quartz mercury vapor lamp (nonluminous). Hot mercury lamps are used for minimal erythema dose (MED) tests and treatments, psoriasis, or dermatological conditions. Cold mercury lamps are used to kill bacteria. Place 1 inch above the skin for infected wounds and ulcers.

Precautions

- Some medications will increase the patient's sensitivity to ultraviolet.
- The eyes should be covered at all times.
- The treating staff should wear protective goggles.
- MED test should be done prior to treatment to determine the patient's ability to tolerate the treatment.

Indications

- Psoriasis
- Dermatological conditions
- Infected wounds
- Decubitus ulcers

Contraindications

- Fresh skin grafts/scars

- Diminished sensation
- Hypersusceptibility to ultraviolet
- Lupus erythematosus

Application

1. Explain the procedure to the patient.
2. Drape the patient, expose the area to be treated, and place patient in a comfortable position. Provide protective goggles for the patient and treating staff. Patient should remove jewelry.
3. Test for minimal erythema dose:
   - Prepare a test strip by cutting out six holes approximately 1 inch apart.
   - Secure the test strip to the treatment area.
   - Place the lamp at a right angle, 30 to 36 inches from the treatment area, allowing the lamp to warm up 5 to 10 minutes.
   - Open the lamp shutter and uncover the first circle for 15 seconds.
   - Continue to uncover each additional circle one at a time for 15 seconds.
   - After all six circles are exposed 15 seconds, turn off the lamp.
4. Determine the dosage for patient.
   - Suberythema dose is the amount of ultraviolet insufficient to cause an effect on the skin—one-half to one-third minimal erythema dose (MED), increase the daily dosage 12% or every other day to 25%.
   - MED is the barely noticeable amount of redness in 6 to 8 hours following treatment and subsiding within 24 hours. Increase dosage 20% daily.
   - Second-degree erythema dose is the reddening of skin, slight peeling and mild itching and burning 4 to 6 hours post-treatment—two to five times MED, so increase 50% every other day as warranted.
   - Third-degree erythema dose is intense reddening 2 hours post-exposure with blistering and exudate. Ten times MED, so apply once every 3 to 4 months.
5. Determine the treatment time and results after the MED test is completed and establish a therapeutic dose. Decide on the frequency of treatments and monitor the area.

WHIRLPOOL

A whirlpool is a water bath in a tank that has an agitator/motor, which circulates the water in the tank. The whirlpool can be used for either heating or cooling. The part to be treated is immersed in the tank. Whirlpools come in a variety of sizes from a small tank to a hubbard tank for full body immersion.

Precautions

- Make sure the whirlpool treatment area is free of water so that a patient does not slip getting into or out of the tank.
- Whirlpool must be grounded for electrical safety.
- Properly clean and disinfect the whirlpool prior to and/or after each treatment.

Indications

- Wound debridement/care
- Arthritis
- Reduce edema—cold whirlpool
- Muscle spasms
- Decubitus ulcers
- Burns
- Pain management
- Preparation for further therapeutic intervention such as exercise or stretching
- Post-surgical conditions

Contraindications

- Hemorrhage

- Malignancy
- Deep vein thrombophlebitis
- Diminished sensation
- Ischemic tissue

Application

General Whirlpools

1. Explain the procedure to the patient.
2. Drape the patient to protect privacy and clothing, expose the area to be treated and place the patient in a comfortable position.
3. Select the temperature of the water for a hot or cold whirlpool.
4. Fill the tank to the proper water level.
5. Add disinfectant to the tank as needed or as indicated by the diagnosis.
6. All staff should follow universal precautions.
7. The room temperature should be warmer than other treatment areas to provide a comfortable treatment climate for the patient.
8. Assist the patient in immersing the part to be treated into the tank. Position the patient as comfortably as possible to avoid pressure points from the tank.
9. Adjust the agitator to the desired position and the amount of intensity of the agitation, direction, and the depth of the agitation.
10. The treatment time is typically 15 to 30 minutes; turn on the whirlpool and give the patient a signaling device.
11. After the treatment is completed, dry and inspect the area. Record your observations.

Hubbard Tank

1. Explain the procedure to the patient.
2. Patient changes into a bathing suit or clothing to protect privacy. In case of a full body burn patient, enclose treatment area with curtains.
3. Treatment room should be warmer then other areas in the clinic to provide a comfortable treatment area for in and out of tank.
4. Select temperature for whirlpool and fill tank.
5. Add disinfectant to the hubbard tank as needed or prescribed.
6. All staff should follow universal precautions.
7. Place the patient on the stretcher and secure.
8. Utilize the hoist or lift to place the patient in the hubbard tank. Position the patient comfortably to avoid pressure points and secure head position if the patient cannot maintain control independently.
9. Remove hoist or lift from tank area and allow stretcher to sit in the bottom of the tank or at the appropriate water level for treatment.
10. Adjust the jets and pressure to the desired position and intensity.
11. Treatment time is 20 to 30 minutes.
12. Staff member should stay with the patient at all times for safety.
13. After treatment is finished, remove the patient utilizing the stretcher and lift.
14. Inspect the treatment area and record in notes.

CHAPTER 18

Orthopedics

MUSCULOSKELETAL DISORDERS/DISEASES

Adhesive Capsulitis

- May also be called a frozen shoulder and results in a joint contracture that involves the entire capsule.
- Occurs after immobilization for long periods or following an injury, sprain, fracture, or surgery. Pattern of restriction may vary in individuals.
- Symptoms include pain, stiffness, and loss of range of motion and strength. Activities of daily living (ADLs) are affected, patient may not be able to dress or fasten clothing behind their back, and may have difficulty getting a wallet out of a back pocket.
- Treatment may include ice, ultrasound, pain-relieving modalities, stretching to increase abduction, external and internal rotation, joint mobilization, strengthening of shoulder muscles, and posture instructions.

Arthrogryposis

- Nonprogressive, congenital disorder of fibrous stiffness in the joints.
- Characterized by rigid joints of the extremities. This is usually symmetrical, "sausage-like"shapeless limbs, and weak or nonfunctioning muscles.
- The following may occur as a result: hip dislocations and contractures of abduction, flexion, and external rotation, clubfeet, and shoulder contractures in abduction and external rotation.
- Treatment may include range of motion exercises, splinting, positioning, activities of daily living training, and use of adaptive devices.

Bursitis

- Inflammation of the bursa. Bursa is a fluid-filled sac found between the tendons and bones to reduce friction between the surfaces. The inflammation may also continue into the surrounding connective tissue.
- Bursitis may occur at the following areas: subacromial, olecranon, subdeltoid, iliopectineal, pes anserinus, prepatellar, and trochanteric.
- May be caused by arthritis, strains, sprains, contusions, excessive exercise, injury, and trauma.
- Treatment may include rest, modalities for healing, phonophoresis or iontophoresis, and ice. Gentle stretching may begin after the acute phase.

Carpal Tunnel Syndrome

- Results from compression of the median nerve where it passes through the carpal bones and the transverse ligament, and carpal tunnel.
- Symptoms occur as a result of the median nerve compression and follow the median nerve distribution to the hand. It may result in atrophy, paresthesia, and loss of digital dexterity and strength. Patient may report burning sensation or numbness in the hand at night.

- Treatment may include immobilization or wrist splinting, education on prevention and activities to avoid (eg, repetitive motion of the hand). Ultrasound may give some relief. Surgery may be necessary after conservative treatment fails to release pressure on the median nerve by releasing the transversal carpal ligament, the flexor retinaculum.

Chondromalacia

- Results in degeneration of the patellar surface. More commonly occurs in young females.
- Symptoms may include patellofemoral pain; tenderness, swelling, grinding or crepitus under the kneecap with movement; aggravated going up and down stairs, running, or jumping; pain with compression of the patella.
- Treatment may include exercises for the quadriceps in extension, ice, rest, patellar taping, straight leg raises, hamstring, and calf stretching.

Colles' Fracture

- A fracture at the radius that occurs within 1 inch from the wrist joint. This wrist fracture is commonly from a fall on an outstretched hand.
- Most common type of wrist fracture.
- Results in displacement of the distal radius.
- Also referred to as a silver-fork fracture, as the displacement is to a dorsal and lateral position to the hand.
- Treatment is casting with physical therapy to follow for regaining range of motion and strengthening following removal of cast; mobilization, training for activities of daily living or return to normal function.

Congenital Dislocation of the Hip

- Present at birth, when the femur is not articulating with the acetabulum. This may occur because of an abnormally shallow acetabulum. More common in females. It may be unilaterally or bilaterally.
- A lower extremity may appear shorter than the other lower extremity.
- Treatment consists of keeping the lower extremity in abduction, flexion, and lateral rotation. This allows the femur to articulate with the acetabulum, causing it to become deeper.

Dupuytren's Contracture

- Contracture involving the palmar fascia of the hand. It results in flexion deformities and loss of finger's normal functioning.
- Most commonly occurs in the ring finger.
- Treatment may include splinting, passive stretching, contract and relax whirlpool, and ultrasound.

Epicondylitis

- Epicondylitis is an inflammation of either the tendon. It is called lateral epicondylitis (tennis elbow) when it affects the extensor tendons where they commonly insert into the lateral humeral epicondyle. It is called medial epicondylitis (golfer's elbow) when it affects the flexor tendons where they commonly insert into the medial humeral epicondyle.
- Symptoms may include pain and tenderness with palpation, swelling, decreased strength and increased pain to resistance, wrist extension for tennis elbow and wrist flexion for golfer's elbow. Weakness of either the wrist extensors or wrist flexors.
- Treatment may include ice, iontophoresis, transverse friction rub, strengthening after the acute phase. A strap may be worn around the forearm distal to the elbow to help move the pressure off the common extensor tendon site and distribute the force more evenly in the forearm/elbow.

Herniated Nucleus Pulposus

- A disorder that occurs in a variety of staging. The nucleus can displace into the vertebral body or in severe cases it may extend into the spinal canal. It can protrude in any area of the spine: cervical, thoracic, and lumbar. It may be a bulge or complete herniation.
- There are four degrees of herniation as follows: intraspongy nuclear herniation, protrusion, extrusion, and sequestration. The herniation tends to develop over time but may occur in severe stages in the case of traumatic injury.

- Symptoms also vary with the individual and the stage of herniation. They may include low back pain in the early stages to loss of feeling and movement of the lower extremity in the latter stages. It may be bilateral lower extremity pain or unilateral. It typically starts at the buttocks and radiates down the lower extremity. It is usually considered to be in the later stages depending on how far down the lower extremity the radiation of symptoms is occurring. It is also true for cervical spine injuries that the further it radiates into the upper extremity down to the hand, the further advanced the injury. It may include pain, burning, numbness, and loss of function.
- Treatment will also depend on the staging of the injury. It may include bedrest, moist heat and traction, McKenzie exercises, postural instructions, Williams' exercises, proper body mechanics instruction, interferential electrical stimulation, and a home exercise program.

Iliotibial Band Friction Syndrome

- Irritation cause by the rubbing of the iliotibial band over the lateral epicondyle of the femur. The iliotibial band is a band of connective tissue that extends from the iliac crest to the knee.
- Symptoms may include tenderness upon palpation to the lateral epicondyle and pain over the lateral aspect of the knee. This syndrome often occurs in runners, especially those who run long distances.
- Treatment may include rest, ice, iontophoresis, evaluation of running shoes and biomechanics, and education on prevention.

Legg-Calvé-Perthes Disease

- The femoral head of the hip will experience vascular necrosis. It is commonly seen in children ages 4 to 10.
- Results in inflammation of the hip or synovitis.
- Treatment may include range of motion exercises and use of braces to keep the femoral head in the acetabulum. The main focus of physical therapy is to prevent joint deformity and maintain motion.

Myositis Ossificans

- Formation of heterotopic bone in soft tissue.
- Muscle tissue is replaced with bone, usually found in the muscles, quadriceps, deltoid, and hamstrings.
- Treatment is determined by whether the disease is in an active stage or inactive stage, determined by x-rays.
- Treatment will be rest if the disease is determined to be active. If the disease is in an inactive stage, the patient may receive heat and gentle exercises. There is no known cure for this disease.

Osgood-Schlatter Disease

- Irritation of the tibial tuberosity.
- Common in adolescents, usually from excessive tensions of the patellar tendon and typically results from overuse of the quadriceps muscles.
- Symptoms may include pain, swelling, and tenderness over the tibial tuberosity; symptoms are typically increased with activity and decreased with rest.
- Treatment may include rest, avoidance of running and jumping activities, and quadriceps stretching and strengthening. If not alleviated through conservative methods, immobilization may be necessary.

Osteomalacia

- A softening of the bones. This is a result of an abnormal bone matrix resulting in loss of calcification.
- Symptoms may include weakness, pain, and fractures.
- Treatments consist of nutritional education, supplemental calcium, and vitamin D intake.

Osteoporosis

- Results in an overall decrease in bone mass or density. Commonly seen in the elderly, sedentary patients, and postmenopausal women.
- Symptoms may include pain, weakness, fractures, and loss of stature.
- Treatment may include estrogen therapy for prevention and management of postmenopausal osteoporosis, heat for temporary pain relief, and active range of motion exercises. It should be noted that hormone therapy carries the risk of endometrial cancer.

Paget's Disease

- A disease characterized by bone destruction and unorganized bone repair.
- The first stage is characterized by softening of the bone. The second stage is a recalcification of the bone. The end stage is thickened and enlarged bones, which may result in deformities.
- There is no known specific treatment program.

Patellofemoral Dysfunction

- The patella fails to track properly in the trochlear groove.
- Instability or pain usually occurs in the first 30° of knee flexion.
- Stair climbing, prolonged sitting, running, squatting, and jumping may aggravate this condition.
- Treatment may include McConnell taping technique, stretching of the vastus medialis and iliotibial band, strengthening of quadriceps through short arc quads, straight leg raises, and possibly backward walking on treadmill.

Piriformis Syndrome

- Short muscle that compresses the sciatic nerve, resulting in sciatic pain but no back pain. Pain may be located in buttocks and radiate down the lower extremity.
- Symptoms are unilateral and not bilateral. May report sharp, burning pain, and sitting may aggravate symptoms.
- Treatment may include ultrasound, piriformis stretching, and instructions in proper posture and body mechanics.

Reflex Sympathy Dystrophy

- Characterized by persistent pain above normal levels and usually follows an injury (eg, a sprain or fracture). Injury is to the afferent pathways and affects the extremities.
- Initial symptoms may show swelling and increased temperature progressing to the skin, which will appear dry, leathery, and shiny.
- Treatment may include contrast baths, electrical stimulation, and range of motion.

Rotator Cuff Tear

- Results in the rupture of the supraspinatus tendon. The tear may vary and in some cases will result in the entire rotator cuff muscle being involved.
- Symptoms will usually include an acute painful shoulder, a clicking or popping sensation, and increase of pain symptoms in shoulder abduction.
- Treatment depends of the level of the tear; rehabilitation may be possible or surgical correction required. Acute stages: apply ice, rest, and prevention of further injury. When stable, progress to isometric exercises to closed chain exercises, shoulder proprioception, scapular stabilization exercises, and shoulder girdle muscle exercises.

Slipped Capital Femoral Epiphysis

- Displacement of the growth plate at the end of the femur.
- Occurs primarily in obese, young adolescent males as a result of hormone changes.
- Symptoms may include the patient exhibiting limited hip rotation, weakness, hip stiffness, and difficulty walking.
- Treatment is usually with orthopedic surgery.

Tendonitis

- An inflammation of the tendon. Tendonitis may typically occur in the following locations: bicipital, supraspinatus, and Achillis' tendonitis.
- Symptoms may include pain upon palpation, tenderness, and edema.
- Treatment may include rest, ice, gentle range of motion, ultrasound, phonophoresis, iontophoresis, stretching, and progressing to strengthening.

Thoracic Outlet Syndrome

- Compression or impingement of nerves and blood vessels. This usually occurs to the subclavian artery as it exits the clavicular-rib region.

- The anterior scalene muscle, scalenus anticus syndrome, or cervical rib could be the cause of narrowing of the thoracic outlet.
- Symptoms may include weakness, paresthesia, and pain.
- Treatment may include spray and stretch for myofascial trigger points, stretching exercises, moist heat, postural instructions, strengthening of scapular stabilizers, neural stretching of scalenes, levator scapulae, and pectoralis minor muscles.

Torticollis

- Spasm of the sternocleidomastoid muscle. May also be called "wry neck."
- Results in contralateral rotation and ipsilateral tilting of the head.
- Symptoms may include muscle spasms, sharp pain, muscle guarding, and limited active range of motion.
- Treatment may include rest and ice for the first 48 hours or acute stage, then progressing to moist heat, gentle active range of motion, manual distraction, stretching, muscle energy techniques, and isometrics.

Total Hip and Knee Arthroplasty

- Arthroplasty is a surgical procedure in which the hip or knee is reconstructed or replaced with a metal or plastic prosthesis.
- This is done secondary to degenerative joint disease, or osteoarthritis or rheumatoid arthritis in which the joint is painful and nonfunctional.
- The type of prosthesis or surgery will vary by the patient's needs and surgical preference.
- General symptoms prior to surgery are severe pain, inability to perform activities of daily living or functional activities, and loss of range of motion and strength.
- Treatment after surgery will again vary according to procedure and prosthesis. It will be determined by treatment protocols and physician preferences to include weightbearing activities, range of motion, strengthening, mobilization, ice, continuous passive movement, and passive/active stretching, as ordered.

SPECIAL ORTHOPEDIC TESTS PERFORMED TO ASSIST IN DIAGNOSIS OF INJURY

Adson's Test

- Test: thoracic outlet syndrome.
- How to perform: the patient takes a deep breath and extends the neck while turning the chin toward the affected side. The therapist palpates the radial pulse and brings the patient's arm into abduction.
- Outcome: the test is positive if there is a decreased or diminished radial pulse.

Allen's Test

- Test: radial/ulnar arterial supply to the hand.
- How to perform: the patient opens/closes the fist quickly several times. Next the patient squeezes the fist as tight as possible. This is to force the venous blood out of the palm. The therapist then occludes the arteries by pressing the radial and ulnar arteries against the underlying bones. The patient then opens his or her hand, which should be a pale color.
- Outcome: the test is positive if the hand does not immediately flush after the therapist releases the pressure on the radial/ulnar artery. This means that the radial/ulnar artery is either partially or completely occluded.

Anterior/Posterior Drawer Test (Ankle)

- Test: ankle instability, anterior for anterior ligaments, posterior for posterior ligaments.
- How to perform: the patient is in a sitting position with the knee flexed. The therapist cups the heel into the hand, stabilizing the leg with the other hand by grasping it above the ankle joint. The therapist attempts to pull the heel anteriorly for anterior drawer sign. For posterior drawer sign, the therapist stabilizes the lower extremity, placing his or her hand on the anterior aspect of the ankle joint, and applying pressure backward.
- Outcome: the test is positive if excessive movement occurs.

Anterior/Posterior Drawer Sign

- Test: anterior/posterior ligament stability.
- How to perform: patient is supine with the knee stabilized in a flexed position and foot flat on surface. The therapist will attempt to pull the lower extremity below the knee either anteriorly or posteriorly.
- Outcome: the test is positive if excessive movement occurs anteriorly or posteriorly.

Apley's Compression Test

- Test: torn meniscus in knee.
- How to perform: patient lies prone on the table with involved knee flexed to 90°. The therapist stabilizes the thigh and applies compression on the heel while applying internal and external rotation alternately to the tibia.
- Outcome: the test is positive if it produces a clicking pain. (note: medial side indicates medial meniscus damage; lateral side indicates lateral meniscus damage).

Apley's Distraction Test

- Test: distinguish between meniscus and ligamentous disorders of the knee.
- How to perform: patient is prone with knee flexed to 90° and the thigh stabilized. The therapist applies traction to the leg while internal/external rotation is applied to the tibia.
- Outcome: the test is positive for ligamentous damage if it produces pain. (note: this will not reproduce pain for meniscus damage).

Apprehension Test

- Test: dislocated patella (subjective test).
- How to perform: patient is in sitting position with knee straight as the therapist attempts to displace the patella laterally.
- Outcome: the test is positive if the patient has a look of "alarm or apprehension" on his or her face. Also look for guarding signs.

Bounce Home Test

- Test: torn meniscus, loose bodies in the knee joint, or effusion.
- How to perform: patient is supine while the therapist cups the heel into his or her hand, bends the involved knee into full flexion, then passively extends the knee.
- Outcome: the test is positive if the patient cannot extend the knee into full extension due to some form of blockage.

Brachial Plexus Tension Test

- Test: brachial plexus injury.
- How to perform: the patient is supine. The shoulder is in abduction with elbows extended and holds this position. The patient externally rotates the shoulder and supinates the forearm, holding just short of onset of pain. The patient then flexes the elbow with the physical therapist supporting the shoulder and forearm.
- Outcome: the test is positive if it produces pain.

Bunnel-Littler Test

- Test: tightness of lumbricales and interossei, which are intrinsic muscles of the hand.
- How to perform: the therapist holds metacarpophalangeal joint in extension (a few degrees), then tries to move the proximal interphalangeal joint into flexion.
- Outcome: the test is positive if one or all of the following occur:
  - The PIP joint cannot be flexed
  - Intrinsic tightness
  - Joint capsule contractures

Compression Test

- Test: neurological pathology in the cervical spine at any level. Examples: neural foramen, narrowing facet joint, disc.

- How to perform: the therapist presses down on the top of the patient's head as the patient maintains a sitting position.
- Outcome: the test is positive if it reproduces pain in the cervical spine or extremity. Note any particular dermatome pattern of pain distribution to determine neurological level of pathology.

Craig's Test

- Test: head of the femur for anteversion/retroversion.
- How to perform: the patient lies prone with the knee flexed 90°. The hip is passively medially and laterally rotated until the greater trochanter is parallel with the examination table. The therapist estimates the degree of anteversion/retroversion.
- Outcome: the test is positive if excessive anteversion/retroversion is measured.

Distraction Test

- Test: determines the effectiveness of traction, which may be used to alleviate pain. This is a complementary test to the compression test, as it is used to obtain the reverse effect.
- How to perform: the patient is supine as the therapist applies manual traction/distraction to the cervical spine.
- Outcome: the test is positive if it alleviates pain, and traction may effectively assist in alleviating the patient's symptoms.

Drop Arm Test

- Test: torn rotator cuff muscles.
- How to perform: the therapist places the patient's arm in abduction and asks the patient to hold arm up.
- Outcome: the test is positive if the arm drops with slight pressure.

Ely's Test

- Test: impingement of the L2 to L4 nerve root level or for tightness of the rectus femoris.
- How to perform: patient lies prone and the therapist passively flexes the patient's knee.
- Outcome: the test is positive if, on knee flexion, the hip flexes on the same side.

Finkelstein's Test

- Test: extensor pollicis brevis and abductor pollicis longus for tendonitis, for deQuervain's or Hoffmann's disease, or for tenosynovitis of the thumb.
- How to perform: the patient makes a fist with the thumb inside the fingers. The therapist stabilizes the forearm and deviates the wrist ulnarly.
- Outcome: the test is positive if it produces pain over the abductor pollicis longus and extensor pollicis brevis tendon of the wrist.

Flexor Digitorum Profundus Test

- Test: determine if the flexor digitorum tendon is intact.
- How to perform: the therapist isolates the distal interphalangeal (DIP) joint through stabilizing the metacarpophalangeal and interphalangeal joints in extension and asks the patient to flex the finger being tested at the DIP joint.
- Outcome: the test is positive if the patient cannot flex the joint because of a cut tendon or denervated muscle.

Flexor Digitorum Superficialis Test

- Test: determine if the flexor digitorum superficialis tendon is intact.
- How to perform: the therapist holds the patient's fingers in extension except for the one being tested and instructs the patient to flex the finger being tested.
- Outcome: the test is positive if the patient cannot flex the finger because the tendon is absent.

Foraminal Compression Test

- Test: impingement in the spinal cord, nerve roots, or dura.
- How to perform: the patient performs lateral flexion to one side. The therapist presses straight down on the head.
- Outcome: the test is positive if it produces pain radiating into the arm toward the flexed side.

Froment's Sign

- Test: ulnar nerve paralysis.
- How to perform: the patient attempts to grasp a piece of paper between the thumb and index finger. The therapist then attempts to pull the paper out.
- Outcome: the test is positive if the terminal phalanx of the thumb flexes.

Galeazzi's or Allis' Sign

- Test: congenital dislocation of the hip in an infant.
- How to perform: the patient is supine with hip and knee flexed.
- Outcome: the test is positive if one knee appears grossly lower than the other knee. The knee that appears lower is possibly dislocated at the hip joint.

Golfer's Elbow Test (Medial Epicondylitis)

- Test: pain reproduced in "golf stroke" or medial epicondylitis.
- How to perform: the patient flexes the wrist while the therapist applies pressure by attempting to force the wrist into extension.
- Outcome: the test is positive if it produces pain at the medial epicondyle site, which is the origin for wrist flexor tendons.

Homan's Sign

- Test: deep vein thrombophlebitis.
- How to perform: the therapist dorsiflexes the patient's ankle while the patient's leg is in an extended position.
- Outcome: the test is positive if it results in pain in the calf region.

Hughston's Jerk Test

- Test: anterior rotator instability.
- How to perform: patient is supine with hip flexed to 45° with medial rotation and the knee flexed to 90°. The leg is extended, maintaining medial rotation and valgus stress.
- Outcome: the test is positive if the therapist feels a jerk at 20° to 30° of flexion from tibia shifting forward, causing a subluxation of the lateral tibia with a jerk.

Hughston's Plica Test

- Test: enlargement of the plica.
- How to perform: patient is supine. The therapist flexes the knee and medially rotates the tibia while pressing the patella medially with the heel of his or her other hand and using the fingers to palpate the medial femoral condyle.
- Outcome: the test is positive if the therapist feels popping of the plica band under the fingers while passively flexing and extending the knee.

Impingement Syndrome Test

- Test: supraspinatus impingement.
- How to perform: patient abducts arm to 90°, then adducts the arm across the chest with internal rotation. Arm must maintain 90° of flexion.
- Outcome: the test is positive if it causes shoulder pain in the supraspinatus region.

Kleiger's Test

- Test: integrity of the deltoid ligament.
- How to perform: patient sits with knee flexed 90°, nonweightbearing on foot. The therapist rotates the foot laterally.
- Outcome: the test is positive if the patient reports increased pain medially and laterally. The therapist may feel the talus displaced from the medial malleolus.

Lachman's Test

- Test: integrity of the anterior cruciate ligament.
- How to perform: patient lies supine. The therapist holds the patient's knee between full extension and 30° of flexion. The therapist stabilizes the patient's femur with one hand while moving the tibia anteriorly with the other hand.
- Outcome: the test is positive if there is soft end-feel when the tibia is moved forward or if there is increased mobility in comparison to the noninjured extremity.

Ligamentous Instability Test (Elbow)

- Test: medial and lateral ligaments of the elbow.
- How to perform: the therapist stabilizes the patient's elbow with one hand and places the other hand above the patient's wrist. The elbow has 20° to 30° of flexion. The therapist applies adduction force on the distal forearm to test lateral collateral ligaments and abduction force to test medial collateral ligaments.
- Outcome: the test is positive if it causes increased pain or laxity.

Lhermitte's Sign

- Test: irritation in the cervical dura.
- How to perform: patient is positioned in long leg sitting. The therapist passively flexes the head and hips (with legs straight) at the same time.
- Outcome: the test is positive if it causes sharp pain down the spine or upper/lower limbs.

McMurray's Test

- Test: torn meniscus in the knee.
- How to perform: the patient is supine. The therapist flexes and extends the knee while applying internal/external rotation.
- Outcome: the test is positive if it produces palpable or audible click during rotation.
  - External rotation: test for medial meniscus
  - Internal rotation: test for lateral meniscus

Noble Compression Test

- Test: iliotibial band friction syndrome.
- How to perform: patient is supine. The therapist flexes the knee and hip 90°. Then, the therapist applies pressure to the lateral femoral epicondyle. The therapist maintains the pressure and passively extends the knee.
- Outcome: the test is positive if the patient complains of pain over the lateral femoral epicondyle.

Ober's Test

- Test: contraction of the iliotibial band.
- How to perform: the patient lies on the unaffected side with the involved leg uppermost; the therapist abducts the leg and flexes the knee to 90°; the hip joint should remain in neutral position.
- Outcome: the test is positive if the thigh remains abducted when the leg is released. Normally the leg would adduct when released.

Ortolani's Click

- Test: congenital dislocation of the hip in infants.
- How to perform: patient's hips are flexed, abducted, and externally rotated.
- Outcome: the test is positive if there is an audible or palpable click during the test.

Patella Femoral Grinding

- Test: arthritis/degenerative changes in the patella.
- How to perform: patient is positioned with the lower extremity in extension. The therapist pushes the patella distally and instructs the patient to tighten the quadriceps muscle.
- Outcome: the test is positive if it causes palpable grinding of surface or pain.

Patrick's or Faber's Test

- Test: pathology in sacroiliac joint or hip.
- How to perform: the patient is supine. The therapist places the foot of the involved extremity on the opposite knee. This places the hip joint in a position of abduction and flexion with external rotation. The therapist places one hand on the flexed knee joint with the other hand on the anterior superior iliac spine of the opposite side, and presses down on each of these points.
- Outcome: the test is positive if the patient complains of pain.

Pelvic Rock Test

- Test: existence of sacroiliac dysfunction.
- How to perform: patient is supine. The therapist flexes the patient's knee and hips. Next, the therapist adducts the hip and rocks the S1 joint by flexion and adduction of patient's hip.
- Outcome: the test is positive if it causes pain in the S1 joint.

Phalen's Test

- Test: carpal tunnel syndrome.
- How to perform: patient places wrists against one another in a flexed position.
- Outcome: the test is positive if numbness and tingling occur along the medial nerve distribution.

Plica Test (Stutter)

- Test: determine whether the plica is interfering with the patellar tracking.
- How to perform: patient lies on the edge of the table with knees at a 90° angle. The therapist places a finger on the patella and instructs the patient to extend knee actively.
- Outcome: the test is positive if the patella jumps or stutters between 45° and 60° of flexion.

Q-Angle Test

- Test: genu valgum by measurement of the Q-angle of the knee.
- How to perform: the therapist measures the angle between the quadriceps muscle and patellar tendon.
- Outcome: normal angle is 13° for male and 18° for female.

Retinacular Test

- Test: retinacula ligament tightness or joint capsule contracture.
- How to perform: the therapist holds the proximal interphalangeal (PIP) joint in a neutral position, then tries to move the DIP joint into flexion.
- Outcome: the test is positive if the joint cannot be flexed.

Shoulder Abduction Test

- Test: cervical extradural compression.
- How to perform: patient is either sitting or supine. The therapist passively performs shoulder abduction so that the patient's hand is right on top of his or her head.
- Outcome: the test is positive if it decreases or relieves symptoms.

Shoulder Depression Test

- Test: encroachment in the foramen or nerve root compression, or adhesions around the dural sleeves of nerve roots.
- How to perform: the therapist flexes the patient's head while applying a downward pressure on the patient's opposite shoulder.
- Outcome: the test is a positive test if pain increases.

Straight Leg Test

- Test: nerve root tension or herniated disc in lumbar spine.
- How to perform: the patient is supine. The therapist slowly raises the foot upward, keeping the knee fully extended. The therapist can also dorsiflex the patient's ankle.
- Outcome: the test is positive if pain is reproduced before 70° is reached, or if aggravated by dorsiflexion of ankle (note: the therapist must rule out if pain is caused by tight hamstring muscles).

Tennis Elbow (Lateral Epicondylitis)

- Test: reproduce the pain in "tennis elbow" or lateral epicondylitis (elbow joint region).
- How to perform: the patient's wrist is in extension. The therapist applies pressure, attempting to force the wrist into flexion.
- Outcome: the test is positive if it produces pain at the lateral epicondyle site, which is the origin for the wrist extensor tendons.

Thomas Test

- Test: hip flexion contractures.
- How to perform: patient's position is supine with the pelvis level and stabilized by the therapist. The therapist then flexes the patient's hip, bringing the thigh up on the trunk. The therapist places one hand in the area of the low back/lumbar spine to determine where the lumbar spine flattens. Further flexion will now occur only at the hip joint. The patient should hold the other leg down on the table. Lastly, the patient extends the hip on the testing leg.
- Outcome: the test is positive if the hip does not extend fully onto the table.

Thompson's Test

- Test: ruptured heel cord.
- How to perform: patient is supine with feet over a ledge, free for movement. The therapist squeezes the calf of the involved leg.
- Outcome: the test is positive if the foot does not plantar flex when the calf is squeezed.

Tinel's Sign

- Test: neuroma within a nerve (elbow joint region).
- How to perform: the therapist taps the area of the nerve in the groove between the olecranon and medial epicondyle.
- Outcome: the test is positive if there is a throbbing sensation down the forearm and/or ulnar distribution in the hand.

Trendelenburg's Test

- Test: muscle weakness in hip abductor, primarily the gluteus medius.
- How to perform: patient is standing. The therapist asks the patient to stand or balance on one leg, then the other. Normally, the pelvis on the opposite side should rise.
- Outcome: the test is positive if the pelvis drops on the opposite side of the stance leg.

Valsalva's Maneuver

- Test: space-occupying lesion (eg, herniated disc). This is a subjective test, and accuracy depends upon the patient's response.
- How to perform: the patient holds his or her breath and bears down as if he or she were moving the bowels.
- Outcome: the test is positive if it increases pain; try to note if the pain has any particular dermatome distribution.

Varus/Valgus Stress Test

- Test: stability of ligaments of the knee.
- How to perform: patient is supine with lower extremity in extension.
  - Varus stress will test lateral ligaments
  - Valgus stress will test medial ligaments
- Outcome: the test is positive if it causes pain.

Vertebral Artery Test

- Test: occlusion of the vertebral artery or nerve root compression in the lower cervical spine.
- How to perform: patient is in a supine position. The therapist passively positions patient's head in extension and side flexion. The therapist rotates the patient's neck to the same side for 30 seconds. Each side is tested separately.
- Outcome: the test is positive if the patient reports having dizziness or nausea.

Waldron's Test

- Test: chondromalacia patellae.
- How to perform: the therapist palpates the patient's knee while the patient does slow, deep knee bends.
- Outcome: the test is positive if crepitus is felt or if pain increases.

Yergason Test

- Test: bicipital tendonitis.
- How to perform: patient supinates the forearm against resistance.
- Outcome: the test is positive if it causes pain in the bicipital groove.

CONVEX/CONCAVE RULE

- The convex/concave rule is important when you are treating a patient with limited motion at a joint. Prior to exercise being used to increase range of motion or mobilization, it is important to understand the rule of the convex/concave surfaces.
- The rule states:
  - When a convex surface moves on a stable concave surface, the sliding of the convex surface occurs in the opposite direction to the motion.
  - When the concave surface moves on a stable convex surface, sliding occurs in the same direction as the motion.
- It is important to note in ovoid joints which surface is convex and which surface is concave so mobilization can be performed in the correct movement.

TERMS

Arthrokinematics: movements between the bones of the joint surfaces (roll, spin, and glide).

Osteokinematics: movement of the bony segments around the joint axis.

Roll: the movement that occurs when the center point of the convex surface contacts the center point of the concave surface, or the center point of the concave contacts the center point of the convex surface.

Spin: the rotation of the concave surface on the linear axis of the convex joint surface, or the convex surface on the linear axis of the concave surface.

Slide: the movement from the same point on the concave surface coming into contact with different points on the convex surface, or the same point on the convex surface coming into contact with the different points on the concave surface.

JOINT END-FEELS

The end-feel is the description of what the joint feels like when it reaches its limit of motion while the therapist is performing passive range of motion. The following end-feel classifications and definitions are according to Cyriax terms.

Bone-to-bone end-feel: hard and abrupt stoppage to the joint motion. This typically occurs when passive range of motion is performed and the bone contacts another bone.

Capsular end-feel: hard, leather-like stoppage with a slight give.

Empty end-feel: a lack of stoppage to the joint. The patient complains of pain during passive range of motion but the therapist feels no resistance to testing.

Spasm end-feel: involuntary muscle contraction that causes resistance to the passive range of motion that the therapist is performing.

Springy block end-feel: rebound movement felt at the end-range of passive range of motion.

Soft tissue approximation: the soft tissue of two bony segments prevents further passive range of motion.

CAPSULAR PATTERNS

Note if the joint's capsule is affected; typically, limitation will occur according to a capsular pattern in the joint. Following are some examples of joints with their capsular patterns:

Joint	Pattern
Glenohumeral	Lateral rotation, abduction, medial rotation
Acromioclavicular	Pain at extreme range of motion
Sternoclavicular	Pain at extreme range of motion
Hip	Flexion, abduction, medial rotation
Knee	Flexion, extension
Cervical spine	Lateral flexion, rotation, bilateral extension
Thoracic spine	Lateral flexion, bilateral rotation, bilateral extension
Lumbar spine	Lateral flexion, bilateral rotation, bilateral extension
Midtarsal	Equal limitations in dorsiflexion, plantar flexion, adduction, medial rotation
Talocalcaneal	Varus
Ankle	Plantar flexion, dorsiflexion
Elbow	Flexion, extension
Forearm	Pronation, supination
Finger digits	Flexion, extension
Wrist	Flexion, extension
Metacarpophalangeal	Flexion, extension
Metatarsals	Extension, flexion

LOOSE-PACKED/CLOSED-PACKED POSITIONS

Loose-packed position: a resting position in which the joint's range of motion is under the least amount of stress. Joint separation occurs because the capsule and ligaments are lax.

Closed-packed position: the position in which the two joint surfaces fit together precisely. The joint surfaces are tightly compressed, and the ligaments and the capsule of the joint are maximally tight.

Joint Position

Facet (spine):
- Loose-packed position: midway between flexion and extension
- Closed-packed position: extension

Glenohumeral:
- Loose-packed position: abduction 55°, horizontal adduction 30°
- Closed-packed position: abduction and lateral rotation

Elbow:
- Loose-packed position: 70° flexion, 10° supination
- Closed-packed position: extension

Wrist:
- Loose-packed position: neutral with slight ulnar deviation
- Closed-packed position: extension with radial deviation

Fingers:
- Loose-packed position: slight flexion
- Closed-packed position: full flexion

Temporomandibular joint:
- Loose-packed position: mouth slightly open
- Closed-packed position: teeth clenched

Hip:
- Loose-packed position: 30° flexion, 30° abduction, slight lateral rotation
- Closed-packed position: full extension, medial rotation, and abduction

Knee:
- Loose-packed position: 25° flexion
- Closed-packed position: full extension and lateral rotation of the tibia

Ankle:
- Loose-packed position: 10° plantar flexion, midway between inversion and eversion
- Closed-packed position: maximal dorsiflexion

Midtarsal:
- Loose-packed position: neutral
- Closed-packed position: maximum supination

Metatarsophalangeal:
- Loose-packed position: midrange
- Closed-packed position: maximum extension

Subtalar:
- Loose-packed position: midrange position
- Closed-packed position: maximal supination

Tarsometatarsal:
- Loose-packed position: midrange position
- Closed-packed position: maximal supination

MOBILIZATION GRADES

GRADE	DESCRIPTION OF MOBILIZATION
One	Small amplitude movement in the beginning of range of motion.
Two	Larger amplitude movement in the midrange of motion.
Three	Large amplitude movement throughout the full available range of motion.
Four	Small amplitude movement at end range.
Five	Thrusting movement done at the anatomical limits of the joint.

PURPOSE OF MOBILIZATION

Grades one and two: typically performed to alleviate pain and maintain joint motions. They are used at the acute stages of a joint sprain or inflammation to guard against development of decreased joint motion, alleviate pain, and promote healing.

Grades three and four: used as the patient progresses from the subacute/acute stage and becomes stable with pain. They are typically utilized to increase the range of motion more aggressively.

Grade five: used to regain all the motion in one manipulation; typically this is done by the physician.

GUIDELINES OF MOBILIZATION

1. Inform the patient of the procedure that you are about to perform and answer any questions the patient has concerning the procedure.
2. The patient and the physical therapist must both be relaxed when performing joint mobilization.

3. The procedure should not be painful, so provide a signal for the patient to tell you if he or she is experiencing any pain during the procedure.
4. Always compare the mobility of the injured side to that of the noninjured side or of one spinal level to the level above.
5. The first treatment should initially be gentle to gauge the patient's response to treatment.
6. When performing multiple mobilizations, always try to perform one at a time and compare it to the other side, then progress to the next mobilization area.
7. After performing the technique, again recheck with the patient to answer any concerns or questions that he or she might have.
8. After performing mobilization, record the patient's range of motion to determine progress.

FRACTURE TYPES

Avulsion fracture: a fracture caused when a strong ligamentous or tendinous attachment forcibly pulls a fragment of bone away from osseous tissue.

Closed fracture: also known as a simple fracture. It is a fracture in which the skin in the area of the fracture is intact.

Comminuted fracture: a break in the bone in which the bone splinters or is crushed, creating numerous fragments.

Compound or open fracture: a break in which the broken end, or ends, of the bone have torn through the skin.

Compression fracture: a break in the bone, especially in a short bone, that disrupts osseous tissue and collapses the affected bone. Bodies of vertebrae are often sites of compression fractures.

Epiphyseal fracture: also called Salter fracture. This fracture involves the epiphyseal growth plate of the long bone, resulting in separation or fragmentation of the plate.

Greenstick fracture: a break in which the bone is bent but fractured only on the outer arc of the bend. Children are particularly likely to have greenstick fractures. Immobilization is usually effective and healing is usually rapid.

Neoplastic fracture: also called pathologic fracture. It is a fracture resulting from weakened bone tissue caused by neoplasm or by a malignant growth.

ISOKINETIC EXERCISES

Advantages

- Adaptability of force throughout range of motion
- Decreased joint compression at high speed
- Capability for variable velocity training and control of velocity
- Efficient loading of muscle throughout entire range; optimal resistance throughout range of motion
- Objective testing and reporting on patient tests
- Safety
- Feedback to patient and therapist on patient's progress
  Note: new isokinetic equipment available on the market allows concentric/eccentric contractions.

Disadvantages

- Poor alignment between anatomical and mechanical axis
- Substitution of accessory muscle for poor stabilization
- Misinterpretation of computer readout/tests
  Note: some manufacturers of isokinetic equipment have greatly improved the ability to align the muscle with the mechanical access. Therefore, this may not be a disadvantage, depending upon the equipment manufacturer.

Purpose of Isokinetic Testing

- Documentation (court cases)
- Screening of athletic injuries
- Objective assessment
- Identification of malingerers
- Development of specific rehabilitation exercises for a variety of conditions based on test results
- Assistance in diagnosis of injuries
- Industrial screening

Contraindications for Testing

- Severe pain
- Instability of joint
- Severe swelling/effusion
- Significantly limited range of motion
- Soft tissue healing
- Sprains

Accuracy of Test Results

Depends on:
- Choosing a test that is reliable and reproducible for retesting
- Calibrating equipment regularly
- Stabilizing the patient, so you are testing only specific muscle groups or joints
- Aligning the anatomical axis joint with mechanical axis
- Educating the patient about the procedure and familiarizing him or her with the equipment
- Consistent verbal communication
- Follow standard testing protocols

ISOMETRIC EXERCISES

Advantages

- Limits joint irritability
- Increases static muscle strength
- Limits swelling
- Limits atrophy
- No equipment necessary
- Allows stimulation of mechanoreceptors

Disadvantages

- Muscle strength limited to range of motion
- No improvement in muscle endurance
- No eccentric work created

ISOTONIC EXERCISES

(Examples: Nautilus, Universal, and free weights)

Advantages

- Concentric/eccentric contraction
- Neurophysiology carryover
- Objective documentation
- Objective muscle endurance
- Objective muscle strength through range of motion
- Affordability and easily available

Disadvantages

- Loads muscle at weakest point
- Uses momentum factor in lifting
- Does not develop force quickness
- Does not develop accuracy at functional speed
- Does not consider velocity of movement

EXERCISE PRESCRIPTION

Variables: each of the following variables must be considered in an exercise program. Sometimes they are abbreviated as FITT.

1. **Frequency** of exercise per day or per week. Usually 3 to 5 times per week.
2. **Intensity** of exercise is based on the amount of resistance used, target heart rate, number of METS prescribed, speed of exercise, etc.
3. **Type** of exercise, whether aerobic, isometric, isokinetic, or using apparatus. Might include jogging, bicycling, and walking.
4. **Time** or duration of exercise session (20 minutes, 1 hour, etc). Usual range is 15 to 60 minutes.

GENERAL TREATMENT—ORTHOPEDIC INJURIES

Following is a sample treatment protocol for post-traumatic synovitis. The purpose of this is to give an example of a treatment protocol. Treatment technique may change depending on certain conditions and a therapist's opinions. For the exam, you need to think in terms of baseline treatment protocol for the general orthopedic condition.

TIME AFTER INJURY	MODALITIES	EXERCISE
24 to 48 hrs	Ice, compression, elevation, high-voltage galvanic	Rest or isometrics
3 to 5 days	Contrast bath, whirlpool, hot packs, high-voltage galvanic	Isometrics, gentle range of motion
5 to 14 days	Whirlpool, hot packs, functional electrical stimulation	Range of motion, strengthening, progressive resistance exercises
3 to 4 weeks if symptoms persist	Less frequent use of modalities	Range of motion, isometrics
>6 to 8 weeks if symptoms persist	To be reevaluated by the physical therapist and physician	

CHAPTER 19

Pediatrics

PEDIATRIC DISORDERS

Asthma

- Unknown cause: possibly stress, fatigue, and trauma. Allergies and exercises may enhance an attack.
- There are two main types of asthma: extrinsic (allergic) and intrinsic (nonallergic).
- Attacks consist of difficulty with breathing, wheezing, inability to get enough air, and/or coughing.
- There are three stages of asthma:
    1. Mild: symptoms will reverse with cessation of activity.
    2. Moderate: patient will be leaning forward attempting to catch his or her breath, audible wheezing and use of accessory muscles for respiration.
    3. Severe: blue lips and fingernails, rib retraction, cyanosis, and tachypnea.
- **Treatment:** improve patterns of breathing, increase exercise endurance and strengthening are long-term goals of rehabilitation. Monitor vital signs of children during treatment and have available medications utilized in case of an attack (eg, have the child or parent bring their inhaler to therapy). Also attempt to have the child exercise in a trigger-free environment.

Athetosis/Ataxia

- Fluctuating tone is present.
- Exaggerated response to stimulus or absence of response to stimulus.
- Typically demonstrates a poor posture.
- Ataxic—loss of distal control of the extremity.
- No consistent response to the same stimulus.
- Decreased proprioception and inability to coordinate movement.
- Slow, writhing, continuous involuntary movement of the extremity.
- Difficulty in timing and sequencing of movement.
- **Treatment:** facilitate normal posture and movement patterns. Repeat activities to reinforce learning; this is secondary to the unreliability of responses.

Brachial Plexus Injury

- May occur to an infant during a difficult birth.
- There are several types of plexus injuries:
    1. Injury to C5 and C6 = Erb's palsy
    2. Injury to C7, C8, T1 = Klumpke's paralysis
    3. Injury to C5, C6, C7, C8, T1 = Erb-Duchenne/Klumpke's
- Results in partial or complete paralysis of the upper extremity, no voluntary movement, as well as possible sensory loss.

- Erb's palsy is the most common type of brachial plexus injury. It is typically from a difficult birth involving a breech delivery or utilization of forceps.
- **Treatment:** initially, rest is recommended. The therapist may recommend the parents to place the upper extremity in a neutral position to protect it. Gentle passive range of motion to prevent loss of range of motion and contractures. This can be accomplished by pinning the baby's sleeve to the diaper. Stimulate active movement and progress (occasionally with splinting) to weightbearing activities as movement is regained.

Cerebral Palsy

- Cerebral palsy is a result of a lesion in the cerebral cortex that is nonprogressive. It results in neuromuscular disorders of voluntary movement and posture. The child may be either passive or stiff and cannot adjust body position.
- This is considered a nonhereditary disease. Although it is classified as a nonprogressive disease, clinical symptoms may change over lifespan.
- Child cannot hold or bring the head into normal position, typically demonstrates a scissors gait, usually has exaggerated reflex responses, and is not self-supporting.
- Other clinical symptoms may include mental retardation, learning disabilities, vision impairments, hearing impairments, seizures, bowel and bladder incontinence, and orthopedic disorders.
- Ataxia results in the child having difficulty with timing and sequencing initiation, irregularity of muscle actions, decreased proprioception, and delays in processing information and completing tasks.
- Cerebral palsy prognosis of mild to moderate cases is good with most living a normal lifespan. Severe cases have a poor prognosis and typically 50% of the children die by age 10.
- Child may be classified as ataxic, spastic (high tone), hypotonic (low tone), or a combination of the two tones.
- **Treatment:** modify tone; either increase or decrease it depending on the child. Facilitate righting reactions, balance reactions, protective reactions, and basic/fundamental movement patterns. Other health care intervention may include orthopedic surgery, drug therapy for infections, and assisting with motor tone, also neurosurgery and family counseling or support groups.

Developmental Dysplasia of the Hip

- Typically affects children younger than 3 years old, and 85% of cases are females. It results in an abnormal relationship between the acetabulum and the femoral head. It can be either unilateral or bilateral.
- There are three types of dysplasia: unstable hip dysplasia, subluxation or incomplete dislocation, and complete dislocation.
- Prognosis is good if found in the first few weeks after birth—it is completely reversible. After latter periods, the deformity worsens and is irreversible, resulting in long-term deformities.
- Tests to determine the above include Ortolani's click test, Galeazzi's or Allis' sign, or Barlow maneuver.
- **Treatment:** typically splinted to maintain the hip in position for normal development of the joint. Von Rosen, Ifeld, and Pavlic designed the commonly used splints. The hip harness and Pavlic harness place the hip in a position of flexion and abduction until the joint capsule tightens.

Cystic Fibrosis

- An inherited disorder affecting the exocrine glands. Excessive secretions from the glands cause an obstruction. The exocrine gland involvement affects the hepatic, digestive, and respiratory systems.
- The majority of mortality cases are a result of lung disease with chronic infection, which causes the loss of pulmonary functioning.
- Typically affects the pancreatic gland, tracheobronchial tree, salivary glands, and intestinal and sweat glands.
- The disease results in salt accumulating in the cells lining the lung and digestive tissue. Parents will report that their child tastes salty when giving them a kiss. The salt causes the surrounding mucus to be abnormally thick in viscosity.
- **Treatment:** exercise programs to assist in clearing lung secretions and providing the child with a sense of accomplishment or positive self image. Chest physical therapy involves postural drainage, chest percussion/vibration, breathing exercises, and improving posture. Drug therapy intervention is often necessary for infections and thinning of mucus.

Down Syndrome

- Down syndrome is a chromosomal abnormality resulting in 47 chromosomes instead of 46. Down syndrome is also called trisomy 21 because the disorder results from an abnormal cell division affecting the 21st pair of chromosomes.
- Infants with the syndrome are small and hypotonic, and their faces have a mongoloid slant to the eyes, depressed nasal bridge, low-set ears, and a large protruding tongue. They are cognitive delayed with short limbs, feet, and hands.
- The motor skills are delay and decrease muscle strength results in a gait pattern of small short steps; increased knee flexion at contact and increased hip flexion posture.
- Congenital heart disease, visual and hearing deficits, musculoskeletal ligament laxity, absence of a kidney, feeding difficulties, and obesity are other associated complications that may be present with Down syndrome.
- The disease may be diagnosed through an amniocentesis during pregnancy.
- **Treatment:** of immediate importance is the prevention of physical problems associated with the disorder, respiratory infections, inadequate nutrition due to feeding difficulties because of the large protruding tongue, positioning difficulties caused by the hypotonicity of muscles and hyperextensibility of the joints. The therapist will treat based on evaluation of the current problem list. This may include postural control, balance, and coordination activities. Teaching the parents a home program for therapy carryover is very important. Long-term goals are to promote optimal motor and mental skills.

Duchenne's Muscular Dystrophy

- An abnormal congenital condition characterized by progressive symmetric wasting of the leg and pelvic muscles. It is also called progressive muscular dystrophy and is the most serious disabling children's disorder.
- Children develop contractures, have difficulty climbing stairs, difficulty getting up from the floor, walking on their toes secondary to anterior tibial and peroneal weakness, contractures, waddling gait, lumbar lordosis, often stumble and fall, and display wing scapulae when raising their arms.
- May also have cardiac murmurs, faint heart sounds, chest pain, and may suffer arrhythmias.
- **Treatment:** there is no successful treatment to stop the progression of the disease. Orthopedic appliances, exercise, physical therapy, medications, and surgery to correct contractures can help preserve mobility. Physical therapy intervention is to prevent contractures, maintain range of motion, and prolong functional capacity, self-care, and teaching the parents a home program. Progression of the disease typically leads to death by age 20.

Muscular Dystrophy

- This disease is characterized by progressive weakness of the muscles and ongoing muscle atrophy. The disease results in progressive deformity and disability.
- Inherited disease with four types of muscular dystrophy: Duchenne's, Becker's, facioscapulohumeral, and limb-girdle muscular dystrophy.
- Becker's muscular dystrophy resembles Duchenne's with a slower progression of the disease, allowing a lifespan into the late 20s. Onset is typically 5 to 10 years of age.
- Facioscapulohumeral muscular dystrophy progression is proximal to distal and most children are active into adulthood with a normal lifespan. They may have periods of progression and remission of the disease. Complications in later life typically involve a loss of walking abilities. Usually occurs at early adolescence but may occur at any age.
- Limb-girdle muscular dystrophy is a slowly progressive disease with mild impairment. Muscular weakness in the upper extremities, winging of the scapulae, and inability to perform activities overhead are symptoms of the disease. Develops in late adolescence and early adulthood.
- **Treatment:** there is no known treatment to stop the progression of the disease. Focus is on preventing muscle contraction, especially in the hip flexors and iliotibial band, facilitating normal motor milestones, and on preventing infections, especially respiratory. Respiratory and cardiac complications are the common reasons for mortality.

Scheuermann's Disease

- The cause is unknown but results in fixed kyphosis that develops between the ages of 12 and 16. The vertebral bodies become wedge-shaped and may affect one or several of the vertebrae, usually at the thoracic spine level. It is also called juvenile kyphosis or vertebral epiphysitis.

- The vertebral bodies are wedged anteriorly and disc lesions develop. The disc lesions are called Schmorl's nodes. Schmorl's nodes are an extrusion of nuclear material through the cartilage plate. The nuclear material goes into the spongy bone of the vertebral bodies.
- **Treatment:** physical therapy involves postural exercises and instruction to prevent permanent disabilities due to kyphosis becoming fixed. Alleviate pain associated with tenderness and stiffness of the spine. Soft tissue and joint mobilization and exercises to strengthen abdomen are recommended. A Milwaukee brace or plaster cast is utilized for immobilization.

Scoliosis

- Scoliosis is an abnormal curvature of the spine.
- May be either:
  1. Structural curves; fixed curves
  2. Nonstructural; functional, flexible curves
  3. More toward the right (more common in thoracic curves)
  4. More toward the left (more common in lumbar curves)
- Most common type is idiopathic (no known cause), or may be congenital in a baby born with a spinal defect. The onset may be at birth, juvenile, or adolescent.
- Mild scoliosis is considered a curvature of less then 20°. This typically does not cause any significant problems for the child.
- Severe scoliosis is considered a curvature of more then 60°. This can create serious problems including, degenerative spinal arthritis, back pain, vertebral subluxation, reduces lung capacity and pulmonary insufficiency.
- Screening of scoliosis now occurs in the school system to focus on early detection of the disease. A scoliometer can be utilized for screening.
- **Treatment:** early detection provides an important element in treating the disease along with the type of scoliosis. Exercises, stretching, and electrical stimulation may be utilized by the physical therapist. No guarantees with treatment but the earlier it's detected and treatment begins, the less likely that surgery will be necessary and long-term results will be good. Surgery is typically necessary in curvatures greater than 45°.

Spina Bifida

- Congenital abnormality; the disorder is a developmental defect in the spinal column, which results in incomplete closure of the vertebral canal. Most typically occurs in the lumbosacral area but may also occur in the cervical and thoracic areas.
- Classifications of spina bifida:
  1. Spina bifida occulta: vertebral arches are unfused, identified externally by a skin depression or dimple, dark tufts of hair, soft subcutaneous lipomas at the site. Does not usually cause neurological dysfunction. Occasionally, foot weakness and bowel or bladder dysfunction.
  2. Spina bifida cystica:
     Meningocele: vertebral arches are unfused with herniation of meninges. No neurological signs of myelodysplasia of spinal cord noted.
     Myelomeningocele: herniation of meninges with abnormal development of the spinal cord. Neurological signs are present and typically involve permanent neurological deficits. This type of spina bifida is also associated with hydrocephalus in 90% of the children.
- **Treatment:** focus on prevention of the deformity and instruct the family in a home program. Facilitate normal motor development, mobility, and passive range of motion. Depending on the seriousness of the disease and a child's age, therapy should be approached cautiously. The child may be highly allergic (eg, allergies to latex) and have a tendency to have fractures.

Talipes Equinovarus

- Congenital deformity of the foot, also called clubfoot. Ninety percent of clubfoot cases are talipes equinovarus, resulting in medial deviation and plantar flexion of the forefoot.
- The foot position is in ankle plantar flexion, inversion, and adduction at the talocalcanea midtarsal joints.
- Talipes calcaneovalgus or calcaneovarus may occur occasionally and is characterized by lateral deviation and dorsiflexion either outward or inward from the midline of the body.

- **Treatment:** the goal of physical therapy is to restore function to the foot through providing correct alignment. The Denis Browne splint is utilized for correction and consists of a curved bar attached to a pair of high-top shoes. The splint may be adjusted to allow for individual abduction of each foot depending on the severity of the disorder. Casting or splinting may also be utilized after birth and as early on as possible for best results. In severe cases, several stages of surgery may be necessary to correct the alignment.

Torticollis

- Neck deformity involving the sternocleidomastoid muscle contracting and causing lateral flexion toward the shorter muscle side and rotation of the chin to the opposite side.
- May be either congenital or a result of trauma/disease. Congenital cases are typically seen after a difficult birth.
- Severe cases include the infant's head flattening on the affected side, shoulder elevation on the affected side, and facial asymmetry.
- **Treatment:** passive stretching exercises for the sternocleidomastoid muscle. Teaching instruction on proper head positioning and handling of the child to the parents. Progression to active range of motion and strengthening techniques. Surgical intervention is seen after 12 months of age and loss of motion greater than 30° of neck rotation. Surgery might also be preformed after failure to correct the deformity with conservative management.

Traumatic Brain Injury

- Brain injury due to mechanical forces that occur from the initial impact. Brain injuries may be open, leaving the brain exposed or closed
- Impairments are dependent upon the severity and location of the initial injury and the secondary brain injury attributed to the processes initiated as a result of the initial trauma.
- Evaluation performed by CT scan, magnetic resonance imaging (MRI), assessment of orientation to time and place, and ability to respond to stimuli performed by behavioral scales (Rancho Los Amigos, Glasgow coma scale), and monitoring intracranial pressure.
- Rancho Los Amigos assesses the behaviors as a function of cognitive recovery. The Glasgow coma scale assesses the level of consciousness in the child.
- Causes for hospitalization or death to the child include falls, automobile accidents, abuse, assault, sports activities like bicycling, and gunshot wounds.
- **Treatment:** stimulate the level of consciousness through sensory stimuli. Improve joint flexibility by positioning and range of motion. Promote motor development with posture and movement activities. Promote strength and stability through manipulation. Rehabilitation goals consist of returning the child to optimal functioning. An interdisciplinary treatment team approach is necessary to accomplish this goal.

SCREENING AND DIAGNOSTIC TESTS

Apgar Scores

An evaluation of an infant's physical condition based on a rating of five factors that reflect the infant's ability to adjust to extrauterine life. This system allows for the rapid identification of infants requiring immediate intervention. It is usually performed 1 minute and a second time at 5 minutes after birth, with the 5-minute total score normally higher than the 1 minute. A score of 0 to 3 represents severe distress, 4 to 7 indicates moderate distress, and a score of 7 to 10 indicates an absence of difficulty in adjusting to extrauterine life.

SIGN	0	1	2
Heart rate	Absent	Slow < 100 beats/minute	> 100 beats/minute
Respiratory effort	Absent	Slow or irregular	Good crying
Muscle tone	Limp	Some flexion of extremities	Active motion
Reflex irritability	No response	Grimace	Cough or sneeze
Color	Blue or pale	Body pink, extremities blue	Completely pink

Alberta Infant Motor Scale

The Albert infant motor scale is an observational assessment to measure gross motor skill maturation. The motor skill maturation is observed and recorded from birth to independent walking. The purpose of this test is to determine if an infant's motor skills are delayed, provide information on mastered skills, and developing skills over a period of time.

Denver Developmental Screening Test II

This test was developed to screen for developmental delays. Originally started in 1967 by Frankenburg and Dodds, it was revised to meet new guidelines and is now called screening test 2. The test screens development in four areas, personal-social, fine motor, gross motor, and language. The test screens from birth to 6 years old.

Gross Motor Function Measure

Designed for pediatric therapists to evaluate children with cerebral palsy or head injuries. The test evaluates gross motor function and how it changes over time or after therapy. The test assesses motor function in five areas: sitting, lying and rolling, crawling and kneeling, standing, and running or walking. The evaluation of the child's ability allows the therapist to plan a treatment program to maximize independent functioning.

Test of Infant Motor Performance

The test evaluates the components of postural and selective control of movement in early infancy. The test was developed for utilization by the occupational and physical therapist.

The test assesses functional activities involving movement in early infancy. This may include movement against the force of gravity, orienting the head and body to listening and looking, interacting with caregivers, and self comfort. The test is for 32 weeks gestational age to 3 1/2 months after full-term delivery.

REFLEXES

Asymmetrical Tonic Neck Flexion (ATNF)

Integrated: 4 to 6 months
Onset: birth
Stimulus: rotation of the head to one side
Response: flexion of skull limbs and extension of jaw limbs

Crossed Extension

Integrated: 1 to 2 months
Onset: 28 weeks gestation
Stimulus: sharp or noxious stimulus to the ball of the foot, extremity test is in extension, and patient is in supine position
Response: withdrawal of extremity tested and extension of opposite lower extremity

Flexor Withdrawal

Integrated: 1 to 2 months
Onset: 28 weeks
Stimulus: noxious stimulus to the ball of the foot in sitting or supine position, lower extremity in extension
Response: the lower extremity tested will withdraw from the stimulus, causing overresponse of hip and knee flexion

Grasp

Integrated: palmar at 4 to 6 months, plantar at 9 months
Onset: palmar at birth, plantar at 28 weeks
Stimulus: palmar pressure to the palm of the hand, plantar to the ball of the foot under the toes
Response: palmar will result in finger flexion, plantar will result in toe flexion or curling

Moro's

Integrated: 5 to 6 months
Onset: 28 weeks gestation
Stimulus: sudden changes in position of the head in relation to the trunk
Response: sudden extension of neck results in flexion and abduction of the shoulders, extension of the elbows, crying followed by extension, adduction of the shoulders and flexion of the elbows.

Protective Extension Reaction

Integrated: persists
Onset: upper extremities 4 to 6 months and lower extremities 6 to 9 months
Stimulus: displace the center of gravity outside the base of support by pushing the body to either side
Response: the upper extremity and lower extremity will extend and abduct to protect from falling toward the side the body being pushed

Startled

Integrated: persists
Onset: birth
Stimulus: loud noise or sudden harsh noise
Response: extension and abduction of the extremities and usually crying

Symmetrical Tonic Neck Reflex (STNR)

Integrated: 8 to 12 months
Onset: 4 to 6 months
Stimulus: flexion or extension of the head
Response: flexion of the head results in flexion of the upper extremities and extension in the lower extremities. Extension of the head results in extension of the upper extremities and flexion of the lower extremities.

Symmetrical Tonic Labyrinthine

Integrated: 6 months
Onset: birth
Stimulus: prone or supine position
Response: prone position results in increased flexor tone and flexion in the upper and lower extremities. Supine position results in increased extensor tone and extension in the upper and lower extremities.

Traction

Integrated: 2 to 5 months
Onset: 28 weeks gestation
Stimulus: grasp forearm and pull up from supine to sitting
Response: flexion of the upper extremities and grasp, the head will lag behind until four to five months of age.

DEVELOPMENTAL SEQUENCE CHART

AGE	KEY DEVELOPMENT
Neonate (0 to 10 days)	In supine position, the head turns to the side due to lack of muscular control May hold head up for 3 seconds in sitting
1 month	Turns head to side Holds head up in prone position Tracks a moving object
2 months	Turns from side to side Sits with complete support and head bobs when sitting Holds object placed in the hand
3 months	Head can be maintained in upright position but will be accompanied by shoulder elevation and a forward head posture Can support some weight in standing with assistance Head can lift to 90° Weightbearing on forearms
4 months	Holds head erect Reaches for object with both hands Starts hand-to-mouth activities Rolls prone to side and supine to side Midline orientation is established Prone pivots
5 months	Head control in supported seating Rolls prone to supine Practices weight shifting, lateral head and trunk righting Equilibrium reactions begin in prone position
6 months	Reaches for object with one hand Completes turning and rolling Independent sitting Ability to extend, flex, and laterally flex head against gravity Prone position with use of shoulder girdle to control weight shift on extended arms and reach forward Bears weight on lower extremities and bounces
7 to 8 months	Sits unsupported for longer periods of time Trunk rotation in sitting Pushes up to four-point position Equilibrium reactions in supine Beginning equilibrium reactions in sitting At 8 months, full equilibrium reactions in sitting
9 months	Locomotion through crawling Pulls to stand from kneeling Can stand alone
10 months	Cruises Gets to stand position through half-kneeling position
11 to 14 months	Twelve months sequence to standing is kneeling, half-kneeling, weight shift forward, squat, then upright Walks but very unsteady Stands without support
15 months	Walks more steady but with a wide base of support May walk backward and sideways
18 months	Continues to improve balance when walking Starts climbing Running-like walk Reciprocal arm swing with heel strike

AGE	KEY DEVELOPMENT
20 months	Climbs stairs with two feet on each step
	Improves running coordination
	Jumps off low steps
2 years	Starts running
	Improves balance
	Decreases pelvic tilt, hip abduction, and external rotation in gait
3 years	Can stand on one foot for short periods
	Can catch a bounced ball
	Gait cycle is established
4 years	Skips on one foot
	Alternates feet when going up and down stairs
	Can walk on tiptoes with control
5 years	Dresses self
	Gross motor control will be more advanced than fine motor control

ADAPTIVE EQUIPMENT FOR CHILDREN

Mobility Equipment

Scooter boards and tricycles are a fun way for children who are physically challenged to have independent mobility and locomotion. The scooter board is a flat, padded board with four casters. The child lays prone and propels through utilizing the hands on the floor. This allows for prone stability and prone mobility work, which is fun for the child. The tricycle can be adapted (eg, back supports or foot straps) to allow the child locomotion through utilization of their lower extremities. Other mobility aids may include specially adapted wheelchairs, walkers, crutches, and orthotic devices.

Prone Standers

Prone standers are used for children who cannot stand upright. The child is placed in a prone position on the stander. The prone stander gives the child weightbearing activity through the upper extremities. This allows the child physiological development changes that occur from weightbearing. The child is placed in the prone position on the stander and the vertical position depends on the child's tolerance and goals of the treatment program. The prone stander also services to provide positive social and psychological experiences for the child. The child is now able to see from an upright position and have peer interaction at an elevated position.

Sidelyers

Sidelyers are utilized for children with a low level of developmental functioning. The child is placed sidelying so that the trunk is symmetrical as possible, head is in alignment neutral to the trunk, and supported, nonweightbearing limbs are free to move, and weightbearing limbs are in a slightly flexed position.

Supine Standers

A supine stander is the opposite of the prone stander and provides an upright position through weightbearing at the trunk and lower extremities. The hips, knees, ankles, and trunk are placed in optimal alignment with support. The angle of the table can be vertically adjusted up to 90°. The child will benefit physiologically and psychologically from the vertical positioning.

CHAPTER 20

Wound Care & Burns

SKIN AND TISSUE

The skin is the largest organ of the body. Its functions include protective covering, regulation of body temperature, aiding in regulation of blood pressure, housing sensory receptors, and synthesizing various chemicals. The skin is composed of the following layers:

Epidermis

- Outer layer of the skin
- Layers are between 0.5 and 1.1 mm in thickness
- Contains striated squamous epithelium cells
- Functions to protect the underlying tissue against water loss, effects of harmful chemicals, and mechanical injury
- Location of the pores and the hair shafts

Dermis

- Binds the epidermis to underlying tissues
- Composed of fibrous connective tissue
- Contains nerves, nerve endings, glands, hair follicles, blood, and lymphatic vessels
- Functions with vitamin D production
- The following are contained in the dermis:
  - Ducts
  - Arrector pili muscles
  - Sebaceous glands
  - Nerves
  - Blood vessels

Subcutaneous Tissue

- A continuous layer of connective tissue beneath the dermis. It comprises an outer, normally fatty layer, and an inner, thin elastic layer
- Composed of adipose tissue
- Anchors the superficial tissue layers to the underlying tissue

SKIN RESPONSE TO INJURY

Burns

- Minor burns will cause the blood vessels to dilate and the tissue surrounding the area to become red
- Response is localized to the injured area in small minor burns

- As burns become more severe in nature, blisters will form in the skin due to fluid being retained underneath the skin
- In severe burns, the protective skin layer will be removed. The wound may heal by filling in or skin grafts may be necessary
- Burns, depending upon the damage, will affect the following systems in the body: renal, respiratory, cardiovascular, gastrointestinal, pulmonary, and immune system.

Wound Healing Response

- There are three phases in the wound healing response: inflammatory, proliferation, and remodeling.
- The inflammatory stage is where you see the cardinal signs of inflammation: calor (heat), rubor (redness), dolor (pain), and tumor (swelling).
- The blood vessels will dilate, becoming red and permeable. The vascular permeability allows fluids to enter the damaged tissues. This is what causes the redness and pain response.
- The proliferation stage results in exudation of the fluid, clustering of leukocytes in the vessel walls, phagocytosis of debri, and deposits of fibrin.
- The remodeling stage results in migration of fibroblasts and development of new normal cells.

CLASSIFICATION OF ULCERS

Stages

1. **Stage one:** destruction is limited to the epidermis and redness may be noted. Nonblanchable erythemia of the skin and a heralding lesion of skin ulceration.
2. **Stage two:** involvement of the epidermis, dermis, and subcutaneous fat; redness, edema, blistering, and hardening of the tissue may be noted. The ulcer is superficial and may appear as an abrasion, blister, or a shallow crater.
3. **Stage three:** full thickness of dermis is involved, and undermining of the deeper tissues may extend down to the underlying fascia. The ulcer is a deep crater that may or may not involve the undermining tissues.
4. **Stage four:** full thickness involves penetrating to the fascia with possible muscle involvement, and there is usually bone destruction.

TYPES OF ULCERS

Arterial Insufficiency Ulcers

Occur secondary to arteriosclerosis obliterans, often in diabetics. Peripheral pulses are weak or absent. Bruits may be heard via stethoscope over peripheral vessels. Bruits are sounds of blood turbulence as a result of narrow vessels. Limb elevation will result in pallor. The dependent position (down) will cause rubor. The ulcers that may form are usually located on the lateral malleolus and toes. Can be very deep and painful. Bed rest with the head of the bed moderately elevated, no smoking, wound care and protective environment are conservative ways of managing these wounds. No external compression is used.

Venous Insufficiency Ulcers

Occur secondary to venous thrombosis, varicose veins, and other venous problems. Peripheral pulses usually are good and edema is present. The ulcers are usually located on the medial side of the ankle. The surrounding skin may be pigmented and indurated. They are often painless and may be extensive but not deep. They can endure for decades. Elevation and compression to control edema is vital. Unna's boot, custom-fitted elastic stockings, and intermittent compression therapy can be helpful. Wound care is performed, however, whirlpool is not helpful. Exercise is permissible if support garments are worn and the part is elevated after exercising.

Diabetic Ulcers

Diabetic ulcers occur as a result of improper glucose metabolism, resulting in a diminished vascular system. Sensory neuropathy may also occur in diabetics, leading to a loss of sensation. Diabetic ulcers result because of repetitive stress and pressure on the skin lacking sensory input. The lack of sensory input results in the patient not protecting the injured area, then the subcutaneous and cutaneous break down. A common area of ulcers to occur is over bony areas, like the medial malleolus, lateral malleolus, and greater trochanter. Diabetic ulcer treatment depends on additional factors outside of physical therapy treatment plans. The patient's nutritional balance, insulin control, glucose levels, and exercise level all integrate with the healing process. These factors must also be working for optimal wound healing in conjunction with physical therapy treatments.

Location of Ulcers

Ulcers may be caused by prolonged pressure over bony areas or possibly from a lack of healing in an area. For example, in a diabetic patient, they most likely occur over bony areas, such as the medial malleolus, lateral malleolus, and greater trochanter. The following are risk factors for a pressure ulcer: friction between surfaces, external pressure on an area, two layers sliding against each other in opposite directions, and softening caused by excessive moisture. There are additional risk factors for patients who have restricted mobility. As a result of restricted mobility, the risk factors are contractures, obesity, and loss of sensation, edema, and decreased muscle tone.

TREATMENT OF THE WOUND

1. Cleansing the wound to promote healing. Whirlpool may be utilized with wounds to remove loosely attached debris and clean the wound bed. Whirlpools should be set up with a sterile technique. Additives, such as antibacterial agents, may be utilized depending on the type of wound. All staff members should wear protective barriers.
2. Debridement of the wound of necrotic or damaged tissue. The necrotic tissues obstruct the formation of granulation and epithelial cells from migrating across the wound. The debridement may consist of a whirlpool with agitation directed at the wound. Debridement may also take place using a scalpel, scissors, and forceps. This is only utilized when it is clear that the tissue is devitalized.
3. Dressings that are removed from the patient should be placed in a biohazard container as per facility policy.
4. Patient's dressing should be reapplied after treatment, utilizing sterile techniques and protective barriers.
5. Pressure-relieving devices, such as foam padding, may be utilized to protect the wound from further pressure and deterioration.
6. Teach weight shifting or turning schedules to the patients, family, and staff for home education programs.
7. Exercises can increase circulation to the area to promote healing. Exercises can also be utilized to prevent contractures, increase muscle strength, and decrease edema.
8. Oxygen, ultrasound, and electrical stimulation may be utilized to increase wound healing.
9. A physician may utilize surgery to remove excessive necrotic tissue and debris.
10. If possible, restoring normal function to the tissue is the final goal.

PREVENTION OF WOUNDS

1. In diabetic cases, provide the patient with the proper education. Also, early intervention will aid in preventing the ulcer from entering the later stages.
2. Check skin frequently for red spots.
3. Patients at risk should at least have a daily skin inspection.
4. Skin should be thoroughly cleaned at the time it is soiled, prevent infection through proper cleaning as soon as possible.
5. Immobile patients should be placed on a frequent turning schedule.
6. Proper position of the bedridden patient and frequent repositioning every 2 hours.
7. Pressure-reducing devices should be utilized. Wheelchair patients should have a doughnut type device. In bed, positioning devices should include pillows and foam wedges. Bedridden patients should use pressure-reducing surfaces, foam, gel, air, or water mattress.
8. Transferring techniques should emphasize reducing friction through utilization of a slide board, trapeze, and hydraulic lifts.
9. At a minimum, maintain current range of motion and mobility. If the patient has rehabilitation potential, try to increase the activity level and mobility.
10. Environment for patients should be stable with little fluctuation to cold/hot temperatures or humidity that creates dry skin.
11. Utilization of lubricants, like creams, can decrease friction between surfaces sliding on one another.

CLASSIFICATION OF BURNS

Superficial Burn

- Minimal thickness
- Affects the epidermis only
- Skin appears red
- Skin surface is dry
- Slight pain
- Minimal edema
- No blistering
- Healing with no scarring

Superficial Partial-Thickness Burn

- Affects the epidermis and possibly the superficial part of the dermis
- Severe pain
- Considerable edema
- Mottled appearance
- Blister formations intact
- Healing with minimal or no scarring

Deep Partial-Thickness Burn

- Damage to entire epidermis, as well as severe damage to the dermis
- Broken blisters
- Wound color a mixed red or waxy white color
- Severe pain or possible loss of pain if nerve endings are damaged
- Moderate edema
- Healing occurs with hypertrophic scarring and keloids

Full-Thickness Burn

- Complete destruction of the entire epidermis and dermis
- Possible damage to subcutaneous fat layer
- Hard parchment-like eschar formation
- No pain
- No blisters
- Severe edema
- White leathery appearance
- Healing tissue only occurs at the edges of the wound requiring skin grafting

Subdermal Burn

- Complete destruction of the epidermis, dermis, and fat layers
- May damage the bone and muscle
- Typically as a result of prolonged contact with a flame, chemical or electricity
- Extensive surgery is required
- Sometimes amputation is necessary

RULE OF NINES

This allows the therapist to determine the percentage of the body burned. The rule of nines was developed by Lund and Brower. The rule of nines is based on dividing the body into sections, which represent 9% or a multiple of 9%. Each area of the body is assigned a specific value, as listed in the following chart:

Body Area	Adults	Children
Head—anterior	4.5%	18%
Head—posterior	4.5%	
Arm—anterior	4.5%	9%
Arm—posterior	4.5%	
Leg—anterior	9%	14%
Leg—posterior	9%	
Chest	18%	18%
Back	18%	18%
Genitals	1%	1%

Graft and Flap Types

Advancement flap: a local flap where adjacent skin is moved to cover the burn without detaching the flap from its existing site.

Allograft: may also be called a homograft; a graft is taken from a donor who is the same species but not identical to the patient. See homograft definition.

Autograft: skin taken from a part of the burn victim's own body.

Biosynthetic graft: a graft that is a combination of collagen and synthetics.

Delayed graft: a graft that is partially elevated, then replaced. It is replaced so that it can be moved to another site.

Free flap: skin tissue that is moved to another site where vascular reconnection is made. The moved skin tissue may also include blood vessels.

Full-thickness graft: consists of all layers of skin but no subcutaneous fat.

Heterograft or xenograft: skin taken from another species. Most often pigskin dressing to speed healing. Temporary grafts.

Homograft: human skin from a donor (often cadaver skin is used).

Isologous graft: donor and patient are genetically identical.

Local flap: movement of skin to an adjacent site. Part of the flap will remain attached to retain its blood supply.

Mesh graft: the donor's skin is cut away from the mesh so it can cover a larger surface area.

Myocutaneous flap: the flap consists of muscle, patent blood vessels, skin, and subcutaneous fat.

Sheet graft: the donor's skin is applied without changing the recipient's site.

Split-thickness skin graft: autograft that is one-half thickness of skin.

Test-tube graft: a biopsy providing epidermal cells that are cultured into smooth sheets of skin. These sheets of skin are then grafted onto the burn area. This is a new procedure utilized for burns that cover the entire body.

Z–plasty: a simple form of the rotational flab where a section of skin is incised on three sides and pivoted to cover the injured area.

Treatment of Burn Patients

1. Sterile whirlpool in order to promote healing. This is done to control infection and aid in loosening the necrotic tissue, making debridement easier. Sterile towels and dressing must also be used post-whirlpool. It is extremely important to maintain a faultless sterile technique so that no cross-infections occur.
2. Reduce dependent edema formation and promote venous return.
3. Proper positioning and splinting to control contractures and edema.
4. Passive range of motion and stretching exercises.

5. Closure of the wound. Grafting as necessary. Physician may utilize medications to assist in controlling infections and pain. Pain relievers may be given 45 minutes prior to treatment to assist with the pain from the treatment program.
6. Active range of motion progressing from therapist assistance to resistive exercise as tolerated.
7. Pressure garments for reducing edema and scar formation.
8. Massage to reduce scarring and tissue contracutres.
9. Increase strength, range of motion, and functioning.
10. Promote independence in activities of daily living and self-care.
11. Proprioceptive and sensation exercises.
12. Referral to counseling or support services (social worker, occupational therapy and vocational counselor) as necessary.
13. Instructions in a home care program to promote burn healing, prevention of infection, prevention of edema and scar formation, and maintenance of normal joint function.

BURN POSITIONING TO PREVENT CONTRACTURES

AFFECTED AREA	POSITIONING
Ankle/foot	Neutral. May use padded footboard or ankle position devices
Knee	Extension with posterior splint, toes pointing toward the ceiling
Hip	Extension/abduction/neutral rotation and toes pointing toward the ceiling.
Shoulder	Abduction/flexion/external rotation—may use clavicle strap or abduction axillary splint
Axillary region	Arm abducted to 90° to 110°
Elbow	Extension and supination. Elbow splinting position in extension with slight degree of elbow flexion
Wrist	Wrist placed in extension with a hand splint
Metacarpophalangeal (MCP) joint	MCP flexion at 90° with a hand splint
Proximal or distal interterphalangeal joint (PIP/DIP)	PIP and DIP are placed in extension with a hand splint
Thumb	Thumb abduction with a hand splint
Web spaces	Finger abduction utilizing web spaces, gauze, or foam
Burn claw hand	MP flexion (70°), IP extension, thumb opposition, wrist extended (15°).
Anterior neck	Hyperextension, cervical brace, no pillows, may have a small towel beneath the cervical spine to promote extension
Posterior neck	Neutral position with no pillow
Circumferential neck involvement	Neutral position toward extension with no pillow

CHAPTER 21

Spinal Cord

TYPES OF SPINAL CORD INJURIES

Anterior Cord Syndrome

Results in damage to the anterior part of the spinal cord. This is an incomplete lesion and sense of light touch, proprioception, and position are usually intact. Bilateral loss of motor function, sensation of pain, and temperature. Typically caused by an injury that causes the loss of function from the anterior spinal artery.

Brown-Séquard's Syndrome

Results in hemisection of the spinal cord. Typically seen after a stab wound or gunshot injury. This is also an incomplete lesion, which typically results in loss of motor function on the same side as the lesion and loss of pain and temperature on the opposite side. It is rare to have a complete hemisection on one side of the spinal cord; it is more likely the patient will have an irregular lesion. Lateral column damage will result in a positive Babinski sign and a loss of proprioception in the dorsal column, vibratory, and kinesthesia senses.

Cauda Equina Injury

Involves the lower end of the spinal cord at the first lumbar vertebra and the bundle of lumbar, sacral, and coccygeal nerve roots that emerge from the spinal cord and descend through the spinal canal of the sacrum and coccyx before reaching the intervertebral foramina of their particular vertebrae.

Central Cord Syndrome

Occurs when there is damage to the central portion of the cord and is an incomplete lesion. Typically greater deficits are found in the upper extremities than in the lower extremities upon evaluation. Hyperextension injuries of the cervical spine typically cause the central cord syndrome.

Complete Lesion

Occurs when the entire spinal cord is severed. It results in no sensation or muscle power below the level of the lesion. Complete lesion is usually the result of severe compression, extensive vascular dysfunction, and transection.

Discomplete Lesion

Signifies that the spinal cord is partially injured, but discomplete. It results from sparing of a small amount of axons in the spinal cord.

Incomplete Lesion

A partial loss of sensation or voluntary muscle power below the neurological level of the lesion. Incomplete lesions are usually the result of edema in the spinal cord and bony protrusion or bone fragments in the spinal cord.

Paraplegia

Injury classification for patients who lose function of both lower extremities. Typically, the injury level is between T1 and L1.

Posterior Cord Syndrome

This is a rare syndrome and typically not seen in spinal cord injuries. It will result in loss of proprioception and a steppage gait. The loss is below the level of the lesion.

Quadriplegia

Injury classification for patients who lose function of all four extremities and trunk. The injury level is between C1 and C8.

Sacral Sparing

Occurs in the sacral area and is an incomplete lesion. Typically, sensation will be intact in the sacral area; however, paralysis and loss of sensation are complete in all other areas below the level of lesion.

SPINAL CORD IMPAIRMENT/CLASSIFICATION SCALES

American Spinal Injury Association Impairment Scale

Grade A: Complete lesion, no sensory or motor function is intact in the S4 to S5 segment level.
Grade B: Incomplete lesion, sensory but no motor function below neurological level. Sensory function is intact through S4 to S5.
Grade C: Incomplete lesion, motor function is intact below the neurological level. Most key muscles below the level have a muscle grade of less then three.
Grade D: Incomplete lesion, motor function is intact below the neurological level. Most key muscles below the level have a muscle grade of three or more.
Grade E: Normal sensory and motor function.

Modified Frankel Classification Scale

Grade A: Complete sensory and motor involvement.
Grade B: Complete motor involvement and some sensory sparing.
Grade C: Motor sparing but is not functional.
Grade D: Motor sparing that is functional.
Grade E: No neurological involvement.

MEDICAL COMPLICATIONS OF A SPINAL CORD INJURY

Autonomic Hyperreflexia

- A distended bladder, distended rectum, or neurological procedures with catheterizations or bladder irrigation generally cause this. This condition can occur in any patient with a lesion above the T5 level.
- Symptoms may include pounding headache, hypertension, sweating above the level of the spinal cord injury, slow pulse, and nasal obstruction.
- The therapist should monitor symptoms. If the above symptoms are seen, the patient should be positioned in sitting immediately to create postural hypotension or decrease the blood pressure. This can be performed only if the patient's spine is stable enough for him or her to be in the sitting position. The therapist should check the catheter and tubing, empty the leg bag if it is full and, depending upon the severity of the symptoms, notify the attending physician or nurse.

Bowel and Bladder Complications

- Urination is controlled by the conus medullaris, and primary reflex control is in the sacral segments.
- Spinal shock and lesions above the conus medullaris result in the bladder being flaccid, absent reflexes, a reflex neurogenic bladder, and reflex bowel. This will result in spasticity, ureteral reflux, voiding complications, and detrusor muscle hypertrophy.
- Lesions at the conus medullaris result in the bladder being nonreflexive, decreased tone of the ureteral sphincter and perineal muscles, and nonreflex bowel.

Heterotopic Ossification

- This is defined as ectopic or hypertrophic bone growth. It is an abnormal occurrence of bone growth in the soft tissue, usually the tendons and connective tissue. Typically, the hip, knee, elbow, and shoulder joints are most frequently involved. The specific cause is unknown, although it appears frequently in spinal cord population, predominantly in males, and unilaterally or bilaterally in the hips. Heterotopic ossification occurs within the first year of injury and below the level of the lesion.
- Symptoms include pain, warmth, and edema.
- Treatment includes stretching and range of motion exercises.

Ulcers or Pressure Sores

- Caused by improper pressure relief or breakdown of the skin and tissue.
- Symptoms may include redness or red spots, and/or skin breakdown.
- Treatment includes teaching the patient the proper pressure relief. The patient needs to be able to relieve ischial pressure, sacral pressure, and greater trochanter pressure. The patient needs to learn weight shifting, independent pressure relief, and repositioning.

METHODS OF BRACING/STABILIZING A SPINAL CORD INJURY

Foot Orthosis (AFO)

A short leg brace designed to prevent the patient from tripping secondary to weak or absent dorsiflexors. This is an L-shaped brace typically made out of plastic.

Halo

An external brace designed to stabilize the cervical vertebrae.

Harrington Rods

Rods placed internally to stabilize either the thoracic or lumbar vertebrae.

Jewett Orthosis

An external method of providing stabilization to the thoracic and lumbar vertebrae. This is a three-point brace that prevents hyperextension, with the three points of pressure on the sternum, lumbar spine, and synthesis pubis.

Knee-Ankle-Foot-Orthosis (KAFO)

A long leg brace that stabilizes the knee and ankle. Brace may be metal or plastic.

Knight-Taylor Orthosis

A method of applying external stabilization to the thoracic and lumbar vertebrae. Typically utilized for fractures above the L3 region.

Scott-Craig Orthosis

A metal KAFO used by spinal cord patients.

Sterno-Occipital Mandibular Immobilization (SOMI)

A method of external stabilization for the cervical vertebrae.

Thoracic-Lumbar-Sacral Orthosis (TLSO)

Any orthosis that provides external immobilization of the thoracic and lumbar spine.

Weiss Springs

An internal stabilization method for the thoracic and lumbar vertebrae.

COMMON MUSCLE SUBSTITUTIONS

The spinal cord patient will use muscle substitution in areas where voluntary muscle activity may not be present or only partially available. Following is the muscle and its typical substitution.

Muscle	Substitutions
Upper trapezius	Levator scapulae
Middle trapezius	Rhomboids, levator scapulae
Rhomboids	Middle trapezius
Serratus anterior	Pectoralis minor and coracobrachialis
Biceps	Brachioradialis
Pectoralis major	Long head of the biceps, anterior deltoid
Triceps	Supraspinatus, infraspinatus, teres minor
Deltoid	Long head of the biceps, long head of the triceps, supraspinatus, infraspinatus, and teres minor
Supinator	Biceps, brachioradialis, external rotators of the shoulder, extensor muscles of the wrist, and supinator muscles of the forearm
Shoulder—external rotator	Supinators of the forearm and extensors of the wrist to rotate the arm with gravity
Shoulder—internal rotator	Pectoralis minor and coracobrachialis
Wrist extensors	Supination of the forearm or externally rotating the shoulder so gravity can extend the wrist
Wrist flexors	Pronating the forearm or internally rotating the shoulder so gravity can flex the wrist
Pronators	Brachioradialis
Latissimus dorsi	Teres major, posterior deltoid, lower trapezius
Abdominals	Neck flexors, pectoralis major and minor, and serratus anterior
Quadratus lumborum	Latissimus dorsi
Oblique abdominal	Latissimus dorsi
Hip flexors	Lower abdominal muscles
Hip extensors	Lower back extensor muscles
Hip abductors	Latissimus dorsi
Hip adductors	Lower abdominal muscles
Hip internal rotators	Lower abdominal muscles
Hip external rotators	Lower back extensors
Knee flexors	Sartorius and gracilis
Quadriceps	Adductor magnus
Inversion of the foot	Medial gastrocnemius
Eversion of the foot	Lateral gastrocnemius

EXPECTED FUNCTIONAL OUTCOME OF SPINAL CORD INJURIES ACCORDING TO LEVEL

Cervical Spine Injuries

C1, C2, C3 Spinal Cord Injury

- Respiration: dependence on a respirator, may use phrenic nerve stimulator during the day.
- Bed mobility: needs a full-time attendant.
- Pressure relief: electric wheelchair with recline backs, dependent.
- Transfers: dependence on caregiver.
- Mobility in the wheelchair: electric wheelchair with sip and puff control may be utilized, seat belt, and trunk support.

C4 Spinal Cord Injury

- Respiration: vital capacity of at least 30% to 50% of the norm.
- Bed mobility: patient is able to direct bed mobility and give occasional minimal assistance.
- Pressure relief: patient is able to direct pressure relief activities or utilize reclining back on wheelchair.
- Transfers: patient is able to direct all transfers, otherwise dependent.
- Mobility in the wheelchair: patient is independent using a motorized wheelchair without hand controls on level surfaces, use breath, sip and puff, chin, or mouth controls.

C5 Spinal Cord Injury

- Respiration: vital capacity of 40% to 60% of norm; patient can assist with bronchial hygiene.
- Bed mobility: patient can give minimal assistance, overhead swivel bar.
- Pressure relief: patient may assist in changing wheelchair position, recline back—otherwise dependent.
- Transfers: patient is able to direct transfers, as well as give minimal assistance, overhead swivel bar, sliding board.
- Mobility in the wheelchair: patient is independent utilizing a motorized wheelchair with hand controls or electric wheelchair with joystick or adopted upper extremity controls.

C6 Spinal Cord Injury

- Respiration: vital capacity of 60% to 80% of norm; possibly independent with bronchial hygiene.
- Bed mobility: independent with side rails.
- Pressure relief: independent.
- Transfers: independent to and from a level surface, patient could give moderate assistance in all transfers, sliding board.
- Mobility in the wheelchair: independent with a manual wheelchair on level surfaces.
- Range of motion: patient is independent.

C7 Spinal Cord Injury

- Respiration: vital capacity of 60% to 80% of norm; independent with bronchial hygiene.
- Bed mobility: independent without special equipment.
- Pressure relief: independent, including wheelchair push-ups.
- Transfers: patient is able to give moderate assistance with transfers to and from the wheelchair and be independent on all level surfaces.
- Mobility in the wheelchair: patient is independent on level surfaces and able to assist on elevation.
- Range of motion: patient is independent.

C8 to T1 Spinal Cord Injury

- Respiration: vital capacity of 60-80% of norm; independent with bronchial hygiene.
- Bed mobility: patient is independent without special equipment.
- Pressure relief: patient is independent, including wheelchair push-ups.
- Transfers: patient is able to give moderate assistance with transfers to and from wheelchair.
- Mobility in the wheelchair: patient is independent on a level surface and able to assist on elevation.
- Range of motion: patient is independent.

Thoracic Spine Injuries

T1 to T5 Spinal Cord Injury
- Respiration: vital capacity of 80% of norm.
- Bed mobility: independent without special equipment.
- Pressure relief: independent, including wheelchair push-ups.
- Transfers: independent to and from the floor.
- Mobility in the wheelchair: independent in a manual wheelchair on all level surfaces and elevations.
- Ambulation: it might be possible for the patient to be independent with bilateral KAFO and the parallel bars.
- Range of motion: independent.

T6 to T8 Spinal Cord Injury
- Respiration: vital capacity of 80% of norm.
- Bed mobility: independent without special equipment.
- Pressure relief: independent, including wheelchair push-ups.
- Transfers: independent to and from the floor.
- Mobility in the wheelchair: independent in a manual wheelchair on all level surfaces.
- Ambulation: supervision with bilateral KAFO and a walker; it might be possible for the patient to be independent with bilateral KAFO and a walker.
- Range of motion: independent.

T9 to T11 Spinal Cord Injury
- Respiration: vital capacity of 80% of norm.
- Bed mobility: independent without special equipment.
- Pressure relief: independent, including wheelchair push-ups.
- Transfers: independent to and from the floor.
- Ambulation: patient is able to use bilateral KAFO and Lofstrand crutches with supervision on elevations and rough terrain.
- Range of motion: independent.

T12 Spinal Cord Injury
- Respiration: vital capacity of 80% of norm.
- Bed mobility: independent without special equipment.
- Pressure relief: independent, including wheelchair push-ups.
- Transfers: independent to and from the floor.
- Ambulation: possible for patient to be independent with bilateral KAFO and Lofstrand crutches on all surfaces.
- Range of motion: independent.

Lumbar Spine Injuries

L1 to L3 Spinal Cord Injury
- Respiration: vital capacity of 80% of norm.
- Bed mobility: independent without special equipment.
- Pressure relief: independent, including wheelchair push-ups.
- Transfers: independent to and from the floor.
- Mobility in the wheelchair: independent in a manual wheelchair on all level surfaces.
- Ambulation: independent with bilateral KAFO and Lofstrand crutches on all surfaces.
- Range of motion: independent.

L4 to L5 Spinal Cord Injury
- Respiration: vital capacity of 80% of norm.
- Bed mobility: independent without special equipment.
- Pressure relief: independent, including wheelchair push-ups.
- Transfers: independent to and from the floor, independent on all level surfaces.
- Mobility in the wheelchair: independent in a manual wheelchair on all level surfaces and elevations.
- Ambulation: independent with bilateral KAFO and crutches or canes.
- Range of motion: independent.

LEVEL, KEY MUSCLES, AND AVAILABLE MOVEMENTS

This chart shows several key muscles and available movements at the neurological level where they add functional outcomes in the patient.

LEVEL	KEY MUSCLES	AVAILABLE MOVEMENTS
C1 to C3	Face and neck muscles: cranial innervation	Talking, sipping, blowing
C4	Diaphragm, trapezius	Scapular elevation, respiration
C5	Biceps, brachialis, brachioradialis, deltoid, infraspinatus, rhomboid major, rhomboid minor, supinator	Elbow flexion and supination, shoulder external rotation, shoulder abduction to 90°, limited shoulder flexion
C6	Extensor carpi radialis, infraspinatus, latissimus dorsi, pectoralis major, pronator teres, serratus anterior, teres minor	Shoulder flexion, extension, internal rotation and adduction, scapular abduction and upward rotation, forearm pronation, wrist extension
C7	Extensor pollicis longus and brevis, extrinsic finger flexion, flexor carpi radialis, triceps	Elbow extension, wrist flexion, finger extension
C8 to T1	Extrinsic finger flexors, flexor carpi ulnaris, flexor pollicis longus, flexor pollicis brevis, intrinsic finger flexor	Full innervation of upper extremity muscles
T4 to T6	Top half of intercostals, sacrospinalis and semispinalis (long muscles of the back)	Improve trunk control, increase respiratory reserve
T9 to T12	Lower abdominals, all intercostals	Improve trunk control, increase endurance
L2 to L4	Gracilis, iliopsoas, quadratus lumborum, rectus femoris, sartorius	Hip flexion, hip adduction, knee extension
L4, L5	Extensor digitorum, low back muscles, medial hamstrings, posterior tibialis, quadriceps, tibialis anterior	Strong hip flexion, strong knee extension, weak knee flexion, improve trunk control

TREATMENT OPTIONS

- **Range of motion:** teach patient self range of motion when injury level allows, positioning to prevent contractures, and self-stretching. Teach patient and family or support personnel to carry over program to home.
- **Strengthening of available movements:** strengthen muscles that are still innervated and provide resistant exercise over time for strengthening and preventing atrophy.
- **Prevention teaching to patient and support system:** teach the patient and support system range of motion exercises, skin inspections, and home safety considerations.
- **Respiratory:** teach bronchial hygiene, assistive coughing, improve respiratory capacity, and breathing exercises.
- **Activities of daily living (ADLs):** assist the patient in performing as many activities of living independently as possible by level of lesion. Teach adaptive devices and fitting for assistance in ADLs.
- **Postural control:** teach proper posture with emphasis on stretching of hamstrings to maintain length. Hamstring length is necessary for transfer, standing, and gait. Correct posture will also assist with pain relief from muscular tightness that may develop.
- **Wheelchair mobility:** assist patients with fitting of wheelchair, wheelchair adjustments, promote wheelchair independence, teach wheelchair independence in all conditions—outdoors and inside. Teach transfers in and out, emergency techniques, and how to get back in a wheelchair in case of falls.
- **Pressure relief:** teach the patient and support system pressure relief techniques.
- **Stability:** teach the patient static balance and control. For example, apply resistance to the head to encourage shoulder stabilization.
- **Orthotic prescriptions:** assist the patient in ordering, fitting, and instructions for orthotics.

- **Cardiovascular endurance:** improve cardiovascular endurance, upper extremity ergonometery and swimming when possible.
- **Transfers:** teach the patient transfer to all surfaces—in and out of cars and bed. Teach patient how to utilize assistive devices for transfer (eg, transfer on sliding boards).
- **Ambulation:** work with the patient toward the goal of ambulation when possible, start with standing tolerance, first supported then unsupported. Functional electrical stimulation can be utilized to stimulate muscles.
- **Support groups:** assist the patient with emotional support when possible and give the patient information on support groups.
- **Referral to other services:** when necessary, facilitate referrals to other services to promote a team approach to the patient's treatment program.

CHAPTER 22

Gait

COMMON GAIT DEVIATIONS

Antalgic Gait (Painful Gait)

The patient will attempt to avoid weightbearing on the involved extremity and shorten the stance phase. Typically, the patient will try to unload the involved extremity when standing in place and they will shift weight to the noninvolved extremity. The patient will demonstrate this gait pattern because of pain in the lower extremity.

Arthrogenic Gait

The patient will elevate the pelvis and utilize circumduction on the involved side during the gait cycle. The noninvolved side will show increased plantar flexion at the ankle. This gait may be demonstrated in patients with hip or knee injury (eg, after cast removal because of stiffness in the joints).

Cerebellar Ataxia

This type of gait is typical for patients with a cerebellar disorder. The gait pattern is unsteady, irregular, wide base of support, and swaying toward the involved lower extremity.

Equinus Gait

Typically demonstrated by patients with an ankle deformity, spasticity of the posterior tibialis, and contractures. The patient will demonstrate excessive plantar flexion during the gait cycle.

Foot Drop or Foot Slap

The patient's foot will "slap" down on the ground. This is done secondary to a weak or absent dorsiflexor. The patient will lift the involved extremity knee high, resulting in the foot drop. This may also be called steppage gait because the patient lifts the involved lower extremity excessively high to clear the foot.

Gastrocnemius-Soleus Gait

During push-off, the patient's heel will not come off the ground, resulting in the involved lower extremity lagging behind the noninvolved. This is done secondary to weakness in the gastrocnemius and/or soleus muscle.

Gluteus Maximus Gait (Hip Extensor Gait)

May also be called extensor lurch. The patient will place the thoracic spine posterior to maintain hip extension during stance. The patient may also show an elevated pelvis on the involved lower extremity to maintain the knee in extension during midstance. This is a compensatory technique for gluteus maximus muscle weakness.

Gluteus Medius Gait (Trendelenburg Gait)

May also be called abducted lurch. The patient will lean over the hip to place the center of gravity over the involved hip, and the pelvis on the noninvolved side will dip during the swing phase. This is a compensatory technique for gluteus medius muscle weakness, congenital hip deformities, coxa vara, and hip dislocations.

Hemiplegic Gait (Flaccid Gait)

This gait is typically demonstrated in patients with one lower extremity shorter then the other, after a stroke, and in cases of deformity in the bones of the lower extremity. The patient swings the involved lower extremity in circumduction, no heel strike, and strike occurs with the forefoot.

Parkinson's Gait

This gait pattern is typical in a Parkinson's patient but may vary with the individual. The patient will demonstrate a slow shuffling gait, difficulty initiating the first movement, loss of reciprocal upper extremity swing, center of gravity forward, increased walking speed because of rapid small steps, may actually be running during gait, and difficulty stopping.

KEY MUSCLES INVOLVED IN GAIT

MUSCLE	ACTION
Erector spinae	Extends and flexes the vertebral column and head Draws the ribs downward
Adductor	Acts to draw a body part toward the axis or midline of the body
Abductor	Draws a body part away from the midline
Gluteus maximus	Acts to extend the thigh
Hip flexors	Hip flexors act to initiate swing, iliopsoas, rectus femoris, gracilis, sartorius, and tensor fasciae latae
Hip extensors	Hip extensors are active during stance to stabilize the lower extremity and control forward trunk movement
Knee flexors	Foot clearance during midswing and assist in shock absorption
Knee extensors	May contribute to forward propulsion and assist in stabilizing the lower extremity during stance
Hamstrings	Most active during the late swing phase; key muscle in deceleration of the lower extremity
Quadriceps	Most active during early stance phase and just before toe-off Quadriceps are involved in forward propulsion of the lower extremity
Anterior tibialis	Most active immediately after heel strike to assist in eccentric lowering of the foot (plantar flexion)
Plantar flexors	Most active to assist initial push-off after heel strike
Gastrocnemius/soleus	Most active in late stance phase in a concentric rising of the heel during toe-off

GAIT PHASES

Stance Phase

Initial Contact

When the heel or another part of the foot touches the ground. It may also be called heel strike. It is the beginning of the stance phase.

Loading Response

The double stance phase when both lower extremities are in contact with the ground. This is also called the footflat phase. It occurs immediately after heel strike and lasts until one lower extremity is lifted for swing.

Midstance

Begins the single limb support; one lower extremity has the total responsibility for supporting the body. It begins when the contralateral lower extremity leaves the ground.

Terminal Stance

This phase is from midstance to just before the contralateral lower extremity contacts the ground. During this phase, body weight moves forward. It is the second half of single limb support and may also be called heel-off.

Preswing

The point after heel-off when only the reference toe is in contact with the ground. It is the second half of the double stance phase. It may also be called toe-off phase.

Swing Phase

Initial Swing

The first phase of the swing phase. It is the point in which the reference toe leaves the ground to when the swing lower extremity is aligned with the stance lower extremity. It may also be considered the point of maximum knee flexion of the swinging lower extremity. The lower extremity is directly below the body. It is also called the acceleration phase.

Midswing

The point from the swing lower extremity being directly below the body to the lower extremity moves forward to a vertical tibial position.

Terminal Swing

From the vertical tibia position and ends when the foot strikes the floor.

GAIT ASSISTIVE DEVICES

Crutches

A wooden or metal staff used to improve stability or relieve weightbearing on the lower extremities. When ascending stairs with crutches, the patient will place the uninvolved lower extremity first and the involved will follow with the crutches. When descending stairs, the involved lower extremity and crutches will go first with the uninvolved following.

Axillary crutches: the crutches are adjustable. They should always be equipped with rubber tips that provide suction, minimizing the possibility of slipping. Axillary pads provide cushion between the top of the crutch and the axilla of the patient and also help keep the crutch tops from slipping. Disadvantages are that they may be difficult to use in small areas and prolonged leaning on the axillary bar can result in vascular or nerve damage.

Measurement: measurement should be performed with the patient standing. The crutch tips should be resting on the floor, about 6 to 8 inches lateral to and forward of each foot. Have the axillary pad in place for measurement. When measuring the patient in the standing position, subtract 16 inches from the patient's height or measure from a point 2 inches below the axilla to a point 6 inches in front and 2 inches lateral to the foot. Measure from the axilla to a point 6 to 8 inches lateral to the heel. The height of the hand grips is determined by measuring from the floor to the hand with the elbow flexed 20° to 30° and with the shoulders relaxed. Verbal instructions should emphasize that the patient should not lean on the crutches in the axillary region.

Forearm (Canadian or Lofstrand) crutches: the crutches resemble a cane except for the presence of cuffs that encircle the forearm and have a hand grip. Forearm crutches are adjustable and constructed of metal. The patient needs good upper limb strength and balance to utilize the crutches. Advantages are that the person can free up the hands without having to set the crutches down. They are less cumbersome and easier to use, especially on stairs. Disadvantages are that they provide less stability than axillary crutches, and some patients find it difficult to remove the hand and forearm from the cuff.

Measurement: measurement of the forearm crutches utilizes the same procedure as measuring the handgrips for axillary crutches. The cuffs are adjustable and should adjust on the forearm without restricting elbow flexion. The cuff height is approximately 4 to 5 inches below the epicondyles of the humerus.

Crutch Gaits

1. **Two-point:** requires more balance from the patient for gait. Opposite crutch and leg are advanced simultaneously.
2. **Three-point, nonweightbearing:** crutches are advanced, then the uninvolved leg, then the crutches.
3. **Four-point:** a slow, stable gait in which one crutch is advanced, followed by the opposite leg (eg, left crutch, right leg, right crutch, left leg).
4. **Partial weightbearing:** toes or ball of involved leg contacts the floor such that the crutches and involved limb are advanced simultaneously and the uninvolved limb is advanced next.
5. **Swing-to and swing-through:** usually used when both lower extremities are involved, such as paraplegia or spina bifida.

Guarding

Level Surfaces

The therapist stands posterior and lateral to the weaker side of the patient.

Stairs

- Ascending: the therapist stands behind and slightly to the side of the affected limb of the patient.
- Descending: the therapist stands in front of and slightly to the side of the patient's affected lower extremity.

Cane

A wooden or metal shaft used to widen the base of support, and improve balance and mobility to an ambulatory but partially disabled patient.

Measuring: the tip of the cane is placed alongside the toes; cane height is measured from the floor to the hand with 20° to 30° of elbow flexion and the shoulder in a relaxed position. Another method of adjusting cane height is by placing the top of the cane at the level of the greater trochanter of the femur.

Standard cane: a small base of support with the point of support in front of the hand. Appropriate only for patients who have good balance and are not required to put a great deal of pressure on the cane.

Quad cane: a wide base of support through four legs projecting from the base of the cane. Disadvantages are that because of the increased size, a quad cane may have to be turned sideways to fit on stairs. Also, a quad cane is awkward to carry when using a handrail. Patients who need more balance and support from the cane use a quad cane instead of a single-point cane.

Gait pattern: cane and involved extremity are advanced simultaneously, followed by the uninvolved extremity. When ascending stairs, the uninvolved lower extremity leads up and the involved lower extremity follows along with the cane. In descending the stairs, the involved lower extremity leads down and the noninvolved follows with the cane.

Walker

The walker has four widely placed, sturdy legs, thereby widening the base of support. It provides lateral and anterior stability and can relieve weightbearing. Walkers may fold and have casters, reciprocal walking mechanisms, or other attachments. A disadvantage is that stair climbing tends to be unsafe, and a walker is awkward to carry while using a handrail.

Measuring: there should be 20° to 30° of elbow flexion; measure from the greater trochanter to a point 6 inches beside the toes. The walker is placed anteriorly or in front of the patient for measuring.

Folding walker: this is a collapsible walker that is easier for traveling and mobility.

Hemiwalker: the handgrip is located in the center for use with patients who utilize one hand for control. This walker is generally used for stroke patients.

Reciprocal walker: patients who utilize a reciprocal gait; this walker is hinged, allowing one side to be advanced at a time.

Rolling walker: this is a walker with wheels that allow for continuous movement. The walker can have either two or four wheels and a hand brake. This is used for patients who benefit from continuous movement (eg, Parkinson's patients who have difficulty initiating movement).

Gait

- **Full weightbearing:** walker first, then one leg, then the other leg is advanced.
- **Partial weightbearing:** walker first, then the involved lower extremity, then the uninvolved extremity is advanced.
- **Nonweightbearing:** walker first, weight shift to arms, then uninvolved extremity is advance.

Amount of Assistance Necessary during Gait by Therapist

Examples:

- Independent: no supervision or assistance required.
- Supervision: no physical contact but visual assistance or verbal cueing.
- Contact guard: hands on the patient for support, and guidance (requires approximately 10% assistance).
- Minimal: hands on the patient for slight assistance (requires approximately 25% assistance).
- Moderate: hands on the patient for active involvement during ambulation (requires approximately 50% assistance).
- Maximal: maximum involvement from the therapist for ambulation (approximately 75% to 90% of activity).

OBSERVATION OF NORMAL RESPONSE CHART

OBSERVATION	NORMAL RESPONSE
Width of base	2 to 4 inches
Center of gravity	2-inch vertical oscillation
Lateral shift of pelvis/trunk	1 inch
Length of step	15 inches
Cadence	90 to 120 steps per minute
Pelvic rotation	4° forward rotation
Arm swing	Opposition with opposite lower extremity
Knee flexion	Comfortable, clear foot
Ankle/foot	Comfortable, clear foot

These are the normally acceptable standards, but they may vary with the individual depending on body type.

CHAPTER 23

Prosthetics & Orthotics

LEVELS OF AMPUTATION

Lower Extremity

- **Hemicorporectomy:** surgical removal of the pelvis and both lower extremities.
- **Hemipelvectomy:** surgical removal of one half (side) of the pelvis and leg.
- **Hip disarticulation:** surgical removal of the femur from the pelvis.
- **Above-knee (AK):** amputation of the leg above the knee joint.
- **Knee disarticulation:** amputation of the knee joint from the femur. The patella is not removed during surgery.
- **Below-knee (BK):** amputation below the knee joint; the knee joint remains intact.
- **Syme's:** amputation of the foot at the ankle joint, including the malleoli; result is a bulbous end on leg.
- **Chopart:** disarticulation at the midtarsal joint.
- **Metatarsal:** amputation through the metatarsal heads.

Upper Extremity

- **Transhumeral:** amputation above the elbow (AE).
- **Transradial:** amputation below the elbow (BE).
- **Elbow disarticulation:** amputation through the elbow joint.
- **Shoulder disarticulation:** amputation through the shoulder joint.

MEDICAL COMPLICATIONS AS A RESULT OF AMPUTATION

Phantom Limb Sensation

The feeling as though the limb is still there. It is a feeling of pressure coming from the amputated limb.

Phantom Pain

This is a burning and/or cramping pain in the amputated extremity. Some patients will report severe pain persisting in the amputated extremity.

Wound Healing

It is necessary for the patient to have good circulation so that the wound will heal and close prior to the patient receiving a prosthesis.

LOWER LIMB DEFORMITIES

- **Anteversion:** femoral neck rotated forward.
- **Calcaneus:** the heel-down position; plantar flexion limitation of the ankle.
- **Coxa valga:** femoral neck shaft angled outward.
- **Coxa vara:** femoral neck shaft angled inward.
- **Equinus:** the toe-down position; dorsiflexion limitation of the ankle.
- **Genu valgum:** tibia is angled laterally, causing the knees to come together or almost touch. Known as "knock knees."
- **Genu varum:** tibia is angled medially, causing the knees to be apart or "bow legged."
- **Hallux valgus:** first metatarsal has an abduction deformity, or "bunion."
- **Internal tibial torsion:** distal aspect of tibia is rotated or twisted medially as compared with its proximal end.
- **Pes cavus:** high-arched or supinated foot.
- **Pes planus:** low-arched foot—"pronated or flat foot."
- **Retroversion:** femoral neck rotated posteriorly or backward.
- **Talipes equinovarus:** ankle and foot are down and in, or "club foot."
- **Valgus heel:** the rearfoot is deviated toward the outside, resulting in a pronated heel. A medial heel wedge (Thomas heel), which elevates the inner border, may help correct this situation.

COMMON GAIT DEVIATIONS WITH PROSTHETIC CAUSES

GAIT DEVIATION	POSSIBLE PROSTHETIC CAUSES
Abducted gait	Prosthesis too long
	High medial wall
	Improperly shaped lateral wall
	Prosthesis aligned in abduction
	Incorrect suspension
Lateral trunk bending	Prosthesis too short
	High medial wall
	Improperly shaped lateral wall
	Prosthesis aligned in abduction
Circumduction	Prosthesis too long
	Socket too small
	Inadequate suspension
	Knee joint stiff
	Tight hip abductors
	Weak hip flexors
Medial whip	Knee bolt alignment too lateral
	Socket too tight
Lateral whip	Knee bolt alignment too medial
Uneven heel raise	Insufficient friction
	Insufficient extension aid
Rotation of foot at heel strike	Too much toe out
	Too much resistance on plantar flexion bumper
	Too much resistance on heel cushion
Foot slap	Not enough resistance on plantar flexion bumper
Terminal swing	Knee extension aid too strong
	Knee friction too soft
Uneven length of steps	Improper socket fit
	Extension aid too weak
	Friction of knee too weak
Vaulting	Prosthesis too long
	Inadequate socket suspension
	Socket too small
	Excessive plantar flexion
	Short residual limb

COMMON GAIT DEVIATIONS WITH PROSTHETIC CAUSES, CONTINUED

GAIT DEVIATION	POSSIBLE PROSTHETIC CAUSES
Lumbar lordosis	Improper shape posterior wall
	Lack of anterior socket support
	Insufficient flexion of socket
Instability of knee	Knee joint too anterior
	Plantar flexion resistance too high
	No limit on dorsiflexion
Pistoning of socket	Poor socket fit
	Weak suspension system
	Knee friction too soft

COMMON GAIT DEVIATIONS WITH ANATOMICAL CAUSES

GAIT DEVIATION	POSSIBLE ANATOMICAL CAUSES
Anterior trunk bending	Hip and knee flexion contractures
	Weak quadriceps muscle
Circumduction	Abduction contracture
	Weak hip flexor muscles
	Weak dorsiflexors
Excessive medial foot contact	Genu valgum
	Pes valgus
	Spasticity, weak invertors
Extensive lateral foot contact	Weak evertors
Hip hiking	Hip extensor spasticity
	Weak quadriceps
Hyperextended knee	Extensor spasticity
	Weak quadriceps
	Loose knee ligaments
Knee instability	Knee flexion contracture
	Weak dorsiflexor muscles
Inadequate dorsiflexion control	Extensor spasticity
	Weak dorsiflexor muscles
Lateral trunk bending	Abduction contracture
	Dislocated hip
	Hip pain
	Weak abductor muscles
Lordosis	Hip flexion contractures
	Weak hip extensor muscles
Posterior trunk bending	Weak hip extensor muscles
Vaulting	Abduction contracture
	Weak hip flexors
Walking wide base of support	Abduction contracture
	Instability or weak abductors
Foot slap	Weak dorsiflexion
Toes first	Weak dorsiflexors
	Spasticity
	Shortened leg

LOWER LIMB PROSTHETICS

Ankle

- **Ankle foot orthosis—AFO:** commonly utilized for drop foot seen in cerebrovascular accidents; prevents plantar flexion during the swing phase of gait. Typically made of L-shaped plastic and consists of a shoe attachment for ankle control. Can have single or double uprights that extend upward from the ankle and attach by a proximal leg band. May limit or lock ankle movement; provides free moving dorsi- or plantar flexion while providing medial/lateral support or assisting dorsi- or plantar flexion with built-in devices. Conventional AFOs with metal uprights are easier to alter as the condition of the patient changes. Molded plastic AFOs are lightweight and cosmetically more appealing. However, they are more difficult to alter as the patient's condition changes or if the patient has reduced sensation. Examples of molded AFOs:
  Solid ankle: no movement, used with severe pain or instability.
  Posterior leaf spring: has a built in dorsiflexion assist. This is not useful in severe spasticity.
  Spiral AFO: primarily for medial/lateral support.
- **Bichannel adjustable ankle lock:** an ankle joint with anterior and posterior channels that can be fitted with springs to assist motion or pins to reduce motion.
- **Dorsi-plantar flexion assist:** assists in plantar flexion of the ankle during the push-off phase of gait.
- **Dorsiflexion stop:** restricts dorsiflexion and allows free range of motion in plantar flexion.
- **Free motion ankle joint:** no restriction on ankle movement.
- **Limited motion stop:** restricts movement for both dorsiflexion and plantar flexion.
- **Plantar flexion stop:** restricts plantar flexion and allows free range of motion in dorsiflexion.
- **Solid ankle:** holds the foot in one position, preventing dorsi- or plantar flexion and varus valgus stress.
- **T straps:** control for varus or valgus at the ankle. Medial strap corrects for valgus and a lateral strap for varus.
- **Upright:** provides some support against inversion/eversion of the ankle. May be single-bar or double-bar upright, also plastic or metal.

Foot

- **Denis-Browne splint:** a bar that connects two shoes and can swivel. Usually used for correction of "club foot" or pes equinovarus.
- **Metatarsal bars:** takes the pressure off the metatarsal heads by building up the sole proximal to the metatarsal heads.
- **Rocker bottom:** builds up the sole over the metatarsal heads and allows more push-off in weak or inflexible feet.
- **Scaphoid pads:** usually support the longitudinal arch and correct for pes planus.
- **Stirrups:** a metal shoe attachment in a brace. Split stirrups allow for shoe replacement, solid stirrups do not.
- **Thomas heel:** a heel with an extended anterior medial border used to support the longitudinal arch and correct for flexible pes valgus.

Knee

- **Adjustable knee lock:** ability to lock the knee joint in flexion, typically at 6° intervals; prevents hyperextension.
- **Drop ring lock:** ability to fully lock the knee joint or allow free motion, depending on the patient's need.
- **Free motion knee joint:** allows unresistive movement in flexion and extension.
- **KAFO (knee-ankle-foot orthosis):** stabilizes the knee and ankle. Many variations of plastic, metal, or supracondylar knee. Consists of a shoe attachment, ankle control, uprights, knee joint, and bands or shells for the thigh and calf. There are a variety of knee joints and locks.
- **KO (knee orthosis):** controls knee motion or provides stability. Some examples are Lenox Hill, Pro-Am, and Don Joy.
- **Lenox Hill brace:** custom fit through a cast impression of the leg; provides stability rotationally, as well as medially/laterally.
- **Oregon orthotic system:** allows for control in sagittal, frontal, and transverse planes of motion. Constructed from a combination of plastic and metal components.
- **Scott-Craig orthosis:** stabilizes the ankle/knee; metal KAFO, typically utilized by spinal cord patients.
- **Swedish knee cage:** prevents hyperextension through one posterior and two anterior straps.

Hip

- **Single axis joint:** allows movement in hip flexion/extension. Typically prevents abduction/adduction and rotation components.
- **Double axis joint:** allows movement and patient control of abduction/adduction, as well as flexion/extension. Patient may have free motion if controlled.
- **Frejka pillow:** keeps hips abducted. Used for congenitally dislocated hips or other conditions with tight adductors.
- **Pelvic band/belts:** assists in holding brace in place. Many variations:
  - Pelvic girdles
  - Unilateral bilateral bands
- **Toronto orthosis** (Scottish rite orthosis—trilateral orthosis): braces utilized for Legg-Calvé-Perthes disease.
- **Van Rosen splint** (Ilfeld splint): utilized in infants for congenital hip dislocation.

SPINE BRACES

- **Cervical collar:** may be soft or rigid. Prevents cervical range of motion. Soft collars provide the minimum amount of control.
- **Boston brace:** molded brace for scoliosis or other back problems below T7 to T9. Worn under clothing and has a more cosmetic appearance.
- **Four-poster orthosis:** provides moderate level of control in individuals with cervical fracture/spinal cord injury. Consists of occipital and thoracic plates with two anterior and two posterior posts to stabilize and prevent movement.
- **Halo orthosis:** provides maximum control for individuals with cervical fracture/spinal cord injury and for postoperative positioning and immobilization after cervical surgery. Four uprights connect from the halo to a thoracic band and is attached to the skull by screws.
- **Jewett brace:** three-point brace that prevents hyperextension. Three points of pressure: sternum, lumbar spine, and symphysis pubis. Used for compression fractures of the spine.
- **Knight spinal brace:** rigid brace utilized for lumbar spine disease.
- **Knight-Taylor spinal brace:** rigid, high-back brace; utilized for fractures above the L3 region.
- **Lumbar corset:** variety of corsets made from canvas or cloth, with or without metal stays. Comes in a variety of sizes.
- **Milwaukee brace:** a cervical, thoracic, lumbosacral orthosis used to help immobilize the torso and neck of a patient for the treatment of scoliosis, lordosis, or kyphosis. Has a molded pelvic section, two posteriors, and one anterior upright.
- **Minerva orthosis:** provides the maximum amount of control of cervical motions. Constructed of a rigid plastic.
- **Parapodium:** an orthotic frame allowing maximal stabilization for activities done in a standing position.
- **Taylor brace:** semirigid brace utilized in thoracic and lumbar spine disease. Can be modified for length and degree of control.
- **Upper extremity orthotics (splints):** numerous varieties constructed of aluminum or thermoplastic materials. May be used for stability, to prevent or correct deformity, enhance motion, decrease pain, or for protection.

UPPER EXTREMITY PROSTHETICS

The majority of upper extremity amputations are the result of trauma. Compression wrapping of the residual limb is required. The amputee may experience phantom limb syndrome, and in some instances severe pain persists.

- **Terminal device:** the component of the prosthesis used to produce holding or prehension. The majority consist of a hook or hand terminal device connected to the amputee by a socket, perhaps with an elbow intervening, and usually with a harness. The overall goal is to provide the lightest and most comfortable prosthesis with the strongest clamping force the amputee can control.
- **Voluntary opening device:** one that is closed at rest and opens with voluntary movement of the amputee. A voluntary opening hand uses a spring and a voluntary opening hook uses one or more rubber bands to provide prehension force. The amputee must overcome the elastic tension to open the device.

- **Voluntary closing device:** one that is open at rest and closed with amputee movement. This is not commonly utilized.
- **Myoelectric device:** activated by the same motions as conventional power systems. This is an externally powered system that utilizes a battery-powered motor to operate the terminal device.

Elbow

- **Below-elbow control system:** to open the voluntary opening terminal device, the amputee moves the glenohumeral joint on the amputated side into flexion. To open the device close to the body, biscapular abduction is used. Closing the device is done by returning to a neutral position.
- **Above-elbow control system:** usually a dual control system of two cables that provides three functions: one cable helps to lock and unlock the elbow by using shoulder depression, abduction, and extension on the amputated side. If the elbow is locked, the other cable will open the terminal device—voluntary opening. If the elbow is unlocked, the cable will flex and extend the elbow joint by using glenohumeral flexion on the amputated side or biscapular abduction. Forearm rotation is done by prepositioning the hand, which stays in place by a friction unit at the wrist.
- **Elbow splints:** immobilizes and protects the elbow. Typically the physician prescribes the degree of angle for optimal healing. Seen with epicondylectomy, ulnar neuropathy, or radial/ulnar dislocation.

Wrist

- **Ulnar/radial gutter:** controls radial/ulnar deviation of the wrist.
- **Dynamic wrist splint:** increases range of motion by providing active assistance with movement.
- **Static wrist splint:** immobilizes the wrist for protection.

Shoulder

- Shoulder splint: the doctor prescribes the position of the patient. Immobilizes the shoulder to promote healing. Utilized with the following:
  - Brachial plexus injuries
  - Muscle tears
  - Rotator cuff
  - Acromioclavicular fracture

Hand

- **Resting hand splint:** static splint for wrist and hand. Typically utilized with arthritic patient; supports hand in functional position.
- **Wrist cock-up splint:** immobilizes the wrist but allows full range of motion in MCP flexion and thumb opposition. Utilized for inflammation and pain.

PROSTHETIC CHECKLIST (LOWER EXTREMITY BELOW KNEE)

- Can patient don and doff prosthesis easily and independently?
- Is patient satisfied with prosthesis?
- Is skin unblemished after wearing prosthesis for 10 minutes?
- Can patient stand comfortable with lower extremity prosthesis?
- Stand with pelvis level?
- Stand with both knees extended?
- Sit comfortably with knee flexed to 90°?
- Kneel comfortably?
- Can ambulate comfortably and quietly?
- Ambulates with adequate suspension?
- Has minimal deviation when ambulating?
- Prosthesis appearance is satisfactory to patient?

PROSTHETIC CHECKLIST (LOWER EXTREMITY ABOVE KNEE)

- Can patient don and doff prosthesis easily and independently?
- Is patient satisfied with prosthesis?
- Is skin unblemished after wearing prosthetic for 10 minutes?
- Stand comfortably?
- Stand with pelvis level?
- Stand with both knees extended and comfortable?
- Sit with knees flexed to 90° and can lean forward to touch shoes comfortably?
- Can ambulate comfortably and quietly?
- Ambulates with adequate suspension?
- Minimal deviation when ambulating?
- Prosthetic appearance is satisfactory to patient?

TREATMENT PROGRAM

- Postoperative dressings
  - Stump wrapping/Ace wraps
  - Stump shrinkers
  - Semirigid dressings
  - Rigid dressings
- Teach patient self skin inspections and warning signs for skin breakdown.
- Contracture prevention
  - Positioning of limb to prevent contractures
  - Teach patient proper positioning and self-stretching exercises
- Desensitizing of the stump
- Strengthening exercises
- Range of motion exercises
- Balance exercises
- Proprioception exercises
- Transfers training
- Gait training
- Wheelchair training
- Activities of daily living training
- Family or support system training
- Referral to support system
- Home exercise program
- Prosthetic training
  - Check out of prosthesis and inspection on delivery
  - Patient's satisfaction with prosthesis and psychological adjustment
  - Teach patient to don and doff prosthesis
  - Teach patient skin inspection prior to and post prosthetic wearing
  - Teach patient transfers with prosthetic on and off
  - Teach patient maintenance of prostheses

CHAPTER 24

Goniometry

NORMAL VALUES FOR THE UPPER EXTREMITY RANGE OF MOTION (ROM)

Shoulder Joint

Flexion 180°, extension 45°
- Axis: center of shoulder joint on lateral side
- Position: supine
- Stationary arm: midline of the trunk (axillary line)
- Movable arm: midline of the shaft of humerus (lateral side)

Abduction 180°, adduction 30°
- Axis: center of shoulder joint on posterior side
- Position: sitting
- Stationary arm: parallel to the longitudinal axis
- Movable arm: midline of the shaft of the humerus

Internal rotation 70°, external rotation 90°
- Axis: olecranon process
- Position: supine
- Stationary arm: perpendicular or parallel to the trunk
- Movable arm: midline between the shaft of the ulnar and styloid process

Horizontal abduction 45°, adduction 135°
- Axis: superior on the acromion process
- Position: sitting
- Stationary arm: horizontal or perpendicular to the trunk
- Movable arm: midline of the shaft of the humerus

Elbow Joint

Flexion 150°, extension 0°
- Axis: lateral epicondyle of the humerus
- Position: supine
- Stationary arm: lateral midline of the humerus
- Movable arm: lateral midline of the ulna

Forearm

Pronation 80°, supination 80°
- Axis: styloid process of the ulna
- Position: sitting
- Stationary arm: anterior and parallel to midline of the humerus
- Movable arm: supination, palmar surface of wrist pronation, dorsal surface of the wrist

Wrist Joint

Flexion 80°, extension 70°
- Axis: lateral side over the styloid process
- Position: sitting
- Stationary arm: parallel to shaft of the ulna
- Movable arm: midline shaft of fifth metacarpal

Radial deviation 20°, ulnar deviation 35°
- Axis: base of the third metacarpal
- Position: sitting
- Stationary arm: midline forearm
- Movable arm: midline along the third metacarpal

LOWER EXTREMITY RANGE OF MOTION

Hip Joint

Flexion 120°, extension 10° to 15°
- Axis: greater trochanter of the femur
- Position: supine
- Stationary arm: parallel to lateral midline of the trunk
- Movable arm: parallel to the shaft of the femur

Abduction 45°, adduction 10°
- Axis: anterior on the anterior superior iliac spine
- Position: supine
- Stationary arm: horizontal across both anterior superior iliac spines
- Movable arm: parallel to shaft of the femur

Internal rotation 35°, external rotation 45°
- Axis: anterior over the center of the patella
- Position: supine
- Stationary arm: perpendicular to the floor
- Movable arm: midline of the tibia

Knee Joint

Flexion 135°, extension 0° to 15°
- Axis: lateral over the midline
- Position: prone
- Stationary arm: aligned with the shaft of the femur
- Movable arm: aligned with the shaft of the fibula

Ankle Joint

Dorsiflexion 20°, plantar flexion 45°
- Axis: just inferior to lateral malleolus
- Position: sitting
- Stationary arm: midline shaft of the fibula
- Movable arm: midline shaft of the fifth metatarsal

Eversion 20°, inversion 35°
- Axis: inversion, lateral side of the head of the fifth metatarsal; eversion, medial side of the head of first metatarsal
- Position: sitting
- Stationary arm: parallel to midline of the tibia
- Movable arm: plantar surface of the metatarsal arch

SPINE RANGE OF MOTION

Cervical Spine

- Flexion/extension 80° to 90°/70°
- Lateral flexion/rotation 20° to 45°/70° to 90°

Thoracic Spine

- Flexion/extension 20° to 45°/25° to 45°
- Lateral flexion/rotation 20° to 40°/35° to 50°

Lumbar Spine

- Flexion/extension 40° to 60°/20° to 35°
- Lateral flexion/rotation 15° to 20°/3° to 18°

CHAPTER 25

Manual Muscle Testing

GRADE LEVELS

- **Zero:** no palpable contraction; no muscle activity detected
- **Trace:** no movement, but palpable twitching contraction felt or observed
- **Poor:** can produce full range of motion in gravity-eliminated position only
- **Fair:** can produce full range of motion against gravity
- **Good:** can produce full range of movement against gravity with strong resistance provided by therapist at the end of range
- **Normal:** can produce full range of movement against gravity with maximal resistance by therapist at the end range

Functional Grades

- **Upper extremity:** requires a fair grade for a muscle to be functional
- **Lower extremity:** requires a fair plus grade for a muscle to be functional

GENERAL CONSIDERATIONS

- Test bilaterally, starting with the noninjured side, secondary to pain, and compare
- Make certain to isolate the muscle you are testing, lining up origin and insertion in same plane
- Palpate the testing muscle to feel for contraction
- Stabilize the proximal part; you must know the proper hand position to isolate the muscle you are testing
- To receive maximum cooperation from the patient, inform him or her of what you will be doing

GRADING SYSTEM ACCORDING TO KENDALL, MCCREARY, AND PROVANCE

0 Zero: no contraction is felt in the muscle

T Trace: no visible movement, but the tendon is visible or slightly contracted

1 Poor -: movement through partial range of motion in the horizontal plane

2 Poor: movement through complete range of motion in the horizontal plane

3 Poor +: movement through complete range of motion in the horizontal plane against resistance or holding in position in response to pressure by the therapist

4 Fair -: in an antigravity position the patient gradually releases from the test position

5 Fair: in an antigravity position the patient can hold the test position with no pressure applied by the therapist

6 Fair +: in an antigravity position the patient can hold the test position with slight pressure applied by the therapist

7 Good -: in an antigravity position the patient can hold the test position with slight or moderate pressure applied by the therapist

8 Good: in an antigravity position the patient can hold the test position with moderate pressure applied by the therapist

9 Good +: in an antigravity position the patient can hold the test position with moderate to strong pressure by the therapist

10 Normal: in an antigravity position the patient can hold the test position against strong pressure applied by the therapist

CHAPTER 26

Posture

Evaluate the patient from the lateral and back views first, then front view if necessary. The front view will allow the patient to realign his or her body to the therapist, presenting a less accurate picture of true posture. The therapist may utilize a plumb line from the ceiling and have the patient stand sideways to utilize the line as a guide for joint alignment.

NORMAL ALIGNMENT: SIDE VIEW

Head

Normal: neutral position
Abnormal: forward head tilt or hyperextension

Scapulae

Normal: flat against the upper back
Abnormal: scapula winging

Shoulder

Normal: neutral position, plumb line falling through shoulder joint
Abnormal: forward or backward shoulders, rounder shoulders

Thoracic Spine

Normal: slightly convex posterior curve
Abnormal: kyphosis, increased flexion, or round back

Lumbar Spine

Normal: slight convex anteriorly
Abnormal: increased lordosis or flattened lordotic curve

Hip Joint

Normal: neutral position, plumb line falling in the center of the joint
Abnormal: flexion or extension

Knee Joint

Normal: neutral position, plumb line slightly anterior to the joint but posterior to patella
Abnormal: hyperextension of the knee or knee joint flexion

Ankle Joint

Normal: neutral position, plumb line slightly anterior to lateral malleolus
Abnormal: plantar or dorsiflexion

NORMAL ALIGNMENT: POSTERIOR/BACK VIEW

Head

Normal: neutral position
Abnormal: rotated or tilted position

Scapulae

Normal: neutral position, level alignment in comparison to each other
Abnormal: elevation or depression of one or both scapulae

Thoracic Spine

Normal: plumb line falls straight through spine
Abnormal: curves in either direction, left or right

Lumbar Spine

Normal: plumb line falls straight through spine
Abnormal: curves in either direction, left or right

Hip Joint

Normal: neutral position, level with each other
Abnormal: rotation or abduction/adduction

Knee Joint

Normal: neutral, straight alignment, proper spaces between knees
Abnormal: knock-knee or bowlegs

Ankle Joint

Normal: slight out-toeing of feet
Abnormal: pronation, supination, or toeing inward

CHAPTER 27

Coordination

EQUILIBRIUM COORDINATION

Static Balance

- Observation of the patient's posture during nonmovement activities (eg, in standing, supine, or sitting)
- Abnormal response is swaying or attempting to overcorrect posture, tremors, or lurching; any excessive movements beyond normal limits

Dynamic Balance

- Observation of the patient's posture while the body is in motion (eg, walking, climbing stairs, walking a straight line, bending, or rolling)
- Abnormal response is excessive swaying, staggering, or postural deviations

NONEQUILIBRIUM COORDINATION

Alternate or Reciprocal Motion

- This tests the patient's ability to reverse movement from agonist to antagonist and back again
- Examples of tests include:
  - Finger to nose
  - Finger to finger
  - Heel to knee to toe
  - Finger opposition
  - Tapping (foot)
- Evaluate the quality of movement, speed, control, and reaction time

Movement Composition or Synergy

- This tests the patient's ability to control movement with several muscle groups acting together
- Examples of tests include:
  - Finger to nose
  - Finger to finger
  - Heel to knee to toe
  - Pointing
  - Walking
- Evaluate quality of movement, control, speed, and reaction time

Movement Accuracy

- This tests the patient's ability to judge distance and speed of voluntary movement
- Examples of tests include:
  - Finger to nose
  - Pointing
  - Heel to knee to toe
  - Drawing a circle
  - Making a figure-eight with foot
- Evaluate quality of movement, control, speed, and reaction time

Fixation or Postural Holding

- This tests the patient's ability to hold a position stationary with parts of the body
- Examples of tests include:
  - Shoulder abduction
  - Shoulder horizontal adduction
  - Lower extremity straight leg raise
- Evaluate to note any tremors or ataxia while holding stationary

FINE MOTOR COORDINATION

- Assess coordination of small muscle groups used for movement
- An example would be instructing the patient to perform thumb to finger opposition

GROSS MOTOR COORDINATION

- Assess coordination of large muscle groups utilized for movement
- An example would be instructing the patient to perform clapping to assess the upper extremity coordination; lower extremity testing has the patient perform alternating knee flexion and extension

GRADING SYSTEM FOR COORDINATION

Rating Scale

0 = patient is unable to perform requested test
1 = patient performs test but with difficulty or errors
2 = patient performs test without difficulty and is error-free

GENERAL PRINCIPLES OF TESTING

The following can be done to determine if it changes the patient's accuracy, quality of movement, endurance, reaction time, and if the movement is steady or tremors are present.
- Test the patient with both the eyes open and the eyes close; start with the eyes open, then test with eyes closed
- Change the speed at which the patient performs the test to determine if accuracy is affected by speed
- Change directions of testing (eg, start on right side, then test left side)
- Have a moving target for the patient
- Perform the test in supine, sitting, and standing
- Time the length it takes the patient to complete the test
- Continue repeating test to determine if there is consistency over time
- Change distance to determine if patient can judge and adapt to changes in distance

COORDINATION TEST

- **Heel on shin:** the patient will slide the heel of one foot up and down the shin of the opposite extremity.
- **Position hold or fixation:** the patient will be asked to hold the extremity in one position (eg, extending the knee and holding it in extension).

- **Finger to finger:** the physical therapist will place his or her index finger out for the patient to touch with the patient also utilizing his or her index finger. The patient will be instructed to touch the tip of the index finger to the therapist's. The therapist will move the position of his or her finger to test patient accuracy, direction of movement and speed.
- **Mass grasp:** the therapist will instruct the patient to open and close the hand; the patient will go from finger flexion to extension. The therapist can instruct the patient to change speeds from slow, normal, to fast to evaluate the patient.
- **Tapping:** the therapist can evaluate the upper or lower extremity. The therapist will instruct the patient to tap the ball of the foot on the floor while maintaining heel contact. In the upper extremity test, the therapist will instruct the patient to tap the hand on the knee while keeping the elbow flexed and the forearm pronated.
- **Pronation and supination:** the patient is instructed to turn the palms up and down, alternating positions while keeping the elbow in 90° of flexion and close to the trunk.
- **Rebound test:** this test can be applied to several muscles groups in the body. For example, the therapist will instruct the patient to place the elbow in flexion and hold while the therapist provides resistance to elbow extension. This results in an isometric contraction, then the therapist suddenly releases the resistance. The normal response is for the biceps to contract or damper the movement of the upper extremity. This is a rebound effect from the biceps on the triceps muscle.

CHAPTER 28

Sensory Testing

PROTECTIVE SENSATIONS

General Considerations

- For all testing on the patient, follow the application of stimulus (eg, a pinprick and patient's response to stimulus). Try to follow a dermatome pattern to determine if sensation is intact.

Pain Sensation

- Test by utilizing a large pinhead to apply the stimulus, either sharp or dull, randomly. Request the patient to respond appropriately to the stimulus—sharp equals sharp and dull equals dull.
- Normal response is correctly distinguishing between sharp or dull sensations. Abnormal response does not distinguish sharp from dull. Note the number of correct versus incorrect responses, as well as the location.

Temperature

- Test by applying test tubes, one with hot water and one with cold water, to the patient's skin. The patient should reply "hot" or "cold."
- Normal response is correctly distinguishing between hot/cold sensation. Abnormal response does not distinguish hot from cold. Note the number of correct versus incorrect responses, as well as the location.

Light Touch

- Test by lightly rubbing a cotton ball or hairbrush designed for testing against the patient's skin; the patient is requested to respond yes or no if he or she feels light touch, as well as to identify location.
- Correct response is both to feel light touch and to identify correct location.

DISCRIMINATIVE SENSATION

Barognosis

- Test by placing an object in the patient's hand and requesting the patient to respond if it is heavier or lighter than the previous object.
- Normal response is correctly identifying an object as heavier or lighter than the previous object.

Deep Pressure

- Test by applying pressure to the patient's skin surface, palm, or sole of foot.
- Normal response is to feel the deep pressure and identify its location.

Graphesthesia

- Test by writing letters or numbers on the patient's skin with a pencil eraser and asking the patient to identify them. Between the drawings, the area should be wiped clean to avoid confusing the patient.
- Normal response is correctly identifying the written letter or number.

Kinesthesia

- Test by moving the patient's extremity up, down, out, or in. The patient is asked to describe the movement by the therapist.
- Normal response is correctly identifying the movement of the extremity by the therapist.

Proprioception

- Test the patient's ability to determine joint position sense by moving the patient's extremity through a predetermined range of motion. The patient is then asked to repeat the movement on his or her own.
- Normal response is correctly duplicating the therapist's movements of the extremity.

Stereognosis

- Test by placing an object, coin, key, or a block in the patient's hand and asking the patient to identify it on the basis of its size and shape.
- Normal response is correctly identifying each object.

Texture

- Test by placing different texture samples—cotton, wool, silk, or leather—in the patient's hand and asking the patient to identify the texture.
- Normal response is correctly identifying the texture.

Two-Point Discrimination

- Test by placing two points of stimulus on the patient's skin and gradually bringing them together until there is one-point stimulus. The patient is asked to determine if there is one point or two points and when they come together to one point.
- Normal response is correctly distinguishing between one or two points.

CHAPTER 29

Vascular Testing

GIRTH MEASUREMENT

- Test for measurement of edema in the extremity.
- Utilize a tape measure to obtain circumference girth measurements. Be sure to note bony landmarks or distance between measurements. You may use a marker that can be easily washed off to mark the extremity in inch(es) increments to assist with accuracy.
- If possible, compare to the unaffected extremity in order to determine normal and abnormal measurements. If both patient extremities are involved, mark individually and record results for future comparison of each extremity to determine improvement.

HOMAN'S SIGN

- Test for thrombosis or thrombophlebitis.
- Test by dorsiflexion of the patient's foot.
- Positive if test produces pain in the calf upon dorsiflexion.

ISCHEMIA AND RUBOR TEST

- Test for arterial insufficiency.
- Test by elevating the upper or lower extremity above heart level and observing the skin color, then placing the extremity in dependent position and observing the skin color again.
- Abnormal result if nondependent position produces pallor and dependent position produces rubor. Always note the time it takes the extremity to turn pale or red; this assists in determining severity.

REACTIVE HYPEREMIA

- Test for the degree to which vascular beds can dilate following mechanical occlusion.
- Test by applying a blood pressure cuff to the extremity and inflating for up to 5 minutes.
- Normal result if skin flushes as refilling of vascular beds occurs after cuff is released. Abnormal result if flushing is absent or delayed.

VOLUMETRIC MEASUREMENT

- Test for edema. This test is best utilized when trying to measure an irregularly shaped area (eg, the ankle or hand). These areas are difficult to measure through girth measurements because of the different angles.
- Test by lowering the extremity to be evaluated into a container of water. The water will then displace into a collection device for measurement of displaced water.
- If possible, measure water displacement of the unaffected extremity to determine normal/abnormal.

Skin Color and Changes

- Assess skin color to assist in vascular evaluation of the patients. Also note any changes in the skin (eg, is the skin leathery, dry, shiny, loss of hair, or pitting edema present).
  Rubor: redness in color. Typically observed in dependent extremity position for patients with peripheral vascular disease.
  Pallor: pale or absent of rosy color. In peripheral vascular patients, this is observed when there is a decrease in peripheral blood flow.
  Cyanosis: bluish color of the skin.
- Assess skin temperature and note in records.

Pulses

- Check pulses to assist with determining vascular status. Note in the medical record if the pulse is present, diminished, or absent.
- In the upper extremity, check the following pulses: carotid, brachial, and radial.
- In the lower extremity, check the following pulses: dorsal pedis, femoral, popliteal, and posterior tibial pulse.
- The following grading system may be utilized for recording:
  2+ = normal
  1+ = diminished
  0 = absent pulse

CHAPTER 30

Health Care System

LEGAL ASPECTS

Liability in Physical Therapy

- The responsibility is with the physical therapist. The physical therapist is directly liable for the physical therapy aide or physical therapist assistant performing under his or her supervision.
- The therapist needs to feel comfortable with the level of training and expertise of the staff members whom he or she is supervising.
- The therapist also needs to monitor and determine the number of staff members he or she can adequately supervise at any one time. This becomes challenging to find a balance under productivity requirements and decreasing payments for services.
- Liability is a reason for thorough documentation, as this is your record of patient care. Accurate and timely documentation during and after care is important.
- The therapist also needs to feel comfortable with the patient diagnosis and requirements for care or refer to another agency for treatment when it is beyond the therapist's qualifications or experience.
- Many areas of liability can be prevented through proper care and precautions.
- A good line of communication between the therapist and patient can prevent many areas of unmet expectations and misunderstanding.
- Professional liability insurance is available and should be obtained if your employer does not provide a policy. It is also an individual choice to obtain and keep a policy in addition to your employer's policy.
- Review your professional liability policies to determine if any exclusion to coverage is listed and if you have a policy that provides funds for your legal defense.

Areas of Liability

- Broken equipment
- Lack of proper maintenance and annual biomedical check
- Failure to give appropriate instructions
- Failure to communicate with the physician
- Water on the floor in the hydro area or an allergic reaction to the chemicals
- Broken electrical equipment
- Burns to a patient from hot pack treatments or electrical stimulation equipment
- Fall off the treatment table or area
- Injury as a result of exercise session
- Failure to check for appropriate diagnosis and for possible contraindications for modalities

Necessary Components in a Malpractice Case

- **Duty of care:** the therapist owes the patient care. The patient is entitled to professional care.
- **Breach of duty:** the therapist did not perform ordinary standards of care that another professional would have performed in similar circumstances.
- **Injury:** injury results from breach of care. The patient is injured as a result of the therapist not following ordinary care procedures.
- **Causation:** patient injury results. There is documented evidence of patient injury as a result of breech of care.

COMMON TERMS

- **Tort:** a private or civil wrong or injury.
  Example: treating a patient without his or her consent.
- **Negligence:** failure to perform ordinary care as another individual would have done in the same circumstances.
  Example: using a modality for a contraindicated diagnosis.
- **Peer review:** a process in which a physical therapist can review a peer's recommendation for care that has been or may be provided. It is possible for the therapist making that decision to be held liable for denial of care or limitation on care procedures.
- **Contributory negligence:** both parties (plaintiff and defendant) are guilty of negligence.
  Example: a therapist who treats a patient inappropriately is guilty of negligence. The patient is guilty of contributory negligence when he or she fails to follow the instructions given by the therapist.
- **Comparative negligence:** both parties are negligent; however one party is more negligent than the other. This determines that the degree of negligence is greater on the part of either the plaintiff or defendant.
- **Statute of limitations:** time limit in which the plaintiff can claim damages.
- **Deposition:** a meeting between you, your attorney, and the opposing attorney. In this meeting, the opposing attorney will ask questions to obtain verbal responses and information prior to proceeding to court.
- **Interrogatories or interrogation:** a list of questions presented by either the defendant or plaintiff that require a written response prior to court. Your attorney usually writes the questions with occasional questions suggested by you.
- **Informed consent:** permission obtained by a patient or his or her legal guardian to begin treatment. Informed consent is typically for specific treatment procedures and is particularly necessary and utilized prior to invasive techniques.
- **Informed refusal:** when the patient refuses treatment or specific treatment recommendations or procedures. The patient should be asked to sign a treatment refusal form if available at your facility. Documentation in the notes is critical, as well as documentation to the physician.
- **Patient confidentiality:** the patient has the right to nondisclosure of information related to his or her care. The patient must sign the appropriate release to have information released verbally or in writing.
- **Licensure:** the process of providing a license to those who are authorized to practice.
  Example: licensing credentials may require passing a state board examination, practical examinations, and education requirements.

LAWS

- It is important to know the laws as they relate to labor, antidiscrimination, and the Americans with Disabilities Act.
- If you are supervising employees, it is also important to be aware of the laws regarding treatment of personnel/employees.

Age Discrimination Act of 1975

Prohibits discrimination against those between the ages of 40 and 70.

Civil Rights Act of 1964 (amended 1978)

Title VI prevents discrimination of job position or promotion based upon race, color, sex, religion, or national origin.

National Labor Relations Act

Public Law 93-360 allows employees the right to organize for collective bargaining or representation.

Section 504 of the Rehabilitation Act of 1973

No otherwise qualified handicapped individual in the United States shall, solely by reason of handicap, be subject to discrimination.

The Americans with Disabilities Act of 1990 (ADA)

Prohibition against the exclusion of people from jobs, services, activities, or benefits based on disability. The ADA is modeled in large part on the Rehabilitation Act of 1973. One major difference is the use of the term "disability" rather than "handicap."

ACCREDITING AGENCIES

JCAHO (Joint Commission on Accreditation of Healthcare Organizations)

A private, nonprofit organization that sets standards and evaluates agencies to assure compliance with standards. A health care team consisting of nurses, physicians, and hospital administrators will review the agency. The evaluation, reviews, and standards are designed to promote high health care quality. Agencies reviewed are hospitals, outpatient surgery sites, urgent care clinics, long-term care facilities, home care, and hospital agencies.

CARF (Commission on Accreditation of Rehabilitation Facilities)

A nonprofit organization that sets standards and evaluates rehabilitation facilities and work-hardening programs.

REGULATORY AGENCIES

OSHA (Occupational Safety and Health Administration)

A regulatory agency created by the department of labor. OSHA evaluates agencies for standards of safety. For example, in an outpatient physical therapy clinic, it would review policies and procedures for handling and disposing of hazardous substances. It also reviews building codes and safety of equipment utilized at the clinic.

HCFA (Health Care Finance Administration)

A federal regulatory agency contracted to administer with the Medicare program. This is accomplished through Medicare's focal intermediate (eg, Blue Cross, Blue Shield, or Traveler's insurance).

AMERICAN PHYSICAL THERAPY ASSOCIATION (APTA)

- The American Physical Therapy Association is the professional membership association available to physical therapists and physical therapist assistants.
- It is highly recommended that you obtain a copy of the following items to review on the professional standards and recommendations.
- The association has developed standards for our profession in several areas:
  - The Code of Ethics and Guidelines for Professional Conduct
  - Guide for Conduct of the Affiliate Member
  - Standards of Practice for Physical Therapy and the Criteria
  - Guidelines for Physical Therapy Practice
  - Guidelines for Physical Therapy Documentation
  - Guidelines for Peer Review

- These items can be obtained through the APTA by contacting the organization at:
APTA
1111 North Fairfax Street
Alexandria, VA 22314
(703) 684-APTA
(800) 999-2782, ext. 3395
www.apta.org

TYPES OF INSURANCE

Automobile insurance: this will cover patients who are injured in an automobile accident. Depending on state law, the coverage may be no fault. Medical coverage may be limited or unlimited.

Commercial: this includes private insurance companies in which patients may participate. The individual, employer, or both pay a premium for insurance. When a claim is filed, the insurance company pays for all or a portion of necessary medical care with certain limitations. In the case of a disability, it pays a percentage of the individual's salary for a period of time if he or she cannot return to work. Typically, patients have some type of deductible and a 80/20 copay system.

Health maintenance organization (HMO): this type of group health care provides a broad spectrum of health services by an organization consisting of physicians. They provide basic and supplemental health maintenance and treatment services. Enrollees prepay a fixed periodic fee that is set without regard to the amount or kind of services received. Often, the individual's employer has contracted for these services as a benefit to the employee. The employees may also partially contribute a portion of their salary for this benefit. Usually the individual and family members covered under an HMO pay a small fixed fee for each routine visit. There may be a limit to the number of treatments for each problem. The HMO may require preauthorization for treatment and a set number of visits per diagnosis. In addition to diagnostic and treatment services, an HMO may offer supplemental services, such as eye care and prescription drugs. Federal financial support for the establishment of an HMO was provided under Title XIII of the 1973 US Public Health Service Act.

Medicaid: Title XIX of the Social Security Act is a state-administered program with some funding from the federal government, which provides health care benefits to primarily the poor and some classes of elderly and disabled. In some cases, Medicaid eligibility can be applied for only after Medicare eligibility has run out, or Medicaid may pay the 20% deductible that Medicare does not cover. Medicaid benefits vary from state to state. The state determines the scope, duration, and amount of patient visits. Preauthorization is needed prior to treatment.

Medicare: Title XVII of the Social Security Act is a federal program that provides funding for the health care of citizens 65 years of age and older. It can also cover certain long-term disabilities such as renal disease requiring dialysis and silicosis (black lung disease), regardless of age.
- Part A: covers inpatient hospital care, inpatient skilled nursing facilities care, home health, and hospice.
- Part B: covers outpatient therapy services whether provided in a clinic, hospital, skilled nursing facility, or at home. It also covers durable medical equipment such as walkers, wheelchairs, or shower seats.

Professional standards review organization: deals with quality and cost control. Prospective payment is the system that provides fixed levels of reimbursement based on a patient's diagnosis. Diagnostic-related groups are a set of categories in a system used by Medicare to standardize diagnoses. A physician must approve any necessary physical therapy under Medicare. These physical therapy services must be of such a level of complexity that the services of a therapist or someone supervised by a therapist (PTA) are required. There is expectation that the patient will improve significantly in a reasonable period of time. Repetitive, preventative, or maintenance programs generally will not be reimbursed under Medicare.

Preferred provider organization (PPO): this is an organization of physicians, hospitals, and pharmacists whose members discount their health care services to subscriber patients. Providers discount fees for service to attract patients and employees trying to control health care costs. Patients may go outside the network of preferred providers, but services are not discounted and they may incur additional expenses.

Workman's compensation: this is a state-administered program that pays health benefits for "injuries that arise out of and in the course of employment." The amount of coverage and reimbursement varies according to the state. Employers only contribute to the fund.

MEDICAL REVIEW

Insurance companies may elect to send physical therapy notes to a peer review panel. The peer review panel may consist of a physical therapist, nurses, or physicians. This is done to determine if the treatment administered was appropriate for the diagnosis and the length of stay was necessary. It is important that the therapist keep thorough and adequate documentation for medical review. This will assist in receiving payment from the insurance company. Also, it is necessary to show objective tests, measurements, and progression of the patient on a week-by-week basis. The medical review panel may deny or adjust reimbursement based upon their estimation of what is medically and reasonably necessary.

UTILIZATION REVIEW

Utilization review can be a current, prospective, or retrospective review of the medical necessity and cost efficiency of services. Auditing and medical records against a written plan of review are then compared to the standards to determine how the medical record complied with the written plan.

PEER REVIEW

Peer review is performed by health care professionals/peers to determine if services are necessary, appropriate, and comprehensive for a patient's condition and diagnosis.

The reviews can be concurrent or retrospective. The primary purpose of peer reviews is for education of health care professionals.

TYPES OF PROVIDERS OF PATIENT SERVICES

Athletic trainer: assists in injury prevention and treatments typically for athletes and of athletic injuries.

Audiologist: evaluates the hearing potential of the patient to determine if there is any hearing impairment.

Case manager: physical therapists may work as case managers. They will focus on discharge planning for the patient. The focus is on planning for the patient to succeed at the next level upon discharge from the program whether that is to home or the next medical treatment level. The case manager may be from a wide variety of backgrounds besides physical therapy.

Chiropractor (DC): chiropractors are licensed by the state board and provide services to patients on an individual basis. They provide services as they relate to the spinal column and nerves. They evaluate the spinal cord and determine treatments typically based on manipulation of the spinal cord. Care may be coordinated with physical therapy.

Home health aide: works in home setting with patients on activities of daily living and supervision of home treatment programs as directed.

Hospice: providers assist in care for dying patients and their caregivers/families, typically in the home setting for patients with less than 6 months to live.

Occupational therapist assistant (COTA): a certified occupational therapist assistant is certified through a national certification exam. They work under the supervision and direction of an occupational therapist in treatment of the patient.

Occupational therapist (OT): licensed by each state to provide services to patients (eg, evaluation, treatment program for orthotic and splint fabrication, hand therapy, work reconditioning program, activities of daily living [ADLs] training, and increased functional performance of patients). May supervise and delegate care to COTAs.

Orthotist: specializes in design and fitting of orthotics (eg, splints, braces, and corsets).

Prosthetist: specializes in design and fitting of prostheses (eg, artificial limbs for amputees).

Physiatrist: a physician whose specialty is physical medicine and rehabilitation. May work in a rehabilitation hospital and coordinate care of patients with disabilities (eg, cerebrovascular accidents). They are certified by the American Board of Physical Medicine.

Physician: a medical doctor in general practice or a specialist (eg, a physiatrist specializing in physical medicine and rehabilitation). The physician provides the diagnosis of the patient's problem and referral to other health care team members. Licensed by state to state, they must pass medical boards and other exams as required by their specialty and state.

Physician assistant (PA): certified through a national certification exam to assist the physician in performing routine care. A PA may specialize in areas of care (eg, orthopedics or pediatrics).

Physical therapist (PT): certified by national examination and licensed state by state. Evaluates patients, develops a treatment plan, goals, and provides care to patients. May supervise and delegate care to a PTA or aide.

Physical therapist assistant (PTA): educated in a 2-year associates program. Licensure necessity varies state to state. Works under the supervision of a physical therapist in the treatment of patients.

Registered nurse (RN): licensed by state and graduated from an accredited program. Must pass a national exam. Works with a physician in the care of patients and as a liaison between other health care team members.

Respiratory therapist: licensed state by state and must pass a national exam. Administers respiratory therapy (eg, pulmonary function tests, exercises, lung volume tests, and administer oxygen as prescribed by a physician).

Speech therapist: specializes in providing care to patients with speech/language impairments.

Social worker: trained in dealing with social, emotional, and environmental problems associated with an illness or disability. A medical social worker is qualified by a master's degree to counsel patients and their families (eg, in a hospital setting, private practice or school).

Vocational rehabilitation counselor: assists in vocational testing, retraining, and job placement for patients.

Site of Providers

Hospital: may consist of an acute care hospital with patient stays typically under 30 days, or a rehabilitation hospital in which the patient stays may be more than 30 days. Ambulation care unit may be within or outside the hospital where patient may be treated typically with 1-day procedures. Patient care is provided in a hospital or at hospital ambulatory center with a physician's order.

Acute care hospital: acute care is for short-term stays at the hospital. This is less then 30 days and often much shorter with 3 to 5 days. The patient typically is in for an acute illness or surgery and is discharged to home or the next level of care. Physical therapy is focus on functional activities of daily living with instruction on home care programs. Family or significant others' involvement in the treatment program is necessary for continuation of care upon discharge.

Rehabilitation hospital: a rehabilitation hospital offers extended stays designed to rehabilitate the patient to his or her full potential. They involve coordination of services (physical, occupational, speech therapy, physician, social, and other services as necessary) to provide a team approach to patient care.

Skilled nursing facility: patients requiring skilled care on an inpatient basis that includes 24-hour nursing care. Patient care is provided in nursing facilities with a physician's order and recertified for services as necessary.

Long-term care facility: patient stays at these facilities are typically longer than 60 days. Patients do not require 24-hour skilled nursing care. Patient has a temporary or permanent disability and is unable or unsafe in caring for self in an independent setting. Patient care is provided in a long-term facility with a physician's order and recertified for services as necessary.

Home care: provider goes into the patient's home to provide care. To qualify for home care the patient must be homebound or unable to travel outside of the home. The therapist and necessary equipment (eg, transfer boards, handrails, cuff weights) are brought into the patient's home. Patient home care requires an order by a physician and recertification to continue services.

Hospice care: provider typically goes to the home or inpatient setting to care for a dying patient. Patient must be certified by a physician for eligibility in the hospice care program. The patient must be classified with a terminal illness, typically with less then a 6-month lifespan.

School system: provider goes into the school to provide services to students with disabilities. Services are ordered by a physician and the provider works by bringing equipment as necessary to the school to assist disabled students to function.

Private practice or outpatient clinics: the patient comes to the provider's location/facility to receive care. A physician's authorization for evaluation and treatment is determined state by state. Private practices may include general care or specialized care to return to work programs, hand care, sports, and orthopedic injuries. The patient pays according to insurance coverage and acceptance of insurance by the facility. Equipment is located at the provider's place of care.

RESEARCH AND EDUCATION

Ethics

The following must be observed for a study to be ethical:
- Informed consent
- Deception should be minimized
- Confidentiality
- Right to terminate experiment
- Debriefing following experiment
- Protection from danger
- Protection from actual harm
- Explanation of results of experiment

Methods of Research

Cross-sectional: interviewing different people over the same time period.

Descriptive research: summarize, record, and analyze. It involves interpretation of the conditions that exist in the research.

Developmental: study over a long period of time (historical research).

Experimental research: described outcome when the variables are controlled and manipulated. Assists with determining the cause and effects in the study groups.

Longitudinal: interviewing same people through lifespan.

Observation: subjective perception of the research.

Questionnaire: standard form that is sent out for participants to answer and return.

Survey: requires one-on-one personal interviews between the research interviewer and the study participant.

Validity

Validity refers to the extent to which a test, instrument, or procedure measures what it is supposed to measure.

INTERNAL VALIDITY	VERSUS	EXTERNAL VALIDITY
Precision control		General
Basic research		Clinical application

TEST–RETEST	VERSUS	INTERRATER RELIABILITY
Consistency over time		Consistency among raters

Types of Validity
- **Construct validity:** the validation of a test based on theory, not statistical analysis.
- **Content validity:** judgmental assessment of how well an instrument measures a trait or body of knowledge.
- **Criterion-related validity:** the extent to which a test agrees with another well-established test.
- **Predictive validity:** related to the ability of a test score to predict some future performance.

Reliability

An instrument is reliable if it consistently measures similar values of the same quantity or quality with repeated application.

Types of Reliability
- **Interrater reliability (intertester):** the degree to which two or more observers agree.
- **Intrarater reliability (intratester):** the degree to which a single individual can replicate his or her measurements and obtain similar results.

Variables

- **Dependent variable:** the outcome that is being studied or evaluated. The change of behavior that results from the independent variable.
- **Independent variable:** the cause or treatment designed to change the behavior of the dependent variable.
- **Intervening variable:** a variable that changes the relationship between the dependent and independent variables but cannot be measured in the study (eg, personal stress or anxiety unrelated to the research experiment).

Research Proposal

The research proposal is the blueprint of the actual project to be performed. It is composed of seven major components:

1. A statement of the project.
2. Significance of the project.
3. Definitions, assumptions, and limitations of the project.
4. Review of all literature related to the research.
5. The hypothesis, which states the questions that the research will be answering.
6. The method of research that will be performed.
7. The time within which the research will be completed.

DEFINITIONS AND COMMON TERMS

Analysis of variance (ANOVA): a parametric test to measure two or more groups or conditions to a selected probability level.

Analysis of covariance (ANCOVA): a parametric test to measure two or more groups or conditions while regulating the effects of intervening variables.

Blind study: subjects are ignorant of actual experiment conditions.

Chi square: a statistical test for an association between observed data and expected data represented by frequencies. The test yields a statement of the probability of the obtained distribution having occurred by chance alone.

Control group: all factors are kept constant.

Correlation coefficient: a relationship between variables, which is measured and expressed using a numeric scale.

Data: collection of observations.

Dependent: hypothetical effect is manipulated by experiment.

Double blind study: administrator and subjects are both ignorant of experiment conditions.

Experimental group: this is the group of participants in the study that receives the new treatment or technique under study.

Hypothesis: a tentative assumption made in order to answer a question. It is an educated guess.

Independent: hypothetical cause is manipulated by experiment.

Intraclass correlation coefficient: a reliability coefficient based on the analysis of variance.

Liability: tortuous conduct that occurs from a break in the contractual relationship.

Mean: the mathematical average of all the scores in the test divided by the number of participants.

Median: the midpoint of the scores; results in 50% of the scores either above or below the median score.

Null hypothesis (HO): a hypothesis that predicts no difference or relationship exists among the variables studied that could not have occurred by chance alone.

Objectivity: assesses the reliability of the research, which should be designed to yield the same results, regardless of who assesses the research.

Research proposal: the blueprint and systematic plan of procedure for the researcher to follow.

Standard deviation of the mean: the difference of the scores from the mean. This is calculated by taking each score and subtracting it from the mean, square each difference, add the squares together, and divide by the number of scores.

Standard error of measurement: the expected number of errors in an individual score.

T-test: a statistical test used to determine whether there are differences between two means or between a target value and calculated mean.

Variable: a measurable characteristic manipulated in the experiment.

EDUCATION

Staff Education

Ongoing staff education is necessary to provide increased clinical knowledge, thereby increasing the quality of treatment available to patients. It also provides increased staff motivation and performance. Staff education should be shared among staff members. For example:

- Inservices of current clinical research provided by the staff
- Vendor inservices of new technology
- Inservices provided to the staff after a team member attends a continued education program outside the facility and reports back to the staff regarding new techniques
- Physician inservices on new surgical treatment options and protocols for rehabilitation
- Home health care agency inservices on available aftercare for patients
- Attendance at regional or national physical therapy conferences
- Attendance at outside workshops—1 day, weekend, or longer programs
- Visitation to other physical therapy facilities to learn of new programs and techniques available

Patient Education

Patient education should start when the patient enters the clinic (eg, upon registration, the patient should be informed of the clinic's hours, scheduling, conditions of appointments/cancellations, and insurance coverage). After the therapist performs the evaluation, the patient should be educated on the results, diagnostic test, treatment care options, assist in developing short- and long-term goals, home program, and provided with educational brochures to explain the condition.

During the treatment session, the patient should be educated on progress, results of treatment, re-evaluation results, and any changes in the treatment plans or goals.

At discharge, the patient and his or her family should be educated regarding the home care program.

Health Care Team Member Education

The physical therapist should educate and review education between health care team members on the patient's diagnosis, condition, changes in condition, treatment program, goals, and discharge planning.

Teaching Methods

Verbal: verbal communication between the physical therapist and patient and team members regarding progress or information relevant to the case. Verbal instructions and cueing during treatment to the patient. Lecturing to a group of patients, team members, or rehabilitation staff.

Visual: Videos of patient's condition, exercises, and proper position. Taping of patient for gait analysis or biomechanics during performance. Visual demonstration of exercises for patients.

Reading: Reading of computerized testing, patient's reports, and the patient receiving and reading educational booklets or articles. Written patient home programs or exercise sheet.

CHAPTER 31

Sample Test Questions

1. A patient comes to the clinic for neck pain with other medical complications. She can't remember the medical diagnosis the doctor told her yesterday at the clinic. She gives you the following description of her symptoms: intense vertigo, occasional unilateral deafness, buzzing or ringing in the ear. What is the medical name for this inner ear disease that affects balance?
   A. Bulging disc C4, C5
   B. Meniere's disease
   C. Otitis media, chronic
   D. Otitis externa

2. This disorder affects bone formation and is transmitted as an autosomal dominant factor. The result is that long bones of the limbs remain short. What is the medical name for this condition?
   A. Osteogenesis imperfecta
   B. Bone tumor
   C. Achondroplasia
   D. Fibrous dysplasia

3. The chart review reveals a patient with a condition known as thyrotoxicosis. This condition is due to hyperthyroidism. An enlargement of the thyroid gland characterizes the disease. What is not another more common name for this disease?
   A. Graves' disease
   B. Primary hyperthyroidism
   C. Secondary hyperthyroidism
   D. Fibrous dysplasia

4. Adrenal cortex hypersecretions can result in many diseases. In this particular one, obesity is the most common feature in the face, trunk, and dorsal spinal regions. The patient often has a "moonface," hypertension, and osteoporosis. Which of the diseases listed below does the above description define?
   A. Cushing's syndrome
   B. Adrenogenital syndrome
   C. Conn's syndrome
   D. Addison's disease

5. There is a special type of electrical stimulation which has a primary purpose of alleviating pain for a patient. There are minimal side effects and the patient can utilize this unit 24 hours a day. What is the name for this type of electrical stimulation?
   A. Transcutaneous electrical nerve stimulation
   B. High-volt stimulation
   C. Low-volt stimulation
   D. Russian stimulation

6. A patient injured the hip adductor muscles in a track race while jumping hurdles. The patient comes to the clinic with pain in the hip adductor muscle group. Which nerves innervate the hip adductor muscles?
   A. Femoral, tibial
   B. Femoral, superior gluteal
   C. Femoral, obturator, tibial
   D. Femoral, obturator, inferior gluteal

7. A 21-year-old female sprains her ankle at a basketball game. You are on the medical staff attending the game. You notice that swelling is beginning as she insists on continuing to play. Which of the following modalities would not decrease swelling?
   A. Ice massage
   B. Cryopressure
   C. Ice towel
   D. Evaporative coolants

8. A patient with inflammation comes to the clinic with evaluation and treatment orders. The physical therapist asks you which of the following modalities could be utilized to place chemical substances into the body with direct current to decrease inflammation?
   A. Myoflex with ultrasound
   B. Phonophoresis
   C. Iontophoresis
   D. Ultrasound

9. You are working with a physical therapist assistant student when performing short-wave diathermy on a 36-year-old female patient. You explain that this treatment is an example of heat transferred by energy. Which term listed below correctly identifies this type of heat transfer?
   A. Conversion
   B. Convection
   C. Conduction
   D. Radiation

10. Your patient is a 56-year-old female, status 3 weeks post left mastectomy. Her chief concern is edema in the left upper extremity. Which of the following would not be appropriate for treatment of this problem?
    A. Isometric exercises
    B. Jobst compression pump
    C. Massage
    D. Whirlpool

11. Your patient is a 44-year-old female with low back pain resulting from no apparent cause/reason. You set her up in traction with a hold period of 40 seconds, and rest period 10 seconds, for 20 minutes at 60 pounds. What type of traction does this best describe?
    A. Autotraction
    B. Gravity lumbar traction
    C. Manual traction
    D. Intermittent mechanical traction

12. Psychology of a patient can play an important role in his or her physical therapy. The physical therapist assistant may treat patients who are in the psychiatric ward of a hospital for a wide range of musculoskeletal conditions. The chart provides the following information: patient may exhibit psychotic behavior, suspicious, resentful, and rigid. What does this description most likely describe?
    A. Hypochondria
    B. Hysteria
    C. Paranoia
    D. Depression

13. As a physical therapist assistant student, you are observing in the psychiatric ward. You are given the following information on a patient: he is pessimistic, irritable, lacks self-confidence, and has a gloomy outlook on life. What would be the most likely diagnosis or problem this patient is experiencing?
    A. Hysteria
    B. Depression
    C. Psychopathy
    D. Schizophrenia

14. An 18-year-old female pregnant with her first child went into premature labor and delivered a baby girl. Labor is defined as premature if it occurs between which weeks of pregnancy?
    A. Between the 30th and 37th week
    B. Between the 28th and 37th week
    C. Between the 24th and 37th week
    D. Between the 20th and 37th week

15. The patient you are working with is a 28-year-old head injury victim of a brutal beating in an alley. The patient clinically demonstrates excessive tone in the limbs, which are resistant to both active and passive movement. Which term listed below would best describe this condition?
    A. Flaccidity
    B. Hypotonia
    C. Hypertonia
    D. Rigidity

16. Your last patient of the day is a spinal cord injury victim whom you are teaching self range of motion. You explain that this will be a very important component in her home program. What is the minimal level this patient can have to perform self range of motion independently?
    A. C7
    B. C8
    C. C5
    D. C4

17. You are treating an electrical burn patient who worked for the power and electric company. After whirlpool and debridement treatments, it is determined that he needs a graft. He receives an autograft. Which of the following best describes the graft this patient received?
    A. Skin applied other than human skin
    B. Pig skin to speed healing
    C. Human skin from a donor
    D. Skin from one part of the body transplanted to another location on the same individual

18. A 26-year-old female is injured in a motor vehicle accident. The injury results in an incomplete spinal cord lesion. The symptoms are paralysis and loss of sensation except in the sacral area. What is the correct term for this injury?
    A. Cauda equina injury
    B. Sacral sparing
    C. Central cord syndrome
    D. Brown-Séquard's syndrome

19. A spinal cord patient is present with the following symptoms: deficits are found more in the centrally located tract and upper extremities than peripherally located in the lower extremities. It is noted in the chart that the spinal cord lesion is incomplete. Which type of injury listed below does this patient most likely have?
    A. Anterior cord syndrome
    B. Central cord syndrome
    C. Brown-Séquard's syndrome
    D. Sacral sparing

20. A 12-year-old male is presented to the clinic with hip flexion contractures. The contractures are secondary to fibrosis where the skin is bound down to the tissue. The physical therapist states that the patient has chronic inflammation of the connective tissue. What is the name of this medical condition?
   A. Chronic contractures
   B. Scleroderma
   C. Fibrositis
   D. Myositis

21. A 12-year-old male is presented to the clinic with hip flexion contractures. The contractures are secondary to fibrosis where the skin is bound down to the tissue. What would be the treatment program for this patient, who has a chronic inflammation of the connective tissue?
   A. Strengthening
   B. Aerobic conditioning
   C. Stretching and flexibility
   D. Isokinetic exercises

22. This plane divides the body into upper and lower parts for the purpose of kinesiology study. Which of the following terms would describe this plane?
   A. Sagittal
   B. Horizontal
   C. Frontal
   D. Rotary

23. This plane divides the body into right and left sides for the purpose of kinesiology study. Which of the following terms would describe this plane?
   A. Frontal
   B. Horizontal
   C. Sagittal
   D. Rotary

24. You are to perform a postural reevaluation of a patient from the side or lateral view, specifically determining normal alignment for the head, scapula, and shoulder. Which of the following is normal alignment?
   A. Head neutral, scapula depressed, shoulder neutral
   B. Head forward, scapula flat, shoulder neutral
   C. Head neutral, scapula flat, shoulder neutral
   D. Head hyperextended, scapula winged, shoulder neutral

25. A spinal cord patient, 2 weeks post motor vehicle accident (MVA), is referred to physical therapy for evaluation and prognosis for rehabilitation. What muscle grade in the lower extremity is necessary for functional performance by this individual?
   A. Fair
   B. Fair plus
   C. Poor plus
   D. Good minus

26. You have an 18-year-old male who crushed his left hand in a sheer press at work. He had tendon surgery on the left index finger. What would be normal range of motion for the distal interphalangeal joint flexion?
   A. 0 to 90°
   B. 0 to 120°
   C. 0 to 80°
   D. 0 to 70°

27. You have a 29-year-old male who was involved in a chemical burn accident at work the previous day. You are instructed to start whirlpool and debridement treatments at 98°F. What would be the correct temperature in Celsius for whirlpool treatment?

A. 36°
B. 50°
C. 25°
D. 30°

28. A patient is a 24-year-old male 2 weeks status post anterior cruciate ligament (ACL) reconstruction surgery. Which of the following treatments is not appropriate at this stage in rehabilitation?
    A. Quad sets
    B. Isometrics
    C. Isokinetics
    D. Straight leg raise

29. Your patient is a 66-year-old male with a history of chronic back pain. The patient also has a history of heart disorders with a pacemaker in place, type unknown. Which treatment is contraindicated for pain relief?
    A. Hot packs
    B. Ultrasound
    C. Pelvic traction
    D. TENS unit

30. In physiology class you are studying electrical stimulation and the body's response. Which of the following terms best fits the definition of minimum intensity of an electrical stimulus to elicit a minimal contraction?
    A. Rheobase
    B. Chronaxie
    C. Anode
    D. Cathode

31. In your physiology class the professor describes the minimal time that a stimulus of twice rheobase stimulates a tissue or strength duration curve. Which of the following terms best fits this description?
    A. Galvanic current
    B. Faradic current
    C. Rheobase2
    D. Chronaxie

32. It is known that a joint in the body can possess only a maximum number of degrees of freedom. How many degrees of freedom is the maximum number that a single joint can possess?
    A. 5
    B. 6
    C. 3
    D. 4

33. Read the following question and answer according to proper kinesiology terminology. Of the following, which is referred to as the muscle group that is noncontracting and passively elongates or shortens to permit the motion to occur?
    A. Antagonist
    B. Prime mover
    C. Agonist
    D. Eccentric

34. Which physics law can be interpreted clinically to mean that the further the infrared light (eg, is moving away from the patient), the greater the decrease in intensity will be?
    A. Joule's law
    B. Ohm's law
    C. Inverse square law
    D. Cosine law

35. The physical therapist requests that you treat a 56-year-old male in the neurointensive care unit. The therapist informs you of the following results regarding this patient: no voluntary movement, lack of response to stimulus, no reflexes, and positive Babinski response. Which most likely describes this patient's condition?
    A. Cerebrovascular accident
    B. Coma
    C. Stupor
    D. Uncooperative patient

36. Gait evaluation reveals an unsteady gait with a wide base of support. The patient has a positive Romberg's sign and watches the ground when ambulating. The patient lands with the heel first, then the toes, creating a double tapping sign. The patient also has loss of position sense in the legs. The area of injury is most likely which of the following?
    A. Posterior column deficit
    B. Basal ganglion
    C. Cerebellum
    D. Corticospinal tract

37. The hip joint is classified as a ball and socket joint. The hip joint has limited mobility but great stability. In a kinesiology study, how many degrees of freedom does the hip joint have?
    A. 1
    B. 2
    C. 3
    D. 6

38. The atlanto-occipital joint axis is an example of which type of lever system found in the body? This type of lever is frequently used for monitoring posture and balance.
    A. First class
    B. Second class
    C. Third class
    D. Fourth class

39. You are studying kinesiology and its mechanical principles as they relate to anatomy. The pull on the brachioradialis and wrist extensors to maintain the position of elbow flexion is an example of which type of lever system found in the body?
    A. First class
    B. Second class
    C. Third class
    D. Fourth class

40. The gait instructor is giving a practical examination of your skills through verbal questions on gait analysis. "During the swing phase, acceleration stage, which muscles remain active throughout the entire stage to help shorten the extremity so it can clear the ground by holding the ankle in a neutral position?"
    A. Tibialis posterior, peroneus brevis
    B. Tibialis anterior, peroneus tertius
    C. Tibialis anterior, peroneus tertius, extensor hallucis longus
    D. Tibialis posterior, peroneus tertius, extensor hallucis longus

41. During the swing phase, deceleration stage, which muscles contract to slow down the swing phase just prior to heel strike, thus permitting the heel to strike quietly in a controlled manner?
    A. Gluteus medius
    B. Gluteus maximus
    C. Hamstring
    D. Quadriceps

42. Your patient is a 4-year-old child who fell off his swing set at home. He has a fracture described as an incomplete fracture. What is the typical name for this fracture, which usually occurs in children?
    A. Open
    B. Closed
    C. Comminuted
    D. Greenstick

43. A patient is an 18-year-old male who was seriously injured in a motorcycle accident. The radiology examination reveals a fracture in which the ends are driven into each other. Of the choices listed below, what is the typical name for this type of fracture?
    A. Comminuted
    B. Impacted
    C. Displaced
    D. Intraarticular

44. On a patient case review, you are asked to look at an electrocardiogram (EKG) of a 46-year-old open-heart surgery patient. Which of the following waves would be the first downward deflection you see when reading the EKG?
    A. T wave
    B. P wave
    C. Q wave
    D. QRS complex

45. We know that the sinus node acts as the cardiac pacemaker of the heart. The sinus node will discharge on impulse to the heart at a certain rate per minute. Which of the following rates does the sinus node discharge?
    A. 100 to 150
    B. 100 to 125
    C. 60 to 100
    D. 80 to 100

46. The sinus node acts as the cardiac pacemaker in the heart. The sinus node is a group of cardiac cells that discharges an impulse. where is the sinus node located in the heart?
    A. Right atrium
    B. Left atrium
    C. Right ventricle
    D. Left ventricle

47. In studying the heart anatomy during dissection in anatomy lab, you locate the tricuspid and mitral valves. These valves also have an additional name because of their position in the heart. Which of the following names is correct for the tricuspid and mitral valves?
    A. Semilunar valves
    B. Atrioventricular valves
    C. Pulmonary valves
    D. Aortic valves

48. You are observing a physical therapist working with a 72-year-old male with pectus carinatum, more commonly known as pigeon chest. Which of the following best describes his condition?
    A. Lower portion of the sternum is depressed
    B. Lateral diameter of the chest is increased
    C. Sternum is displaced anteriorly, increasing anterior-posterior diameter
    D. Sternum is displaced posteriorly, increasing anterior-posterior diameter

49. You are treating a patient in the neurointensive care unit. The patient is unresponsive to stimuli and you determine that he is comatose. You observe the following posture at the patient's bedside: supine, the lower extremities are plantar flexed and internally rotated, and the upper extremities are positioned in shoulder adduction, elbow flexion, and wrist flexion. Which of the following best describes the posture you observed in this patient?

A. Hemiplegia
B. Decerebrate rigidity
C. Decorticate rigidity
D. Spasticity extensor

50. The patient is unresponsive to stimuli and you determine that he is comatose. You observe the following posture at the patient's bedside: supine, the lower extremities are plantar flexed and internally rotated, and the upper extremities are positioned in shoulder adduction, elbow flexion, and wrist flexion. Based on this information, where has the injury most likely occurred?
A. Corticospinal tracts
B. Midbrain
C. Pons
D. Diencephalon

51. Several muscles in the body have dual innervation, which is innervation by more than one nerve. Which of the following muscles does not have dual innervation?
A. Flexor digitorum profundus
B. Flexor carpi ulnaris
C. Flexor pollicis brevis
D. Lumbricales

52. A 16-year-old soccer player enters the emergency room with an anterior tibialis muscle injury sustained during practice. The patient has significant bruising and discoloration in the area. Which nerve innervates the anterior tibialis muscle?
A. Lateral plantar
B. Superficial peroneal
C. Tibial
D. Deep peroneal

53. A patient is 5 days post arthroscopic surgery on the medial aspect of the right knee. Which of the following ligaments would provide the patient's medial stability of the right knee?
A. Medial collateral ligament
B. Medial meniscus
C. Anterior cruciate ligament
D. Medial meniscus and medial collateral ligament

54. In your gross anatomy class, the professor asks you to dissect the muscles that attach to the ischial tuberosity. Which group of muscles listed below attaches to the ischial tuberosity?
A. Biceps femoris, semitendinosus
B. Semimembranosus, biceps femoris
C. Semimembranosus, biceps femoris, semitendinosus
D. Semimembranosus, semitendinosus

55. You are reevaluating the glenohumeral joint of a 33-year-old female. The patient has received 2 weeks of physical therapy for a frozen adhesive capsulitis. Which of the following muscles does not attach to the greater tuberosity of the humerus?
A. Supraspinatus
B. Teres minor
C. Teres major
D. Infraspinatus

56. A 12-year-old male has injured his wrist extensors in a farming accident. All of the wrist extensors are injured at their common origin. What is the common origin of the wrist extensors?
A. Lateral epicondyle
B. Medial epicondyle
C. Olecranon fossa
D. Medial supracondylar line

57. You are studying neuroanatomy in physical therapist assistant school. The neurology professor presents the following question to the class: "At what vertebral level does the spinal cord end?"
    A. S1
    B. S2
    C. L5
    D. L2

58. A patient enters the clinic with a prescription from a prominent neurological surgeon. Due to illegible handwriting you are unable to read the complete diagnosis of the patient. You can make out the first part, which states Lou Gehrig's disease. Next to this there is some continual scrolling. Which of the following is another name for Lou Gehrig's disease?
    A. Parkinson's disease
    B. Amyotrophic lateral sclerosis
    C. Hodgkin's disease
    D. Marfan's syndrome

59. A 32-year-old female enters the emergency room with a knife injury to the spinal cord. The patient is referred to physical therapy for a comprehensive evaluation of the spinal cord injury. Medical history determines that the knife has caused a hemisection of the spinal cord. Of the following, which syndrome may be seen after a knife-type injury to the spinal cord that resulted in hemisection?
    A. Marfan's syndrome
    B. Amyotrophic lateral syndrome
    C. Cerebellar syndrome
    D. Brown-Séquard's syndrome

60. During an internship in the neuro unit at a major university hospital, the physical therapist asks you to perform the test for reflex C5. Which of the following should be tested to determine the reflex at level C5?
    A. Elbow extension
    B. Triceps
    C. Biceps
    D. Brachioradialis

61. A patient enters the clinic with generalized muscle atrophy and decreased reflexes. Upon testing the triceps reflex, you notice a decreased response. In writing your evaluation you state that the triceps reflex tests which of the following levels?
    A. C5
    B. C6
    C. C7
    D. C8

62. A patient enters the clinic with a prescription for direct current electrical stimulation. Upon reading the order, you notice that the patient's diagnosis is Bell's palsy. Of the following, which nerve would you determine to be injured in this patient?
    A. Trigeminal
    B. Trochlear
    C. Facial
    D. Vagus

63. You are reevaluating a patient with a repetitive motion injury from work. You have tested the patient's pronation/supination of the forearm and wrist flexion/extension. Which of the following muscles does not assist in pronation of the radioulnar joint?
    A. Brachioradialis
    B. Flexor carpi radialis
    C. Pronator quadratus
    D. Flexor carpi ulnaris

64. In your examination of a patient for shoulder pain, you attempt to palpate the lesser tuberosity of the humerus. Which of the following muscles attach to the lesser tuberosity of the humerus?
    A. Teres major, supraspinatus
    B. Teres minor, subscapularis
    C. Teres minor, infraspinatus
    D. Subscapularis

65. A 49-year-old male sustains a flexor tendon laceration of the right hand. As a result, the flexor digitorum profundus has permanent nerve injury. Which nerve or nerves innervate the flexor digitorum profundus?
    A. Ulnar
    B. Median
    C. Median, ulnar
    D. Median, radial

66. A physical therapy patient performs scapular movement. The patient can isolate and move only the levator scapulae and rhomboid muscles. What action would take place for scapular movement?
    A. Medial rotation downward
    B. Lateral rotation upward
    C. Adduction
    D. Depression

67. A butcher at the meat shop is responsible for processing meat packaging. In the process of carving the meat, he injured the second and third digits of his hand. The hand surgeon reports that the nerves in the second and third digits have been permanently injured. Which nerve/nerves would be injured with this patient?
    A. Ulnar nerve
    B. Median nerve
    C. Radial nerve
    D. Ulnar/median

68. A triathlon participant enters the clinic with limitations of flexibility of the tensor fasciae latae muscle. The physical therapist places this patient on a flexibility program designed to minimize injuries over the course of his athletic participation. This program includes the tensor fasciae latae, whose origin is which of the following?
    A. ASIS (anterior superior iliac spine)
    B. PSIS (posterior superior iliac spine)
    C. Iliac crest
    D. Greater trochanter

69. You are studying hip ligaments in your gross anatomy class in physical therapist assistant school. Which of the following is classified as the Y-shaped ligament of the hip?
    A. Pubocapsular
    B. Ischiocapsular
    C. Pubofemoral
    D. Iliofemoral

70. A 49-year-old construction worker injures his foot in a work-related accident. The injury involves the navicular tubercle of the left foot. Which of the following muscles attaches to the navicular tubercle?
    A. Anterior tibialis
    B. Posterior tibialis
    C. Hallucis longus
    D. Gastrocnemius

71. Your patient injured the knee ligaments, a basketball player who is in physical therapy for ligament laxity. Which of the following knee ligaments prevents anterior displacement of the tibia on the femur?

A. Anterior cruciate ligament
B. Posterior cruciate ligament
C. Medial collateral ligament
D. Lateral collateral ligament

72. A patient enters the clinic with a history of chronic temporomandibular joint (TMJ) dysfunction. When observing the patient, you notice he has great difficulty in chewing. Of the following, which nerve would be responsible for chewing?
A. Trigeminal
B. Facial
C. Accessory
D. Vagus

73. When studying upper motor neuron lesions in neuroanatomy, you determine that which of the following is not a characteristic typically seen with this type of lesion?
A. Muscle atrophy
B. Spasticity
C. Hyperreflexia
D. Babinski's sign

74. A 26-year-old triathlete has just completed a competitive event in swimming, biking, and running. The patient has extreme muscle fatigue after this event. Which of the following most likely builds up in the body, causing muscle fatigue?
A. Glycogen
B. Lactic acid
C. Fatty acids
D. Glucose

75. A patient is participating in a pulmonary evaluation in the respiratory therapy department. You are observing this evaluation as a part of your physical therapist assistant student internship. How would you best describe the amount of air left over after maximum expiration?
A. Dead air space
B. Forced inspiratory volume
C. Expiratory reserve volume
D. Residual volume

76. During cardiac rehabilitation a patient presents a heart rate of 60 beats per minute. The heart rate will occasionally fluctuate anywhere from 55 to 60 beats per minute. Which of the following would best describe this heart rate?
A. Sinuscardia
B. Tachycardia
C. Bradycardia
D. Normal in athletes

77. A patient during cardiac rehabilitation has a heartbeat best described as tachycardia. When writing your notes you would state tachycardia is a heart rate/beats per minute of which of the following?
A. Under 60
B. Above 60
C. Above 100
D. Above 80

78. A patient undergoes open heart surgery at a prestigious heart hospital. The patient is being evaluated 1 day postoperative for possible placement in the acute inpatient cardiac rehab program. His blood pressure reading indicates hypertension. Which of the following readings would be considered indicative of hypertension?

A. 120/80
B. Above 120/80
C. Above 140/90
D. Under 120/90

79. A 26-year-old marathon runner comes to you for additional training. His goal is to reduce his marathon running time by 5 minutes in the next Boston Marathon. As part of his training and education, you are explaining the benefits that he will receive from aerobic exercise. Which of the following is not a benefit from aerobic exercise?
A. A decrease in serum lipid levels
B. An increase in HDL levels
C. An increase in aerobic capacity
D. A decrease in aerobic capacity

80. You are doing a reevaluation of a patient who has signs of inflammation in the right knee. The right knee is very swollen, warm, and red in color. You are concerned that this patient might possibly have torn the anterior cruciate ligament. Which of the following is not a cardinal sign of inflammation?
A. Rubor
B. Calor
C. Tumor
D. Pallor

81. A patient is assigned to you by the physical therapist. The physical therapist is concerned that the patient might have suffered an injury to the nerve crossing the anatomical snuffbox. Of the following nerves, which would you need to test?
A. Radial
B. Median
C. Ulnar
D. Musculocutaneous

82. A 15-year-old basketball player enters the clinic for a sports medicine evaluation following a twisted ankle in practice yesterday. Evaluation reveals that the ankle is swollen with limited range of motion. However, good ligament stability is present. The ligament most commonly injured in an ankle sprain is which of the following?
A. Anterior talofibular
B. Calcaneonavicular
C. Posterior navicular
D. Anterior tibiofibular

83. In studying the anatomy of the spine, you learn the various components of the vertebrae, as well as the discs. The discs consist of fibrogelatinous pulp. What is the fibrogelatinous pulp in a disc called?
A. Anulus fibrosis
B. Vertebral foramen
C. Nucleus fibrosis
D. Nucleus pulposus

84. The neuroanatomy professor lectures on the divisions of the brain. The brain is divided into three major divisions. Which of the following is not one of the three major brain regions?
A. Brainstem
B. Midbrain
C. Cerebellum
D. Cerebrum

85. A patient is resting quietly in bed when you arrive to begin passive range of motion exercises. What is the name of the nervous system responsible for controlling internal functions under quiet conditions?

A. Sympathetic
B. Parasympathetic
C. Autonomic
D. Preganglionic

86. In physiology class you are studying the fight or flight responses of the nervous system. In preparation for fight or flight responses, which system is activated?
A. Sympathetic
B. Parasympathetic
C. Autonomic
D. Postganglionic

87. The structures in the body perform certain functions. For example, one structure regulates the temperature of the body. Of the following, which structure controls body temperature and appetite responses?
A. Pons
B. Medulla
C. Hypothalamus
D. Adrenal glands

88. It is important to understand the anatomy of a muscle to accurately treat a patient's condition. Which of the following is defined as connective tissue surrounding a muscle that projects beyond the ends of the muscle fibers and becomes cordlike?
A. Aponeurosis
B. Fascia
C. Myofibril
D. Tendon

89. A patient fell in the clinic on a flight of stairs while practicing crutch training. The patient fractured the patella or kneecap. The patella or kneecap is classified as what type of bone?
A. Long
B. Short
C. Irregular
D. Sesamoid

90. In pulmonary class you are studying respiration and pulmonary function. Which of the following best defines respiration?
A. Gas exchange in the lungs
B. Gas exchange secondary to pressure differences
C. Transfer of gases between body cells and the environment
D. Ventilation of the lungs

91. A pregnant patient is advised to avoid Valsalva's maneuver during her pregnancy. What effect listed below does Valsalva's maneuver have?
A. Increase in intrathoracic pressure
B. Decrease in intrathoracic pressure
C. Pressure remains the same, no effect
D. Increase in inspiration needs

92. You are attending a neurology inservice given by a leading neurologist in the hospital. The neurologist describes the junction between neurons. Which of the following is the neurologist describing?
A. Ranvier's nodes
B. Synapse
C. Schwann cells
D. Stellate cells

93. You are attending an inservice on neurology. The instructor is lecturing on mechanoreceptors. The function of mechanoreceptors can best be described by which of the following?
    A. Response to chemicals in which they come into contact
    B. Response to light falling upon the retina
    C. Response to temperature changes
    D. Response to mechanical deformation of tissue

94. You are studying physiology in the physical therapist assistant program at school. You are currently studying muscle physiology. The professor asks you what thick filaments in the sarcomere are called. Which of the following is the best answer?
    A. Actin
    B. Myosin
    C. Myofibril
    D. Z band

95. A 34-year-old female pulled her gluteus muscles while reaching over and lifting a heavy box at work. This resulted in a muscle strain that requires physical therapy. Which of the following is the origin for the gluteus muscles?
    A. Pubis
    B. Ischium
    C. Ilium
    D. ASIS

96. You are treating a 21-year-old track and field star for a pulled muscle. The main muscle that the physical therapist tells you to focus on is the tibialis posterior. Which of the following is the correct insertion for the tibialis posterior muscle?
    A. Sesamoids
    B. Calcaneus
    C. Navicular tuberosity
    D. Peroneus tubercle

97. Your patient is a 36-year-old factory worker who comes to physical therapy secondary to a crushing injury of the right hand injured in a molding press. The patient reports to physical therapy for evaluation and treatment. The physical therapist has instructed you to begin treatment to reduce edema and assist in alleviating pain while regaining range of motion. You are palpating the carpal bone, which articulates with the thumb. Which of the following would you most likely be palpating?
    A. Trapezium
    B. Trapezoid
    C. Hamate
    D. Triquestrium

98. In studying physiology you are discussing where adenosine triphosphate (ATP) is made through oxidative phosphorylation. Which of the following is the location for the powerhouse of the cell where ATP is made through oxidative phosphorylation?
    A. Mitochondria
    B. Cytoplasm
    C. Ribosome
    D. Nucleus

99. You are a physical therapist assistant observing an all-day wrestling tournament as one of the medical personnel on duty in case of injuries. You emphasize to the wrestlers that it will be important during the day to consume fluid, as the gymnasium is extremely hot and fatigue may result. The body consists of which of the following percentages of water?
    A. 25%
    B. 40%
    C. 50%
    D. 70%

100. You are treating a patient with medial epicondylitis of the elbow. The patient informs you that he is an avid golfer and participated in a weekend tournament at a local golf club. He comes to the clinic complaining of pain, inflammation, and tendonitis in the medial epicondyle region of the elbow. You are palpating behind the medial epicondyle region of the elbow for pain and tenderness. Of the following, which is the nerve that lies behind the medial epicondyle of the elbow?
     A. Ulnar
     B. Median
     C. Radial
     D. Brachial

101. You are in physiology class studying the difference between erythrocytes and leukocytes in the body. Each one has a primary function to perform so that the body functions normally. Which of the following is a primary function of erythrocytes in the body?
     A. Transport oxygen
     B. Carry iron
     C. Produce calcium
     D. Produce red blood cells

102. You are studying for a final exam in physiology class. Which of the following would best describe the white cells of the body, which act as the body's defense against infection?
     A. Erythrocytes
     B. Agglutinins
     C. Leukocytes
     D Antibody serum

103. A patient is referred to physical therapy with a ruptured Achilles' tendon. The patient reports that he was mowing the lawn and was going down a steep incline when he felt a sharp, sudden pain in the left heel region. The physical therapist reports that the patient has ruptured his Achilles' tendon. Which of the following would be the proper location for the Achilles' tendon insertion?
     A. Cuboid
     B. Calcaneus
     C. Talus
     D. First metatarsal

104. An 80-year-old female reports the following history: she was at the mall shopping when she stepped onto the escalator and twisted her left ankle. She is now referred to physical therapy and the physical therapist instructs you to perform strengthening programs to the lateral ligament of the ankle. Of the following ligaments, which would you not be rehabilitating?
     A. Calcaneofibular
     B. Anterior tibiofibular
     C. Posterior talofibular
     D. Anterior talofibular

105. You have a patient referred to physical therapy secondary to Bell's palsy. You are to instruct the patient in a series of facial muscle exercises designed to increase and maintain function. The therapist instructs you to work on the muscle whose function is to draw the angles of the mouth downward. Which of the following would you emphasize for this treatment program?
     A. Levator anguli oris
     B. Buccinator
     C. Orbicularis oris
     D. Platysma

106. You are studying abnormal reflexes in neurology class. You are now focusing on the reflex called the flexor withdrawal. The flexor withdrawal integration level is spinal. Where would the stimulus be applied to test the flexor withdrawal?

A. Sole of the foot with lower extremity in extension
B. Sole of the foot with lower extremity in flexion
C. Forefoot with the lower extremity in extension
D. Forefoot with the lower extremity in flexion

107. You are studying the symmetric tonic neck reflex (STNR). The STNR integration level is the brainstem. The physical therapist assistant places the patient's head in the extended position. Which of the following would be the normal response to this stimulus?
A. Upper extremity flexion and lower extremity extension
B. Upper extremity extension and lower extremity flexion
C. Extension of both upper and lower extremities
D. Flexion of both upper and lower extremities

108. You are testing for the tonic labyrinthine abnormal reflex. The integration level is the brainstem and there is no stimulus required. The response the patient will demonstrate will depend upon his or her positioning. You position the patient in prone when testing. Which of the following would the patient demonstrate?
A. Increased extensor tone
B. Increased flexor tone
C. Increased extensor tone in the upper extremities and increased flexor tone in the lower extremities
D. Increased flexor tone in the upper extremities and increased extensor tone in the lower extremities

109. You are testing the positive support reaction. The integration level is the brainstem. Which of the following would be the stimulus you would be using in testing the positive support reaction?
A. Have the patient bounce the patient several times on the soles of the feet but allow no weightbearing
B. Have the patient bounce the patient several times on the soles of the feet with weightbearing
C. Push the patient backward and forward in sitting
D. Push the patient side to side in sitting

110. You are testing the tonic labyrinthine reflex of a patient. You have positioned the patient supine. Which of the following would you consider to be a positive response to this position?
A. Increased extensor tone
B. Increased flexor tone
C. Increased extensor tone in the upper extremities and flexor tone in the lower extremities
D. Increased flexor tone in the upper extremities and extensor tone in the lower extremities

111. You are testing a patient for the negative support reaction. The integration level for the negative support reaction is the brainstem. You bounce the patient several times on the soles of the feet but you do not allow him to bear weight. Which of the following would you anticipate as the patient's response?
A. Increased extensor tone in lower extremities
B. Increased extensor tone in upper extremities
C. Increased flexor tone in lower extremities
D. Increased extensor tone in upper extremities

112. You are testing for the tonic labyrinthine reflex on a specific patient. You have previously tested the prone and supine lying positions. The last position to be tested is the sidelying position. Which of the following will occur when the patient is positioned sidelying when testing for tonic labyrinthine reflex?
A. Increased extensor tone
B. Increased flexor tone
C. Increased flexor tone in sidelying limbs and extensor tone in nonweightbearing limbs
D. Increased extensor tone in sidelying limbs and flexor tone in nonweightbearing limbs

113. You have a pediatric patient referred to physical therapy. The patient is 5 months old. You want to test several reflexes of this patient. The stimulus you utilize for the first reflex is a sudden movement to cause a startle reaction in the patient. Which of the following are you most likely performing?

A. Grasp reflex

B. Protective extension reaction

C. Protective reaction

D. Moro's reflex

114. You are to test the pediatric reflexes on a specific patient. The reflex that you will be testing will be the grasp reflex. Which of the following statements is an incorrect statement regarding the grasp reflex?

A. Involves stimulus to the palm of the hand

B. Involves placing an object in the palm

C. Occurs at 3 to 6 months of age

D. Occurs at 6 to 9 months of age

115. You have a patient referred to physical therapy with cerebral palsy. Which of the following does not describe what you would typically observe in a cerebral palsy child?

A. The child may be either passive or stiff

B. The child cannot adjust body position

C. The child can hold or bring his or her head into a normal position

D. The child may be classified as either spastic or ataxic

116. A patient is referred to physical therapy with an order from a local podiatrist. The podiatrist lists the diagnosis as tarsal tunnel syndrome in the right foot. The physical therapist asks you what nerve is compressed as a result of tarsal tunnel syndrome. Which of the following would be a correct response?

A. Posterior tibial nerve

B. Medial plantar nerve

C. Lateral plantar nerve

D. Anterior tibial nerve

117. You are observing a patient with tarsal tunnel syndrome from approximately 50 feet away in the clinic. You observe the patient from the anterior and posterior views. In your notes you record that the patient, upon ambulation, demonstrates calcaneus valgus. Which of the following would be a correct description of calcaneus valgus?

A. Excessive plantar flexion of the foot

B. Excessive dorsiflexion of the foot

C. Excessive inversion of the foot

D. Excessive eversion of the foot

118. You are working with an inpatient that has congenital dysplasia of the right hip. The patient previously had limitations in specific ranges of motion as a result of congenital dysplasia. Which of the following would show the greatest limitation in movement for this patient?

A. Hip flexion

B. Hip adduction

C. Hip abduction

D. Hip rotation

119. A patient is referred to physical therapy with a fracture to the left femur. The physical therapist informs you that the patient has an angle of inclination below 110° in the upper femur. Which of the following would be a disorder of the upper femur in which the angle of inclination is below 110°?

A. Coxa valgus

B. Coxa vara

C. Transient synovitis

D. Osteitis pubis

120. A patient is referred to physical therapy with a diagnosis of spondylolisthesis. Your supervising physical therapist asks you to best describe the term spondylolisthesis. Which of the following would be a correct definition?

A. Slipped disc in the lumbar region

B. Compression fracture in the lumbar region

C. Adherent nerve root syndrome

D. Gradual slipping of one vertebra over another

121. A patient is referred to physical therapy secondary to neck pain. Upon observation, you notice that the patient has a deformity of the neck that causes rotation and tilting of the head in the opposite direction. When writing your SOAP notes, which of the following would be the best term to utilize in describing this patient's condition?

A. Disc calcification

B. Disc herniation

C. Cervical strain

D. Torticollis

122. A patient is referred to physical therapy secondary to low back pain. The patient's chief complaint is pain on the right low back region. The patient is concerned and has previously received treatment from a chiropractor. The patient informs you that the chiropractor told him that his right leg is one-quarter of an inch shorter than his left leg. You determine that true leg length measurements should be performed on this patient. Which of the following areas will you measure for true leg length?

A. PSIS to medial malleolus

B. ASIS to medial malleolus

C. PSIS to lateral malleolus

D. ASIS to lateral malleolus

123. In performing massage on a patient it is important to know the difference between an indication and a contraindication for massage. Which of the following is not a contraindication for performing a massage on a patient?

A. Hematomas

B. Herniated disc

C. Phlebitis

D. Myositis—nonacute

124. You are working in the burn unit of an acute care hospital. A patient is referred to physical therapy with a burn located in the hip region. The physical therapist performs the initial debridement and instructs you to position the hip so that the patient will not develop a contracture. Which of the following would be the correct positioning for this patient?

A. Flexion

B. Adduction

C. Flexion and adduction

D. Extension and abduction

125. Your last patient of the day in a specialty burn unit has an anterior neck burn. This patient has already received treatment to emphasize decreasing chances of contractures and to promote healing in the area. It is now your responsibility to place this patient in a position to minimize contractures. Which of the following would be the correct positioning?

A. Flexion

B. Rotation

C. Extension

D. Hyperextension

126. You are performing a study of burn patients. In this particular study, both the subject and the administrator are ignorant of experiment conditions. What is this type of study called?

A. Dependent study

B. Independent study

C. Blind study

D. Double blind study

127. In your burn research project, you have several different people testing and measuring range of motion in the patients. You are especially concerned with testing consistency among the raters. Which of the following terms relates to testing consistency among raters?
    A. Test-retest
    B. Validity
    C. Interrater reliability
    D. Face validity

128. You are a physical therapist assistant consulting with a local YMCA on exercise prescriptions for fitness patients. Which of the following components would not need to be included in an exercise prescription?
    A. Intensity of exercise
    B. Duration of exercise
    C. Frequency of exercise
    D. Time of day to exercise

129. The patient is referred to physical therapy secondary to a complication of diabetes. The diabetes has affected the nerves and the patient is having difficulty with ambulation secondary to nerve involvement in the lower extremities. Which of the following is this condition most commonly called?
    A. Neurorrhaphy
    B. Neuropathy
    C. Polyneuropathy
    D. Neurosis

130. A patient is referred to physical therapy. While you are recording her treatment she talks to you regarding her condition. The patient reports that she is in a serious stage of her condition, as her organs are affected by the disease. The patient reports that her condition originally started as thickening of the skin in the subcutaneous tissue, which then eventually affected the organs. The patient is currently in physical therapy for a home exercise program specifically designed for range of motion and to prevent contractures as much as possible. Which of the following would most likely be the condition of this patient?
    A. Dermatomyositis
    B. Scleroderma
    C. Fibrinoid necrosis
    D. Granulomatosis

131. You are treating a 53-year-old woman bedside in the hospital. The patient has been referred for training with a walker to be utilized to go from the bed to the bathroom and back. You notice the patient is in a state in which the act of breathing is causing distress to the patient. Which of the following best describes the state in which the act of breathing will cause distress to the patient?
    A. Syncope
    B. Hypoxia
    C. Dyspnea
    D. Hypercapnia

132. A patient comes to physical therapy for further instructions on crutch ambulation. Upon observation, you notice that the patient moves the left crutch first, then the right leg, then the right crutch, then the left leg. Of the following, which type of crutch gait have you most likely observed?
    A. Three-point gait
    B. Two-point gait
    C. Swing-through
    D. Four-point gait

133. You are treating a patient who has had a left-side cerebrovascular accident (CVA) approximately 6 weeks ago. The patient requires assistance in plantar flexion of the ankle during the push-off phase of gait. Which of the following braces would be most appropriate in planning this patient's treatment program with the physical therapist?

A. Dorsi-plantar flexion assist
B. Dorsiflexion assist
C. Dorsiflexion stop
D. Free motion ankle joint

134. A nursing home patient is sent to physical therapy for evaluation of a decubitus ulcer. Upon evaluation, the physical therapist notices that the full thickness of the dermis is involved as well as the underlying tissues. Further evaluation determines that the ulcer may be protruding into the muscles. Given the information above, how would you classify the ulcer stage?
A. One
B. Two
C. Three
D. Four

135. You are working with a neurological patient and are concerned about promoting stability. You and the physical therapist plan a treatment course that includes proprioceptive neuromuscular facilitation (PNF) patterns to increase and promote stability in this patient. What type of PNF pattern listed below would be most appropriate?
A. Traction
B. Contract-reflex
C. Slow reversal
D. Approximation

136. You are a physical therapist assistant providing medical coverage at a high school basketball game. One of the players is injured and begins hemorrhaging. You notice that there is oozing and a gradual seeping of blood from the wounded area. It is easy for you to control the bleeding through elevation of the injured area and applying direct pressure over the wound. Which of the following is the type of hemorrhaging that this patient is most likely experiencing?
A. Arterial hemorrhage
B. Venous hemorrhage
C. Capillary hemorrhage
D. Internal hemorrhage

137. You are an educational instructor in a physical therapist assistant program. You explain to the class that scores on testing are going to be compared to standard deviation of the mean. What percentage of students taking your examination would you expect to score within plus and minus one standard deviation of the mean?
A. 68%
B. 70%
C. 72%
D. 50%

138. A patient is sent to the physical therapy department with a burn on the right lower extremity from the posterior thigh to below the knee. The patient needs to be positioned to prevent contractures of the knee. Which of the following should be immediately implemented into this patient's treatment program?
A. Exercises to increase the strength of the hamstring muscles
B. Posterior splint with emphasis on extension
C. An anterior splint with emphasis on flexion
D. A whirlpool for wound care

139. A patient is referred to the physical therapy department status post total hip replacement. The orders read "partial weightbearing utilizing a walker." Which of the following would be the most appropriate pattern given the above information?
A. Walker first, then involved lower extremity, then uninvolved extremity is advanced.
B. Walker first, then one leg, then the other leg is advanced.
C. Walker first, then uninvolved lower extremity, then involved lower extremity is advanced.
D. Uninvolved extremity, then the walker, then the involved lower extremity is advanced.

140. Patients with respiratory problems typically have a particular breathing pattern. The patient's breathing pattern can be described as follows: increasing then decreasing in depth, periods of apnea interspersed with somewhat regular rhythm. The patient is critically ill and in the intensive care unit. Based on this information, which of the following breathing patterns listed below does this patient most likely have?
    A. Biot's
    B. Orthopnea
    C. Apneusis
    D. Cheyne-Stokes

141. It is important to be ethical when performing a research study. Which of the following should take place first for a study to be ethical?
    A. The patient should be informed that he or she has the right to terminate the experiment at any time.
    B. The patient should be debriefed following the experiment.
    C. The end results of the experiment should be explained to the patient.
    D. The patient should sign an informed consent document.

142. A patient is referred to physical therapy with a cervical and vertebral disc disorder. The patient reports no previous history of cervical pain. She had a flare-up approximately 2 weeks ago, so she went to see her neurologist. The neurologist has ordered intermittent cervical traction daily along with moist heat, ultrasound, and massage. Note that the patient has no structural abnormalities and slight tenderness to pressure at this time. In implementing this patient's treatment program, which of the following would be the most appropriate set-up of traction?
    A. Cervical traction starting at 8 lbs
    B. Cervical traction starting at 16 lbs
    C. Cervical traction starting at 20 lbs
    D. Cervical traction starting at 10 lbs

143. You are performing a manual muscle test on a patient with a rotator cuff injury. You have tested the teres minor and determined that the patient has 20% strength. The patient demonstrates 100% strength on the uninjured side. Of the following, which muscle grade would you assign in your notes?
    A. Poor minus
    B. Poor
    C. Poor plus
    D. Trace

144. In implementing a treatment program for a patient who has had a nonsurgical operation for an ACL reconstruction, which of the following would be the most appropriate exercise to initiate in the beginning stages of rehabilitation?
    A. Full range isokinetics for knee flexion and extension
    B. Straight leg raises, six repetitions, with maximal weight
    C. Stair machine
    D. N-K table full range of motion, six repetitions, with maximal weight

145. You are treating a nursing home patient with a stage-three ulcer on the greater trochanter of the left hip. You are requested to instruct the nursing staff on what would be the most appropriate course of action to avoid future ulcers in other residents. Which of the following would be the most appropriate response?
    A. You are too disgusted to go to the nursing home and they will have to find another therapist.
    B. You should change the patient's position in bed to relieve weight on bony prominences every 24 hours.
    C. When lying in bed, the patient should be given a donut cushion to support bony prominences.
    D. The patient should be checked frequently for red spots and turned in bed at least every 2 hours.

146. You are a physical therapist assistant providing coverage for a small acute care hospital. During the course of the day, one of the patients is found down on the floor in the physical therapy treatment room. You rush to his side and determine that the patient is unconscious. What is the first thing you should do in examining the unconscious patient?

A. Check breathing and, if breathing is impaired, clear the airway and, if necessary, proceed to give mouth-to-mouth resuscitation.
B. Start with the head and determine first if there is any bleeding or fluid coming from the nose, ears, eyes, or mouth.
C. Check for shock.
D. Since the victim is unconscious, have someone call 911; then proceed to check the airway, breathing, and pulse.

147. You are planning on collecting data on a patient with a diagnosis of a torn meniscus. Which of the following tests would be appropriate to use for this patient when he comes to the physical therapy department?
A. Apley's compression test
B. Anterior drawer test
C. Lachman's test
D. Posterior drawer test

148. You implement a gait treatment program for a patient emphasizing the muscle group responsible for deceleration of the limb. You notice through gait observation that the patient is having a problem decelerating the unsupported limb. Which of the following muscles would be emphasized in this patient's treatment program?
A. Quadriceps group
B. Hamstring group
C. Gastrocnemius
D. Anterior tibialis

149. Your patient is a 36-year-old male who tore his anterior cruciate ligament skiing downhill in the winter. After much consideration, the patient and surgeon decided to take a nonsurgical rehabilitation course. What functional level would you expect for this patient as the outcome of physical therapy treatment?
A. The patient will be able to participate at all activity levels in various sports.
B. The patient will have to avoid further athletic events for a period of 3 years.
C. The patient will be able to participate in light activities or sports with the assistance of bracing.
D. The patient will have to avoid all athletic events for 1 year.

150. You are treating a patient status post anterior cruciate ligament surgery. The orthopedic surgeon has developed a plan of care for this patient with a specific protocol. Initially, the patient is to receive closed-chain kinetic rehabilitation. Of the following exercises, which would be appropriate to start with this patient?
A. Isokinetic with extension blocked minus 20°
B. Straight leg raises in all planes
C. Stair machine
D. Short-arc quads

151. You are participating in a track and field event on a hot summer day in July. The temperature is extremely hot with high humidity. The physical therapist that is participating with you becomes severely dehydrated and, with exposure to the severe heat, goes into shock. Your colleague falls to the ground and needs immediate attention. Which of the following is the first step of action that should be taken with your colleague?
A. After a fall, you should first check for any wounds to see if bleeding is present.
B. Body temperature should be reduced by placing cold towels or cloths on your colleague.
C. Body position should be arranged with the head and trunk higher than the limbs.
D. If available, oxygen should be administered.

152. You are working in the spinal cord unit with a C6 spinal cord patient. Your functional outcome for this patient is for him to be able to perform independent bed mobility with side rails. In the treatment program, which of the following muscles would you most likely emphasize?
A. Pectoralis major
B. Neck musculature
C. Scapula musculature
D. Biceps muscle

153. A patient is being discharged from the hospital to her home. To provide for continuity of care, the patient will continue to receive home physical therapy for total knee replacement. As the physical therapist assistant, which of the following would be the appropriate action for you to take to assure the patient's continuity of care?
    A. Refer the patient to a home health physical therapist whom you have heard good reports.
    B. Report to the patient's home yourself and treat him or her on the side, away from the hospital.
    C. Provide the social worker a report on the patient's status.
    D. Telephone the physical therapist who will be continuing to see the patient at home and give the therapist an update on the patient, as well as a report on the appropriate exercises you have been performing, including any protocols.

154. You are treating a patient who has the following clinical features: muscle twitching and cramping in the lower calf, spasms in the gastrocnemius muscle, and heavy sweating. Which of the following heat disorders is this patient most likely experiencing?
    A. Heat cramps
    B. Heat syncope
    C. Heat exhaustion
    D. Heat hyperpyrexia

155. A patient has an impingement syndrome of the right rotator cuff. You are to implement a therapeutic exercise program with the physical therapist to consist of increasing range of motion, as well as strengthening. The patient is in an acute stage, reporting pain at a 6 to 7 level on a scale of 1 to 10, 10 being severe. Which of the following exercises would be the most appropriate to begin?
    A. Isokinetic exercise
    B. Walking on a finger ladder from 0 to 140°, 20 repetitions
    C. Resistive active movement from 0 to 160° with the therapist providing resistance
    D. Therapy in a stretching program below 90° specifically for supraspinatus and teres minor

156. You are a physical therapist assistant teamed up with a physical therapist and a physical therapy aide in an outpatient clinic. As a team, you work with a set of 12 to 15 patients together daily. Mrs. Smith comes in for physical therapy requiring hot pack, ultrasound, traction, and massage. Which of the following of these activities would not be appropriate to delegate to the physical therapy aide?
    A. Hot pack
    B. Ultrasound
    C. Traction
    D. Massage

157. You have a pediatric patient whose symmetrical tonic reflex must be checked. You provide the test stimulus by flexing the patient's head. Which of the following best describes a positive reaction to this test stimulus?
    A. The arms will flex and the legs will extend
    B. The arms will extend and the legs will flex
    C. The arms will flex and the legs will flex
    D. The arms will extend and the legs will extend

158. A patient comes to the clinic with burns on the left anterior arm and left anterior leg. You have scheduled sterile whirlpool debridement and preparation of dressings for this patient. Utilizing the Rule of Nines and assuming this patient is an adult, what would be the specific value for the percentage of burns suffered by this patient?
    A. 4.5%
    B. 9%
    C. 13.5%
    D. 18%

159. A patient is sent to you for bracing as a result of a fracture at the level of T10 to L1. The physical therapist recommends a rigid high-back brace for stabilization. Which of the following braces listed would be most appropriate to plan for this patient?

A. Lumbar corset
B. Taylor brace
C. Knight Taylor spinal brace
D. Jewett brace

160. You are working in the physical therapy department with a child who has suffered burns on the left arm and left leg. Utilizing the Rule of Nines, which of the following specific values listed below would correctly describe the percentage of the body burned?
    A. 13.5%
    B. 23%
    C. 18%
    D. 36%

161. You are observing the gait deviation of an individual who just had a below-the-knee prosthesis on his amputated leg. You notice that when the patient is walking in the parallel bars, he has a medial whip to his gait. Which of the following would be the first appropriate component to check on this patient?
    A. Remove the prosthesis and check for red sores
    B. Check the resistance on the plantar flexion bumper
    C. Check to see if the socket is appropriately fitted
    D. Check to see if the knee bolt alignment is too lateral

162. You are observing the gait of another individual with a prosthetic. In observing the gait, you notice that the socket has a poor fit and appears to have a weak suspension system, and the knee friction is too soft. Which of the following would be the most likely gait deviation that you would observe?
    A. Lateral whip
    B. Rotation of the foot at heel strike
    C. Instability of the knee
    D. Pistoning of the socket

163. You are performing a gait reevaluation on a patient who has injured his right lower extremity. In evaluating the patient's gait, you notice that he will not bear weight on the injured extremity. When ambulating, he takes a short step to transfer weight to the uninjured side as quickly as possible. Which of the following types of gait would best describe this patient's symptoms?
    A. Steppage gait
    B. Foot slap
    C. Antalgic gait
    D. Abducted lurch

164. You have a patient suffering from low back pain secondary to a posture disorder. The patient enters the clinic bent over, with weight shifted laterally to the right. Your short-term goal is to instruct this patient so that he is independent in proper posture and body mechanics. The patient has very limited time and needs to receive moist heat, ultrasound, and traction. The patient is going to be seen daily for 2 weeks. On which day should proper posture be introduced?
    A. Day 1
    B. Day 2
    C. Day 3
    D. Day 6, after the patient is pain-free

165. In implementing a cardiopulmonary-pulmonary program for a chest physical therapy patient, which of the following positions is most appropriate for the middle lobe?
    A. Patient is sitting in a chair leaning forward approximately 20° to 30°, resting on pillows.
    B. Patient is in prone position, rotated a half turn upward, with the bed elevated 18 inches, chest tilted 20°.
    C. Patient is prone with pillows under the stomach.
    D. Patient is in left sidelying position, rotated backward a half turn, with the bed elevated 14 inches.

166. When observing a stage-three decubitus ulcer of a patient, which of the following would be the least important to note in the progress notes?
    A. The size of the wound
    B. Temperature
    C. Hip muscle strength
    D. Drainage and color

167. You are implementing an exercise program with a physical therapist for a patient who is rehabilitated after right shoulder pain. Which of the following would you suggest in a treatment program of a patient to assist in instructing him or her in functional training and carryover?
    A. Isokinetic rehabilitation
    B. PNF movements
    C. The shoulder wheel
    D. Dressing and undressing activities

168. You are presenting an inservice on the advantages and disadvantages of the following exercises: isometric, isokinetic, isotonic, and eccentric contractions. You inform the group that some of the disadvantages of this particular exercise are that the muscle strength is limited to range of motion, there is no improvement in muscle endurance, and no eccentric work is created. These disadvantages best describe which of the following classifications of exercise?
    A. Isometric
    B. Isotonic
    C. Isokinetic
    D. Free weights

169. In further explaining the different types of exercises, you state that the advantage of this form of exercise is that it allows for variable velocity training and control of the velocity. Which of the following classifications of exercise are you now describing?
    A. Nautilus
    B. Universal
    C. Free weights
    D. Isokinetics

170. You are analyzing a patient's cardiopulmonary-pulmonary status at the physical therapy department. You notice during chest physical therapy that percussion sounds dull with wheezing and crackles upon auscultation. These clinical signs are most likely associated with which one of the following lung pathologies?
    A. Atelectasis
    B. Pulmonary edema
    C. Pneumonia
    D. Pneumothorax

171. You have a cardiac patient 3 days postoperative referred to the cardiac rehab program. The physician refers the patient to physical therapy for the physical therapist to evaluate and develop a treatment program. Of the following, which treatment program would be appropriate for this patient at this stage?
    A. Ambulating 200 yards in a 5-minute period with no EKG changes in symptoms
    B. Lower extremity ergometry x 15 minutes
    C. Lower extremity ergometry x 30 minutes
    D. Upper extremity ergometry x 15 minutes

172. You are performing a treatment program for a neurological patient. The physical therapist assistant moves the patient's extremity through a predetermined range of motion. This motion is shoulder flexion and extension. Then the patient is requested to repeat the movement on her own. Which of the following are you most likely performing on this patient?
    A. Kinesthesia
    B. Proprioception
    C. Graphesthesia
    D. Barognosis

173. You are reading the medical chart of a patient status post myocardial infarct. Included on the patient's chart is an electrocardiogram. The electrocardiogram shows an absent P-wave. This would be indicative of which of the following abnormalities?
    A. Ischemia
    B. Infarct
    C. Ventricular arrhythmia
    D. Pericarditis

174. A 25-year-old female 6 days post-cesarean delivery is to receive training in proper posture and body mechanics. Which of the following would be the proper instructions for body mechanics for a post-cesarean patient?
    A. Whenever sitting, the patient should avoid hard chairs because they have poor back support.
    B. When standing, the patient should relax the abdominal muscles in order not to place any strain upon them.
    C. When bending over, the patient should keep a flattened lordotic curve in the low back and a wide base of support with legs parallel.
    D. When getting up from a lying position, the patient should roll over to the side, swinging the legs over the edge, and get up slowly.

175. You are treating a patient who comes to physical therapy complaining of lower thoracic pain. Upon palpation, you notice no significant structural or muscular problems. You decide to test the patient's reflexes, particularly the upper abdominal reflex. Which of the following levels listed below are you testing?
    A. Thoracic 10, 11, 12
    B. Thoracic 8, 9, 10
    C. Thoracic 5, 6, 7
    D. Thoracic 9, 10, 11

176. A patient is in the clinic being treated for low back pain. You place the patient on a hot pack for 20 minutes. You instruct the patient to call you if he feels too warm. You leave the room to dictate a short note about the patient. Upon leaving the room, you hear a crash and return to find the patient on the floor, not breathing. Which of the following would be the first procedure to perform in a cardiopulmonary resuscitation?
    A. Prior to performing CPR, call code blue.
    B. Go over to the patient and begin CPR by opening the airway and tilting the head back.
    C. You have let your CPR certification lapse so you call another therapist who is certified to come over and begin CPR.
    D. Immediately begin mouth-to-mouth with five breaths in the patient.

177. Which of the following modalities would be most appropriate to implement in a treatment program for back pain in the following patient: patient is a 24-year-old female, 2 months into her pregnancy. Patient has a long-standing history of chronic back pain as a result of an automobile accident 6 years ago. Patient currently is reporting acute pain across the low back when sitting, standing for long periods of time, and driving.
    A. Rest in a sidelying position, supported with pillows between her knees.
    B. Moist heat for 20 minutes in a sidelying position.
    C. Ultrasound pulsed at 2.0 watts per centimeter squared.
    D. Alternate knee to chest exercises.

178. A truck driver is sent to physical therapy with a diagnosis of Bell's palsy. The patient related that he has been driving for 3 days continuously for periods of 12 to 14 hours on the road. The patient reports that he kept his window rolled down so that he could get fresh air to keep himself awake. What type of treatment program listed below would be most effective for this patient?
    A. DC (direct current) electrical stimulation to the motor points
    B. Iontophoresis for the inflammation
    C. High-volt electrical stimulation
    D. Massage

179. The physical therapist is performing an inservice on proper body mechanics to a group of physical therapist assistants. Which of the following best describes the domain in education that deals with motor skills?
    A. Cognitive
    B. Affective
    C. Psychomotor
    D. Motor skills

180. You are treating a patient who is complaining of right shoulder pain. The patient has been diagnosed with a frozen adhesive capsulated shoulder. Which of the following would describe the capsular pattern of the glenohumeral joint?
    A. External rotation, abduction, internal rotation
    B. External rotation, internal rotation, abduction
    C. Internal rotation, abduction, external rotation
    D. Abduction, external rotation, internal rotation

181. You are implementing a treatment program for bed mobility on a C4 quadriplegic. You have instructed the patient in the importance of maintaining normal range of motion, the importance of checking for pressure sores, and monitoring respiratory status. You now are especially concerned with strengthening the muscles of the patient. You want the patient to be able to move from supine to sitting and back using an electric bed. In implementing a strengthening program, which of the following would you be emphasizing?
    A. Neck musculature
    B. Triceps
    C. Wrist extensors
    D. Shoulder depressors

182. You are treating a pediatric patient with cystic fibrosis. The patient suffers from excessive secretions. The patient was diagnosed with cystic fibrosis through a sweat test administered by the physician. Which of the following would be an appropriate treatment program for this patient?
    A. Breathing exercises
    B. Breathing exercises and postural drainage
    C. Medication therapy should be ordered by the physician
    D. Chest physical therapy

183. In treating a 36-year-old patient for hip pain, you notice, when measuring range of motion, that the patient demonstrates a capsular pattern in the hip. Which of the following best describes the capsular pattern that this patient most likely demonstrates secondary to inflammatory process of the hip?
    A. Extension, abduction, internal rotation
    B. Flexion, abduction, internal rotation
    C. Flexion, adduction, internal rotation
    D. Internal rotation, flexion, abduction

184. You have been working with a patient who demonstrates equilibrium coordination deficits during treatment. Which of the following tests would be important to evaluate the equilibrium coordination of this patient?
    A. Observe the patient's posture while the body is in motion.
    B. Have the patient perform finger-to-nose and finger-to-finger tests, and evaluate the quality of movement.
    C. Test the patient's ability to judge distance and speed of movement by drawing a circle.
    D. Evaluate the quality of movement control and speed with the patient pointing.

185. You are treating a 16-year-old male diagnosed with chondromalacia, degeneration of the patellar surface. The patient is very active and participates in football, basketball, and baseball. Of the following, which exercise would you recommend in this patient's treatment program?
    A. Quadriceps exercise in extension
    B. Short arc quads
    C. Isokinetic, limiting extension to -30°
    D. Exercise bike

186. You are going to perform a grade-one mobilization on a glenohumeral joint of a 26-year-old patient. Mobilization should not be performed when the joint is in a closed-packed position. Which of the following answers best describes a closed-packed position of the glenohumeral joint?
    A. Adduction, external rotation
    B. Extension
    C. Abduction, internal rotation
    D. Abduction, external rotation

187. A patient is referred to physical therapy for sensory testing. The physical therapist has requested that you evaluate the protective sensations of the patient and recommend a treatment program to enhance them. Which of the following would be the most appropriate test to perform on this patient?
    A. Deep pressure
    B. Proprioception
    C. Two-point discrimination
    D. Light touch

188. The physical therapist recommended that you develop a treatment program to enhance a patient's protective sensations. Which of the following would be the most appropriate to recommend as a treatment option?
    A. Use test tubes, one with hot water and one with cold water.
    B. Treat the patient using sharp and dull to enhance stimulation.
    C. Have the patient hold an object in the hand and try to determine the weight.
    D. Use a cottonball and rub lightly against the patient's skin.

189. You are treating a neurological patient in a rehabilitation unit. You are treating the patient according to the theories of Brunnstrom. Which of the following would be an appropriate treatment emphasis according to Brunnstrom?
    A. Limb synergies are a necessary intermediate stage of recovery and the patient should be encouraged to use limb synergy patterns.
    B. Patient should learn diagonal patterns of movement.
    C. Do not reinforce abnormal patterns of movement.
    D. Do not use associated reactions.

190. You are fabricating an orthotic for a patient with a left foot disorder. The patient has a diagnosis of pes planus. The patient will require a longitudinal arch for support and to correct the pes planus. Which of the following shoe modifications would most likely be prescribed for this patient?
    A. Thomas heel
    B. Rocker bottom
    C. Scaphoid pads
    D. Metatarsal bars

191. You are implementing a treatment program for a patient who has a noncemented total hip replacement. You are to implement the treatment program considering the patient's ambulation requirements while in the hospital and leaving the hospital. The patient will require an assistive device for gait activities. In implementing this treatment program, how long can you anticipate that this patient will require an assistive device for gait?
    A. 2 weeks
    B. 1 month
    C. 8 weeks
    D. 3 months

192. You are a physical therapist assistant who has been sent out to consult with a nursing home secondary to ulcers on the ischial tuberosity of several patients. Upon entering the nursing home you begin to observe the patient. You notice redness, edema, blistering, and hardening of the tissue. The inflammation has extended into the fat layer and there is superficial necrosis. Which of the following stages in characterized by such symptoms?

A. Stage one
B. Stage two
C. Stage three
D. Stage four

193. You are implementing a treatment program for a patient who needs to improve his gait pattern. You reevaluate the patient's gait and notice that the patient is having difficulty in initiating the swing phase of gait. Which of the following muscles would be most appropriate to emphasize in this patient's rehabilitation?
    A. Hamstring group
    B. Quadriceps group
    C. Gastrocnemius
    D. Anterior tibialis

194. A patient comes to the clinic complaining of severe pain following a sprain that occurred approximately 3 months ago. The patient reports that the pain is persistent and above the normal level that he had typically experienced on previous sprains. The patient has had recurring ankle sprains for the past 3 to 4 years. The patient reports that typically the sprain heals and goes away in approximately 1 to 2 weeks. Initially, he had swelling and increased warmth in the ankle. The patient reports that in the past 2 months he has noticed that the skin has appeared shiny and leathery around the ankle. In planning this patient's treatment program with the physical therapist, which of the following would be most appropriate?
    A. Range of motion exercises
    B. Contrast baths, electrical stimulation, and range of motion
    C. Whirlpool treatments
    D. Therapeutic exercises consisting of an ankle progressive resistive exercise machine

195. You are implementing a treatment program for a patient who is 1-day post cesarean delivery in the OB/GYN ward of the acute care hospital where you work. Which of the following would not be an appropriate exercise program on day 1?
    A. Diaphragmatic breathing
    B. Huffing
    C. Pelvic floor exercises
    D. Leg slides

196. On performing a musculoskeletal reassessment of a patient, you particularly note the end-feel of the glenohumeral joint. The end-feel can be characterized as a hard, leather-like stoppage at the end of range of motion. There is full normal range of motion of the shoulder with a slight give at the end. Which of the following best describes the end-feel of this particular patient?
    A. Bone-to-bone end-feel
    B. Capsular end-feel
    C. Empty end-feel
    D. Springy block end-feel

197. The physical therapist is evaluating a patient with a cerebrovascular injury that presents the following symptoms: decreased balance, ataxia, decreased coordination, and a decreased ability for postural adjustment. These symptoms would best describe which of the following cerebrovascular accidents?
    A. Right hemisphere
    B. Left hemisphere
    C. Brainstem
    D. Cerebellar

198. You are assisting in planning the diet of a runner for a prolonged low-intensity running event. You are determining the number of calories required in the conversion process for energy for the runner. The number of calories required is different for protein, carbohydrates, and fats. One gram of carbohydrate yields 4 calories. How many grams of fat would yield 9 calories for this runner?

A. 1
B. 2.25
C. 3
D. 4

199. A physical therapist is practicing in a rural setting and supervising a physical therapist assistant and a physical therapy aide. The physical therapist will be off for 1 day to attend a continuing education course on preventing low back pain in OB/GYN patients. While the physical therapist is away, the physical therapist assistant will be able to perform all the following duties except?
A. Carry out modified treatment programs
B. Supervise the physical therapy aide
C. Evaluate new patients
D. Write progress notes

200. A physician has performed a test on a patient to determine the intensity of a current required to produce a minimal muscle contraction. This test results in a graph plotting the excitability of the muscle against a set of measured duration. Which of the following tests does this best describe?
A. Strength duration curve
B. Electromyogram
C. Nerve conduction velocity
D. Chronaxie

201. You are performing a respiratory assessment on a patient for a chest physical therapy program. When reading the chart, you are looking at the values of testing performed by the respiratory therapist. One of the particular values that you are noting is the amount of air that can be forcibly expired by the patient after maximum inspiration. Which of the following was the respiratory therapist evaluating?
A. Forced expiratory volume
B. Forced inspiratory volume
C. Inspiratory capacity
D. Tidal volume

202. You are treating a 16-year-old male status post ACL reconstruction on the right knee. The patient was injured in summer practice for the upcoming football season. The patient has responded very well to physical therapy and is aggressively rehabilitating the right knee. It is the patient's goal to return to the football team in time for the play-offs in December. Based on the above information, what would be an appropriate time to implement a therapeutic exercise program consisting of isokinetics?
A. 8 weeks postoperative
B. 12 weeks postoperative
C. Check with the referring physician's protocol
D. 6 weeks postoperative so the patient can return to football in time for the play-offs

203. You are treating a 40-year-old woman with a diagnosis of frozen adhesive capsulitis of the right shoulder. The patient comes to the clinic on day 1 complaining of acute pain and limited range of motion. You begin mobilization to reduce pain and at least maintain joint motion. Which of the following grades of mobilization would be best implemented at this stage in the rehabilitation?
A. Grade one
B. Grade three
C. Grade four
D. Grade five

204. You are working with a 16-year-old high school cross-country runner. Which of the following effects would occur through aerobic exercise in a cardiopulmonary training program for this patient?
A. Resting heart rate increases
B. Cardiac output decreases
C. Tidal volume decreases
D. Resting heart rate decreases

205. You and the physical therapist are planning a treatment program for a neurological patient. You and the PT have determined that to achieve the best neurological rehabilitation you will be using exteroceptive stimulation techniques. Which of the following is not an example of this technique?
A. Prolonged icing
B. Quick stretch of the muscle belly and tendon
C. High-frequency vibration
D. Rhythmic stabilization

206. You are treating a patient with a prosthesis in the gait laboratory of the physical therapy department. During observation, you discover that the patient's prosthesis is too long and the socket is too small. It also appears to have an inadequate suspension. Which of the following gait deviations would this patient most likely demonstrate?
A. Lateral trunk bending
B. Medial whip
C. Circumduction
D. Lateral whip

207. You have treated a patient with neck pain for 2 weeks. Today she returns to the clinic complaining of acute cervical spine pain. On a scale of 1 to 10, 10 being unbearable pain, the patient reports pain at level 9. Active range of motion for flexion is limited to approximately 25% of movement. Manual muscle testing, using the break test method, reveals a fair minus grade of cervical flexion. In writing a progress note, you identify the patient's short-term goals. Which of the following would be an example of a short-term goal for this patient?
A. Patient will be able to demonstrate proper posture and body mechanics.
B. Patient will decrease pain level from a 9 to a 7 in a 1-week period.
C. Manual muscle test will reveal strength increase from a fair to a normal grade.
D. Patient will be able to independently perform a home exercise program.

208. You are performing mobilization on a patient to decrease pain and increase range of motion. It is the patient's first time in the rehabilitation department and you thoroughly explain what to anticipate from the mobilization. You begin by mobilizing the involved side first and comparing it to the uninvolved. Which of the following would not be an absolute contraindication to performing mobilization on this patient?
A. Active inflammation
B. Active infection
C. Hypermobility
D. Recent fracture

209. In implementing a prenatal care program for a patient, which one of the following elements may not be included in her physical therapy regimen?
A. Relaxation training
B. Kegel exercises
C. ADL modifications
D. Valsalva's maneuver

210. The physical therapist is testing the reflexes of a pediatric patient. In testing, the patient demonstrates a startle response when his head suddenly drops backward unsupported. In addition to the startle response, the patient's arms extend and abduct. Which of the following reflexes is most likely being tested?
A. Moro's reflex
B. Protective reflex
C. Landau reflex
D. Equilibrium

211. You are treating a patient who has suffered a second-degree collateral ligament injury. The patient injured the knee as a result of a lateral hit to the knee during football practice. The patient is currently 2 days post injury. Which of the following would be the recommended treatment for a second-degree medial collateral ligament injury?

A. Crutch ambulation with toe-touch weightbearing
B. Swimming x 20 minutes, flutter kick only
C. Exercise bike x 15 minutes
D. Whirlpool for range of motion

212. You are a physical therapist assistant (PTA) who is going to give an inservice to another PTA on the APTA code of ethics as it relates to a PTA. Which of the following would not be an APTA code of ethics standard relating to the physical therapist assistant?
A. Physical therapist assistants are to provide services under the supervision of a physical therapist.
B. Physical therapist assistants accept the responsibility to protect the public and profession from unethical, incompetent, or illegal acts.
C. Physical therapist assistants make judgments that are commensurate with their qualifications.
D. Physical therapist assistants may independently carry out any procedures in physical therapy.

213. You are performing isokinetic testing on a patient status post hip injury. Utilizing standard testing protocols, which of the following would be the first consideration for isokinetic testing?
A. Test the uninvolved side first
B. Have the patient do warm-ups
C. Educate the patient
D. Look up the appropriate testing protocols

214. You are implementing a treatment program for a 26-year-old female who is approximately 2 months away from delivering a baby. The patient has been sent to the clinic for low back pain. In implementing a treatment program, which of the following exercises would not be appropriate for this patient to perform?
A. Diaphragmatic breathing
B. Pelvic floor exercise
C. Partial curl-ups
D. Postural instructions

215. You read the following in the patient's chart: the patient responds appropriately and has an intact dermatone distribution for the anterior thigh. However, below the knee level at the lateral aspect crossing the knee to the medial aspect into the half greater toe, the patient cannot distinguish between sharp and dull. Given this information, which of the following is most likely the level of dermatome involved?
A. L1
B. L3
C. L4
D. S1

216. This case study involves a spinal cord patient. The patient has the following functional outcomes: vital capacity is 80%, patient is independent with floor to wheelchair transfers, patient can perform gait with bilateral knee-ankle-foot orthosis (KAFO) and a walker. Based on this information, which is probably the level of lesion of this patient?
A. T1 to T5
B. T9 to T12
C. L4 to L5
D. T6 to T8

217. You are collecting data on a patient with a complaint of foot and ankle pain. You are observing the ability of the patient to adduct, plantar flex, and invert the foot. Which of the following muscles listed below are you observing?
A. Tibialis anterior
B. Tibialis posterior
C. Peroneus longus
D. Peroneus brevis

218. You are a physical therapist assistant student who is studying the classes of levers in kinesiology. The instructor describes one class of lever in the following way: a common example is a seesaw, or in the body, an example would be the atlantooccipital joint. With the information given above, which of the following is most likely the class of lever described?
    A. First-class lever
    B. Second-class lever
    C. Third-class lever
    D. Fourth-class lever

219. You are treating a patient with an anterior thigh bruise on the right lower extremity. You notice considerable discoloration 6 inches above the knee. The patient is tender to palpation and swelling is present. You attempt to perform manual muscle testing of the quadriceps muscle. The patient does not have complete range of motion secondary to edema. You can palpate a contraction upon testing, but the patient is in severe pain. Given the information above, what would be the most appropriate response to define the muscle testing grade for this patient?
    A. Zero
    B. Trace
    C. Poor
    D. Fair

220. The physical therapist has ordered whirlpool and debridement to assist in the healing process of a patient with a 2-day-old wound injury. The patient has inflammation as a result of the injury. The layered skin that has been damaged is composed largely of fibrous connective tissue. The nerve fiber and blood vessels are located in this area. Which layer of the tissue has been damaged based on the above description?
    A. The epidermis
    B. The dermis
    C. The subcutaneous layer
    D. Adipose cells

221. The patient comes to the clinic with an injury to the skin as a result of exposure to excessive heat. Which of the following will be the first response to this type of skin injury?
    A. The fluids will seep into the damaged tissue.
    B. The blood vessels will become dilated and more permeable secondary to inflammation.
    C. Phagocytic cells will remove dead cells and debridement of the area will occur.
    D. Blood clotting will occur.

222. A 33-year-old female is referred to the clinic by a local dentist with a diagnosis of TMJ. The physical therapist requests that you perform a treatment. During the treatment you are monitoring the patient's ability to open and close her jaw. Which of the following muscles would you be evaluating during observation of the patient's ability to open the jaw?
    A. Pterygoideus medialis muscle
    B. Pterygoideus lateralis muscle
    C. Temporoparietalis muscle
    D. Masseter muscle

223. A patient is referred to physical therapy status post fracture to the left wrist joint. The physical therapist has ordered mobilization to the joint to assist with increasing movement. In order to perform mobilization, it is necessary to know what type of joint you will be treating. Which of the following best describes the radial carpal articulation of the wrist joint?
    A. Condyloid joint
    B. Hinge joint
    C. Pivot joint
    D. Saddle joint

224. A patient reports to physical therapy with a diagnosis of a fracture on the right humerus. He informs you that the fracture occurred at the midshaft of the humerus as a result of falling down a flight of steps. Given the information above, which of the following nerves would most likely be damaged secondary to this injury?
    A. Median nerve
    B. Subscapular nerve
    C. Ulnar nerve
    D. Radial nerve

225. A 22-year-old male was involved in an automobile accident in which he was a passenger pulled out of a burning car. As a result, the patient suffered a brachial plexus injury to the terminal branches of the lateral cord. Which of the following muscles would you not expect this patient to be having a problem with?
    A. Biceps
    B. Coracobrachialis
    C. Deltoid
    D. Pectoralis major

226. A patient is a 26-year-old male patient status post arthroscopic surgery. The physical therapist requests that you reevaluate the muscles that insert into the pes anserinus. You have the patient flex the knee and medially rotate the leg while the knee is flexed. Of the muscles listed below, which are you not evaluating?
    A. Gracilis
    B. Sartorius
    C. Semimembranosus
    D. Semitendinosus

227. A patient has a lesion in the tibial nerve. Which one of the following muscles would not be affected by this condition?
    A. Flexor hallucis longus
    B. Peroneus tertius
    C. Flexor digitorum longus
    D. Tibialis posterior

228. The physician has sent a patient to the clinic for a brace, which will assist in controlling knee rotation and adduction. Which of the following ligaments was most likely injured?
    A. Anterior cruciate ligament
    B. Posterior cruciate ligament
    C. Medial collateral ligament
    D. Lateral collateral ligament

229. A patient comes to the clinic secondary to a right ankle sprain. The patient reports that he was playing basketball when his foot landed on another player's foot, causing a severe twisting injury. The patient has been diagnosed as having an injury that resulted from an inversion sprain. Which of the following ligaments would least likely need to be rehabilitated with this patient?
    A. Anterior talofibular ligament
    B. Calcaneofibular ligament
    C. Deltoid ligament
    D. Posterior talofibular ligament

230. In a class on clinical pathology, the professor asks you what lupus erythematosus, scleroderma, and dermatomycosis have in common. They can best be grouped together as which of the following?
    A. Acute infections
    B. Acute bacterial diseases
    C. Collagen vascular diseases
    D. Circulatory disorders

231. In clinical pathology the professor describes a pathological disease that involves the arteries and veins of the lower extremity. The symptoms are inflammation, venous thrombosis, and ischemia of the feet. Which of the following diseases is being described by the professor?
    A. Raynaud's disease
    B. Thromboangiitis obliterans
    C. Thrombophlebitis
    D. Pitting edema

232. You receive an order from an inpatient physical therapy department for range of motion and strengthening to both upper extremities and the left lower extremity. Upon arriving at the patient's bedside, you notice that the patient has the right lower extremity in balance skeletal traction. Which of the following areas has this patient most likely fractured?
    A. Patella
    B. Femur
    C. Tibia
    D. Lateral malleolus

233. The patient is sent to physical therapy secondary to a lower extremity injury. Reading the patient's past medical history you note that the superficial peroneal nerve has been damaged. Which of the following muscles would be emphasized in your treatment program?
    A. Tibialis anterior
    B. Peroneus tertius
    C. Peroneus brevis
    D. Extensor hallucis longus

234. You are in cardiology class studying the difference between cardiac muscle versus skeletal muscle. It is known that the cardiac muscle is physiologically different from skeletal muscle. Which of the following statements best describes this?
    A. It has no bony attachments
    B. The actin and myosin filaments produce a different type of striation
    C. It does not develop a length-tension relationship
    D. It divides into atrial and ventricular proportions

235. While studying cardiology you are learning about cardiac output. Cardiac output refers to the amount of blood pumped by the heart in a specific time period. Which of the following best describes cardiac output?
    A. Blood pumped by the heart in a 24-hour period
    B. Blood pumped by the heart in 1 hour
    C. Blood pumped by the heart during a 60-second period
    D. Blood pumped by the heart during an 8-hour period

236. In a class on cardiology, the professor is lecturing on Sterling's law of the heart. Which of the following best sums up Sterling's law of the heart?
    A. Stretching the heart muscle will cause it to weaken.
    B. Stretching the heart muscle will result in decreased cardiac output.
    C. Stretching the heart muscle will increase the vigor of contractions.
    D. Exercise which is extremely vigorous and prolonged may stretch the heart beyond its limits.

237. The cardiac chamber experiences both a period of contraction and a period of relaxation. Which of the following would best describe the relaxation phase of the cardiac chamber?
    A. Diastole
    B. Systole
    C. Syncope
    D. Tachycardia

238. You are performing cardiac rehabilitation with an acute patient and he experiences severe heart failure. Which of the following symptoms will not be exhibited by this patient?
    A. Decrease in normal cardiac output
    B. Hypertrophy
    C. Higher than normal cardiac output
    D. High-end diastolic pressure

239. You are working with a patient who has a stroke volume and pulse pressure, which are small. Which of the following lesions would the patient most likely have?
    A. Atrial sclerotic disease
    B. Mitral stenosis
    C. Congestive heart failure
    D. Myocardial infarct

240. You are studying the signs and symptoms of congestive heart failure. Which of the following would not be a sign or a symptom of congestive heart failure?
    A. Pitting edema
    B. Excessive fluid in the intercellular space
    C. Stenosis
    D. Orthopnea

241. A 43-year-old male executive has a myocardial infarction. He is brought to the emergency room of the hospital where you work. His myocardial infarction is in a frequent location for patients. Which of the following is the most frequent location for a myocardial infarction to occur?
    A. Left atrium
    B. Left ventricle
    C. Right atrium
    D. Right ventricle

242. You are treating an 83-year-old patient whose diagnosis is a CVA. Which of the following is the most common cause of a CVA in older adults?
    A. Aneurysm
    B. Hemorrhaging
    C. High blood pressure
    D. Thrombosis

243. You have a patient in cardiac rehabilitation. You are monitoring the patient's EKG wave with the physical therapist. You notice an irregularity of the P wave in the patient while he is exercising on the treadmill. The P wave of the EKG corresponds to which of the following?
    A. Atrial repolarization
    B. Atrial depolarization
    C. Mitral repolarization
    D. Mitral depolarization

244. You have a patient who is on medication for chronic congestive heart failure. In reading the chart you note that the patient is taking digitalis. Which of the following actions of digitalis would be common on a patient with chronic congestive heart failure?
    A. A decrease in heart rate
    B. An increase in heart rate
    C. A decrease in the strength of the contraction
    D. No effect on heart rate

245. You are treating a pulmonary patient bedside for passive range of motion. There is no edema noted in this patient's lower extremities. However, the patient is developing an acute pulmonary edema. Given this information, which of the following types of heart diseases would this most likely indicate?

A. Left atrial
B. Left ventricular
C. Right atrial
D. Right ventricular

246. Rheumatoid arthritis can cause many symptoms in the later stages. Which of the following symptoms would most likely be common in a patient with rheumatoid arthritis for a long duration?
A. Radial deviation of the fingers
B. Enlargement of Heberden's nodes
C. Ulnar deviation of the fingers
D. Increased muscle strength

247. A patient is recently admitted to the hospital emergency room after falling down the stairs at home. This 62-year-old female complains of pain in her left groin and gluteal area. You observe that the left hip is in flexion, adduction, and internal rotation. Which of the following is the patient most likely suffering?
A. A gluteus maximus strain
B. A dislocated hip
C. A fractured femoral head
D. An adductor muscle strain

248. A patient is referred to you from the arthritis center. The patient has a diagnosis of osteoarthritis. Which of the following would differentiate osteoarthritis from rheumatoid arthritis?
A. Bones are involved rather than the joints
B. Weightbearing joints are involved
C. Osteoarthritis is a systemic disease
D. There are acute inflammatory signs and symptoms

249. A patient comes to the clinic with a complaint of severe knee pain. During the physical therapist's evaluation, you observe that the knee joint is extremely swollen and warm. Upon testing, the tibia can be displaced posteriorly on the femur. There appears to be considerable pain and instability of the knee joint during evaluation. Which of the following structures is most likely involved?
A. Anterior cruciate ligament
B. Posterior cruciate ligament
C. Medial meniscus
D. Lateral meniscus

250. A patient is sent to physical therapy with orders for mobilization to the shoulder. More specifically, the physical therapist calls you and notifies you that he wants inferior glide performed to the humeral head. Which of the following positions should the shoulder be placed in to perform this?
A. Abduction to 5°
B. Abduction to 10°
C. Abduction to 20°
D. Abduction to 30°

251. You are observing the patient's ability to flex and fully extend the knee. Which of the following muscles is responsible for unlocking the knee from a full extension position?
A. Biceps femoris
B. Gastrocnemius
C. Popliteus
D. Semitendinosus

252. A patient comes to the clinic suffering from second-degree burns. The injury occurred approximately 1 day ago and the patient is in the initial stage of wound repair. Wound healing typically occurs in four stages. Of the following stages, which is the patient most likely in?

A. Differentiation
B. Migration
C. Mobilization
D. Proliferation

253. A patient is evaluated in a nursing home for an ulcer in the greater trochanter. The wound destruction is described in the following way: it involves full thickness of the dermis and undermining of the deeper tissues and the muscle is slightly involved. There is no bone destruction. Given this information, which of the following stages would best describe this ulcer?
A. Stage one
B. Stage two
C. Stage three
D. Stage four

254. As the process of age takes place, there are changes in the neurological system. Which of the following would not be a process of aging?
A. Toxication of the meninges
B. 20% reduction of blood flow
C. Increase in ventricular size
D. Reduction of nerve conduction velocity

255. An athlete will be participating in competition on an extremely hot afternoon. It will be important that the athlete receives plenty of hydration during the prolonged softball tournament. Water comprises what percentage of weight in the human body?
A. 30%
B. 40%
C. 50%
D. 70%

256. A patient is sent to physical therapy to be set up on an exercise program to assist in weight loss. The patient has knee problems, which he feels are due to his overweight status. Which of the following exercise programs would best help this patient lose weight?
A. Exercise of short duration and high intensity
B. Exercise of low intensity and long duration
C. Prolonged and strenuous exercise
D. Intermittently strenuous exercise

257. In a class on physiology of exercise, you are studying the energy needed for muscle contractions. Which of the following statements is false in regard to energy for muscle contractions?
A. Energy is produced during aerobic metabolism
B. Energy is produced during anaerobic metabolism
C. Energy may be stored as cretin phosphate
D. Energy is derived from ATP

258. Your patient is a 23-year-old male who has been on bed rest for 20 days as a result of an acute infection with severe complications. You are sent up to start performing rehabilitation to assist this patient in recovery. Which of the following would not be a physiological effect of 20 days of bed rest for this patient?
A. The recovery period would take almost as long as the exercise period
B. The patient would suffer considerable loss of bone and mineral content
C. There would be a small decrease in the maximum of oxygen consumption capacity
D. The patient would experience loss of stamina and fatigue

259. In clinical pathology class, you are studying the causes and different types of diabetes. Which of the following is the primary stimulus to insulin secretion in the body?

A. Blood levels of hormones

B. Increased blood glucose levels

C. Decreased blood glucose levels

D. Increase of glycogen

260. Which of the following timeframes is the most susceptible time for injury to the fetal cardiovascular system? It is during this timeframe that the fetal cardiovascular system produces most congenital defects.
A. Third month
B. Sixth month
C. Between the 21st and the 40th days
D. Between conception and the 20th day

261. You are teaching an OB/GYN lecture to a group of physical therapist assistant students. You have set up a sample content of how the course will proceed. You also have included unit objectives for the lecture and lab practical. Which of the following would be considered a unit objective?
A. The introduction that explains the role of the physical therapist assistant in OB/GYN care
B. To demonstrate the three principles of body mechanics
C. An explanation of anatomy and physiology during pregnancy
D. Theories on labor and delivery

262. A professor is presenting a lecture on the advantages and disadvantages of the following exercises: isometric, isokinetic, isotonic, and eccentric contractions. The professor informs the class that some of the disadvantages of this particular exercise are that it loads muscle at the weakest point and the momentum factor in lifting. These disadvantages best describe which of the following classifications of exercise?
A. Isometric
B. Isotonic
C. Isokinetic
D. Free weights

263. A patient is seen in physical therapy and has a disturbance in his static equilibrium. When testing the patient, you have him stand perfectly still and instruct him to close his eyes. Upon doing this, the patient wavers from side to side and starts to fall, but you catch him and help him sit back down on the mat. Which of the following tests has most likely been performed on this patient?
A. Labyrinthine righting reflex
B. Romberg's sign
C. Babinski's sign
D. Chronic labyrinthine test

264. A neurological lesion has occurred in the frontal lobe of the cerebral hemisphere of a previous patient. This patient is to receive physical therapy in a couple of weeks. Which of the following would most likely be affected in this patient?
A. Vision
B. Sensory perception and interpretation
C. Personality and speech
D. Hearing and comprehension of speech

265. An 18-year-old male tests positive for shoulder dislocation. This patient may have complications as a result of this shoulder dislocation. Which of the following would most likely be involved if the patient were to have complications?
A. Axillary artery
B. Axillary nerve
C. Radial artery
D. Radial nerve

266. A patient reports to physical therapy for evaluation of his hand. Upon evaluation of the patient's right hand, the physical therapist notices atrophy involving the muscles of the thenar eminence. Which of the following would you most likely suspect would be injured?
    A. Median nerve
    B. Axillary nerve
    C. Ulnar nerve
    D. Radial nerve

267. A patient reports to physical therapy with a diagnosis of a lesion in the lateral cord of the brachial plexus. Which of the following would you most likely detect upon treatment of this patient?
    A. Paralysis of the biceps, coracobrachialis, and the finger flexors
    B. Paralysis of the deltoid
    C. Paralysis of wrist extension
    D. Paralysis of the hand

268. A patient is referred to physical therapy for ultrasound. You perform ultrasound on the patient 1.5 watts per centimeter squared for 8 minutes. On which of the following sites would you be able to perform ultrasound on this patient?
    A. At a fracture site
    B. Over the spinal cord
    C. Over healed scar
    D. Over the epiphyseal plate

269. You are performing physical therapy on a patient status post CVA. The patient is having difficulty with trunk control and transfers from supine to sit and left to right sidelying. In performing PNF techniques on this patient, which of the following would be best to utilize to assist this patient?
    A. Hold and relax
    B. Rhythmic initiation
    C. Rhythmic stabilization
    D. Slow reversal hold

270. In studying the pulmonary system of a patient, you are discussing the site of gas exchange in the pulmonary system. Which of the following is the most likely site of gas exchange?
    A. Alveoli
    B. Bronchi
    C. Brachialis
    D. Trachea

271. The first level of respiration is due to a muscular force. Which of the following would be the primary muscular force for respiration?
    A. Diaphragm
    B. Abdominals
    C. Intercostals
    D. Intercostals and abdominals

272. The skin is the first defense mechanism by the body against infection. Which of the following is not a reason why the skin is such an important barrier?
    A. Sweat glands secrete chemical toxins to certain bacteria.
    B. Membranes covered with sticky mucus may sweep away particles by ciliary action.
    C. Moisture within the cells tends to slow down invading pathogens.
    D. Sebaceous glands secrete chemicals that are toxic to certain bacteria.

273. You are attending pulmonary class and discussing measurements of pulmonary function. Certain volumes of air have been designated with specific names. These names represent part of the pulmonary function test, which may be done to assess a patient's pulmonary condition. Which of the following best describes the amount of air that can be forcibly exhaled at the end of normal expiration?

A. Functional residual capacity
B. Expiratory reserve volume
C. Residual volume
D. Tidal volume

274. You are performing passive range of motion on a pulmonary patient. What effect will passive range of motion have on this patient's pulmonary ventilation?
    A. No effect
    B. An undetermined effect
    C. A response proportional to the number of joints involved in passive range of motion
    D. A response proportional to the speed and duration of exercises administered

275. In teaching the pathology of the pulmonary system, a professor describes a condition in which pathological changes occur in the lung tissue as a result of matter being inhaled. Which of the following would be the medical term for this condition?
    A. Pneumoconiosis
    B. Asthma
    C. Bronchitis
    D. Emphysema

276. You are treating a patient in the intensive care unit with a diagnosis of meningitis. You note that the patient's breathing pattern has a slow rate, shallow depth, apnea periods, and irregular rhythm. Of the following breathing patterns, which is demonstrated by this patient?
    A. Biot's
    B. Apneusis
    C. Orthopnea
    D. Cheyne-Stokes

277. You are working with a physical therapy patient who exhibits extreme defense mechanisms. In reading the patient's medical chart you see that there was a psychiatric consult that showed that the patient was experiencing symptoms of paranoia. Which of the following would most likely be the defense mechanism noticed in a paranoid patient?
    A. Projection
    B. Regression
    C. Rationalization
    D. Anger

278. Your patient is a 53-year-old obese female. She injured her right lower extremity in an automobile accident 3 months ago. The physician's order stated "increase range of motion and alleviate pain." Which of the following would be the maximum loose-packed position of the knee joint to perform mobilization?
    A. 5° knee flexion
    B. 10° knee flexion
    C. 25° knee flexion
    D. 35° knee flexion

279. A client has been positioned on his side. The physical therapist assistant would anticipate that which of the following areas would be a pressure point in this position?
    A. Sacrum
    B. Occiput
    C. Ankles
    D. Heels

280. You are providing a continuing education inservice on the necessary elements for a physician's prescription to be acceptable. You have had problems within the department of several PTAs treating patients with prescriptions that have been lacking information. Which of the following best describes the minimum amount of information that should be included in a physician's prescription?

A. Diagnosis, date, precautions, treatment, and physician's signature
B. Diagnosis, frequency of treatment, as well as an "eval and treat" order
C. Physician's signature, diagnosis, and date
D. Physician's signature, diagnosis, date, and modalities

281. A patient comes to the clinic with an order for a knee evaluation. Evaluation reveals the following: the patient is walking on his toes and exhibits foot inversion with forefoot adduction and plantar flexion. Given this clinical picture, which of the following would this patient most likely have?
A. Talipes calcaneovalgus
B. Talipes valgus
C. Talipes equinovarus
D. Talipes calcaneus

282. A patient is referred to physical therapy status post below-elbow amputation. The patient has a very short below-elbow amputation and you need to teach control of her prosthesis. Which of the following motions would you utilize to teach the patient to control her prosthesis?
A. Shoulder flexion
B. Scapular protraction
C. Shoulder extension
D. Scapular retraction

283. A patient has had an amputation that has resulted in removal of one leg above the ankle joint. The result is a bulbous end on the leg above the ankle joint. Which of the levels of amputation listed below would this patient most likely have experienced?
A. A below-knee joint amputation
B. A Chopart amputation
C. A metatarsal amputation
D. A Syme's amputation

284. A patient is a 59-year-old male who suffered a third-degree, full-thickness burn as a result of a chemical accident. Which of the following would be the healing characteristics expected for this patient?
A. Healing within 3 to 7 days, no scarring, no pigment changes
B. Healing less than 3 weeks, minimal scarring, pigment changes
C. Healing greater than 3 weeks, scar formation may occur, may need grafting
D. Requires grafting

285. A patient is referred to physical therapy for gait evaluation with a prosthesis. Upon observing the patient on the parallel bars, you notice that he is demonstrating a gait deviation of lateral trunk bending. Which of the following would be the most likely anatomical cause of lateral trunk bending?
A. The prosthesis is too short
B. The prosthesis is too long
C. Abductor muscles are weak
D. The prosthesis is in abduction

286. You are observing a patient with a prosthesis who shows instability of the knee. Which of the following would most likely not be a possible prosthetic cause for instability of the knee?
A. The knee joint is too anterior
B. Plantar flexion resistance is too high
C. There is no limit on dorsiflexion
D. Plantar flexion resistance is too low

287. In a research project during your senior year at school, each student is assigned a different method of research on what percentage of time the physical therapist assistant in private practice spends on clinical practice versus administration functions. You perform your research by sending out standardized forms to 100 physical therapist assistants in private practice in your state. You request that the physical therapist assistants fill out and answer all the appropriate questions and return the forms to you to correlate the answers and report on them. Which of the following best defines the method of research that you are utilizing?

A. Cross-sectional
B. Developmental
C. Questionnaire
D. Survey

288. You are reading the section on infection control policies in the policy and procedure manual at your new job. Of the following, which would not be an example of an infection control policy?
A. Universal precautions should be followed with each and every patient, regardless of diagnosis or condition.
B. Hand washing should occur at the beginning of the day and at the end of the day.
C. Infectious medical waste should be placed in a container labeled "only for medical waste."
D. Whirlpool should be cultured at least annually or after usage by a patient with an infectious disease.

289. A 23-year-old female is referred to physical therapy with a diagnosis of a lesion in the upper trapezius. The physician has referred the patient for evaluation and treatment as appropriate. As a physical therapist assistant, what results would you expect to see if an individual has a lesion in the upper trapezius?
A. Shoulder abduction would be weak
B. There would be no upper rotation of the scapula possible
C. The scapular retraction would be weak
D. The scapula would be rotated downward, which may result in subluxation of the sternoclavicular joint

290. A patient is referred to physical therapy secondary to pain in the right elbow. The physician notes upon x-rays that it appears there is a tear in the annular ligament. Which of the following would you expect as a result of a tear in the annular ligament?
A. Ulnar nerve entrapment
B. Valgus stress on the lateral collateral ligament
C. Dislocation of the head of the radius
D. A tear in the biceps muscle

291. In class you are studying the elbow joint and optimum force output. Which of the following would be the position for elbow flexion in terms of the greatest advantage of optimum force output?
A. 120° of elbow flexion
B. Flexion supination
C. Midposition or semiprone
D. 90° of elbow flexion

292. In anatomy class, you are studying the tendinous cuff muscles, also called SITS (supraspinatus, infraspinatus, teres minor). Which of the following does the combined action of the tendinous cuff muscles produce?
A. Abduction of the shoulder
B. External rotation of the shoulder
C. Pulling of the humerus upward and outward
D. Depression of the head of the humerus

293. Your patient is a 26-year-old paraplegic. You are observing the patient standing with braces for a prolonged time. For the paraplegic, prolonged standing with braces in a lordotic position may result in which of the following?
A. Stretching of the hip flexors
B. Stretching of the hip extensors
C. Stretching of the hip extensors and iliofemoral ligament
D. Stretching of the ischial femoral ligament

294. You are performing light touch to determine the sensory level of a spinal cord injury patient. When you move the brush along the patient's chest in a vertical manner, the patient states that he does not feel any stimulus as the brush reaches the level of the umbilicus. Which of the following would be the best estimate of the level of lesion for this patient?
A. T2
B. T4
C. T10
D. T12

295. You are a physical therapist assistant giving instruction on skin care to a 65-year-old female who is a below-knee amputee. Upon observation, you notice that the patient's opposite lower extremity toes are dark and discolored with mild atrophic changes in the nails. You also note that there is some mild swelling of the foot and ankle. Which of the following would you most likely suspect?
    A. The presence of thrombophlebitis
    B. Chronic venous insufficiency
    C. The patient will lose her remaining lower extremity within a few months
    D. Lymphedema

296. Your patient is a 65-year-old female who is a below-knee amputee. The patient suffers from chronic venous insufficiency. The patient has discolored and atrophic changes in the nails of the opposite extremity. Which of the following would be appropriate activities to recommend for this patient?
    A. Wearing of support hosiery, patient education on foot care, active exercises of the distal extremity, and elevation of the foot in bed.
    B. Patient education on foot care, a regular walking program, and Burger-Allen exercises.
    C. Jobst intermittent compression and sleeping with the leg in a position of dependency.
    D. Education on foot care, bed rest, and anticoagulant therapy.

297. You are testing a patient's nonequilibrium coordination. You ask her to run her right heel from her left kneecap down her left shin to the ankle and back to the knee again. The patient can touch her kneecap fairly accurately but cannot keep the heel of the right foot on the tibia during the up and down motion. These results describe which of the following?
    A. Dysmetria
    B. Dysdiadochokinesia
    C. Barognosis
    D. Dyssynergia

298. You are in anatomy class studying motions of the wrist. It is known that the motion that the wrist produces is actually a combination of several motions at several different articulations. Which of the following would best describe the axis of motion for the radial and ulnar deviation?
    A. It lies in the coronal plane through the lunate
    B. It lies in the sagittal plane through the trapezoid
    C. It lies in the sagittal plane through the capitate
    D. It lies in the coronal plane through the capitate

299. You are performing a test on a patient for hip flexor length. The extremity being tested abducts and remains slightly flexed when lowered to the table. Which of the following would you most likely suspect of muscle tightness?
    A. Psoas major
    B. Tensor fasciae latae
    C. Semitendinosus
    D. Rectus femoris

300. You are working with a patient in the pulmonary wing of the hospital. You are observing the patient bedside, noting a particular pattern of breathing. The patient appears to be gasping for breath, and on occasion her shoulders and thorax rise on inspiration and her abdominal wall is retracted. Which of the following would you most likely suspect, given this patient's pattern of breathing?
    A. She suffers from barrel chest
    B. She is a paradoxical breather
    C. She is an upper chest breather
    D. She has had a lung removed

301. On a pulmonary patient you decide to measure normal expansion at the xiphoid process. Which of the following would be the normal value for expansion when measured at the xiphoid process?
    A. 5 to 10 cm
    B. 5 to 10 inches
    C. .5 to 1 cm
    D. .5 to 1 inches

302. You are in rheumatology class studying degenerative joint disease. The instructor asks you where Heberden's nodes are most frequently located as a result of degenerative joint disease. Which of the following is the correct answer?
   A. Distal and proximal interphalangeal joints of the fingers
   B. Distal and proximal interphalangeal joints of the fingers and toes
   C. Distal interphalangeal joints of the fingers
   D. Distal interphalangeal joints of the toes

303. Your patient is a 24-year-old female who comes to physical therapy complaining that she has been experiencing abnormal movement and pain since her fourth month of pregnancy. It is known that during pregnancy the hormone relaxin can lead to abnormal movements and pain for the patient. Which of the following would most likely be the location of pain in this patient?
   A. Left hip joint
   B. Bilateral hip joint
   C. Lumbar sacral joint
   D. Sacroiliac joint

304. Your patient is a 5-year-old female with a diagnosis of a herniated disc between vertebrae C6 and C7. During a conversation with the physician, he informs you that the patient has a C7 nerve root impingement. Upon testing this patient, you expect weakness in all the following motor activities except which one?
   A. Wrist flexion
   B. Finger flexion
   C. Finger extension
   D. Elbow extension

305. You are a physical therapist assistant who has been instructed by the physical therapist to lead an exercise group of 20 geriatric patients at the community center. The physical therapist suggests that you emphasize areas that typically show reduced range of motion for geriatric patients. Which of the actions listed below would not be an emphasis of your program?
   A. Hip flexion
   B. Hip extension
   C. Pectoralis muscle stretch
   D. Chin glides, chin tucks

306. You are a physical therapist assistant teamed up with a physical therapist conducting a cardiac rehabilitation session for 10 patients. The therapist receives a phone call and must leave the room to speak with a physician concerning one of the patient's programs. Which of the following would be the most appropriate response for the physical therapist assistant?
   A. Terminate the exercise session and send the patients back to their rooms.
   B. Temporarily terminate the exercise session while awaiting the therapist's return.
   C. Continue the exercise program with less strenuous exercises.
   D. Continue the exercise program as previously outlined by you and the physical therapist.

307. A patient is sent to physical therapy with a dermatological disorder of psoriasis. The treatment order suggests ultraviolet as a course of treatment for this patient. Prior to beginning the treatment, you need to determine what will be an effective dosage for this patient. You perform the test under the supervision of the physical therapist and tell the patient to notify you when he starts to notice some redness. The patient reports that 6 to 8 hours post-treatment he noticed a slight redness but had no peeling, blistering, or inflammation. He barely noticed that the ultraviolet had taken place. Which of the following dosages were performed on this patient?
   A. Minimal erythemal dosage
   B. Second degree erythemal
   C. Third degree erythemal
   D. Fourth degree erythemal

308. You are a physical therapist assistant practicing in a rural setting with a physical therapist. Due to a family emergency, you will be unable to work at the clinic the next day. You have 16 patients scheduled for physical therapy between you and the physical therapist. What would be the most appropriate response to care for these patients?
    A. Reschedule the patients for your return to work the next day.
    B. Have the physical therapist treat all the patients utilizing your progress notes from the prior week.
    C. Call the physical therapy department some time the next day to inform them of what treatments the patients should receive.
    D. Provide a thorough summary of each patient and leave it at the department for the physical therapist to begin with the next morning.

309. A patient returns for physical therapy treatments after the weekend complaining of acute back pain. You notice that the back pain increases from the low back and down the right posterior aspect of the lower extremity. You perform a range of motion assessment, and repeated flexion severely increases this patient's pain. In implementing a treatment program for this patient, which of the following would be the most appropriate initial exercise initially to recommend to the treatment team?
    A. Williams' exercises
    B. McKenzie exercises
    C. Prone lying x 15 minutes
    D. Proper posture and body mechanics instruction

310. A 70-year-old patient enters the clinic requesting physical therapy services immediately for low back pain. The patient was previously seen by you and the supervising physical therapist in the clinic on several different occasions for low back pain. The patient presents you with a prescription that is over 30 days old. Which of the following would be the most appropriate response to this patient?
    A. Since the patient has a prescription signed by a physician with appropriate orders, treat the patient and schedule on the supervising physical therapist's agenda.
    B. Inform the patient that the prescription is 30 days old; consequently, it has expired. Therefore, the patient will have to obtain a new prescription from the physician.
    C. Since the patient has been seen on multiple occasions and is well known to you, treat the patient yourself with the previous treatment plan.
    D. Call the physician to request a verbal approval over the telephone to treat the patient and consult with the supervising physical therapist.

311. You have a workman's comp patient who has been treated three times a week for 2 weeks, receiving moist heat to the cervical paraspinal, right scapular muscle, upper trapezius, and right anterior shoulder, followed by ultrasound to the right cervical paraspinals. The patient has also received soft tissue massage to the bilateral cervical paraspinal, upper trapezius, and upper thoracic paraspinals. The patient continues with complaints of elevated pain. In continuing this patient's treatment program, which of the following would be the most appropriate response?
    A. The patient has been treated only 2 weeks, so continue with 2 more weeks of physical therapy.
    B. The patient is a workman's comp patient and most likely a malingerer, so discharge him from physical therapy.
    C. Contact the supervising physical therapist to suggest changes in the treatment program.
    D. Since the patient is not showing significant progress, he really does not need a physical therapist assistant's attention; therefore, the physical therapy aide should take over this patient.

312. You are treating a patient status post knee surgery. You are setting up short- and long-term goals for this patient. Note that when the patient originally came to physical therapy, his range of motion was zero to 73°, and strength for knee extension was 3+/5, knee flexion 3-/5. Which of the following is the best example of a long-term goal?
    A. Patient should be able to perform left knee flexion 90°
    B. Increase strength from 3+/5 to 4/5 for knee extension
    C. Increase range of motion to 125° of flexion
    D. Patient should be able to increase strength from 3-/5 to 3+/5 for knee flexion

313. You are assisting in implementing a cardiopulmonary-pulmonary treatment program for an inpatient at the hospital. You need to perform chest physical therapy to the left lingular aspect of the upper lobe. Which of the following listed below would be the appropriate positioning for this patient?
    A. Patient is in right sidelying position, rotated backward one-quarter of a turn with the bed elevated 14 to 18 inches.
    B. Patient is in left sidelying position, rotated backward one-quarter of a turn with the bed elevated 14 to 18 inches.
    C. Patient is in prone position with the bed elevated 14 inches and a pillow placed under the abdomen.
    D. Sitting in a chair, the patient leans forward to approximately 20°, resting on pillows.

314. You are providing an education program to an industry in which repetitive motion injuries are commonly seen. To assist in decreasing repetitive injuries within this company, which of the following would be the most important concept to emphasize?
    A. Instruct the employees in proper warm-up procedures
    B. Instruct the employees in strengthening exercises
    C. Provide the company with isokinetic testing and results on each employee
    D. Provide posters on proper body mechanics

315. You are treating a patient for juvenile arthritis. The patient has severe pain and inflamed joints. The physician is concerned that the severity of the disease may destroy the growth plates in the child. Which of the following treatments would be the best choice for this patient in physical therapy?
    A. Ultrasound
    B. Diathermy
    C. Physician intervention, which requires that typically the patient is placed on high doses of aspirin
    D. Range of motion exercises, home program taught to the patient and family

316. A patient is sent to physical therapy with a burn on the posterior aspect of the elbow. The patient has low pain tolerance and was admitted to the hospital in the early morning. It is afternoon and the patient is sent down for physical therapy. You have limited time to see this patient, as your schedule is full. The physical therapist performs the examination and presents the patient to you for treatment. Which of the following would be the most appropriate treatment program to begin therapy?
    A. Active range of motion emphasizing flexion
    B. Active range of motion emphasizing extension
    C. Passive range of motion emphasizing extension and positioning of the elbow in full extension
    D. Whirlpool

317. You are to perform mobilization on the glenohumeral joint of a patient with a painful (R) shoulder. You wish to increase abduction of the shoulder and provide pain relief. Which of the following would be the correct mobilization technique for this patient?
    A. Inferior glide
    B. Posterior glide
    C. Anterior glide
    D. Anterior glide—mobilization level 4

318. You are working with a patient for a neurological problem as a result of an arterial occlusion in the brain. The patient is conscious and demonstrates ataxia with severe coordination problems, no hemiplegia or loss of sensation, and hemiparesis is present. Which of the following arteries has most likely been occluded in the brain?
    A. Middle cerebral artery
    B. Posterior cerebral artery
    C. Cerebellar artery
    D. Vertebral artery

319. You are treating a patient status post total hip replacement. You notice in the patient's chart that she has received a cemented total hip replacement. Which of the following is not an advantage of a cemented hip?

A. It allows early weightbearing
B. Surgeons report a 90% success rate
C. There is less postoperative pain
D. It requires less bone tissue removal

320. You are treating an inpatient at a local hospital status post left cerebrovascular accident (CVA). The patient is to return home in approximately 2 weeks and you are working on transfers into and out of a vehicle. Which of the following would be the most important to implement in this patient's treatment program?
A. Notify the patient's family that the patient will be leaving the hospital in 2 weeks. Request that they come in to learn how to perform transfers into and out of a vehicle.
B. You have a modified vehicle within the rehabilitation program. Have the patient practice transfers into and out of that vehicle.
C. Instruct the patient that he or she will be returning home in 2 weeks, so it is extremely important to concentrate on transfer techniques and cooperate 100% with you.
D. Obtain a handicapped parking permit for this patient.

321. You have a 40-year-old female who attends physical therapy for severe pain in the posterior region of the right shoulder and upper trapezius. The patient reports numbness and tingling in the right upper extremity and you suspect possible thoracic outlet syndrome. The patient is treated with moist heat, ultrasound, and massage for 2 weeks with no effect. You are collecting data for the physical therapist. Which of the following tests would be best to utilize to confirm your suspicions?
A. Drop arm test
B. Apprehension test
C. Adson's test
D. Tinel's sign

322. A patient is referred to physical therapy with an open wound on the lateral malleolus of the right ankle. The patient is a spinal cord patient who has developed this wound through improper pressure on the ankle. The physical therapist wants to use a lamp to assist in killing the bacteria in the wound and for wound healing. In implementing this patient's treatment program, which of the following lamps would be utilized?
A. Hot mercury lamp
B. High-pressure mercury vapor lamp
C. Low-pressure mercury vapor lamp
D. Ultraviolet lamp

323. You are treating a patient with a job-related injury who has a registered nurse (RN) assigned to his case through a vocational rehabilitation service. The office manager tells you that the RN case manager is on the phone and has questions about the patient's treatment, progress, and attendance, and requests permission to watch the patient perform during physical therapy. Which of the following would be the first appropriate response?
A. Since the patient is on workman's compensation, permit the RN to come in and observe the patient's treatment. Answer all her questions prior to observation or treatment.
B. Check the patient's file and see if a consent release form has been signed prior to speaking with the RN.
C. Notify the RN that she can come in and watch the patient only after the patient completes a signed release form.
D. Ask the patient if he minds having the RN come in to observe.

324. You are treating a patient in the neurological unit of a rehabilitation hospital that follows the theories of Bobath. Which of the following would be a treatment emphasis with a neurological patient using the theory of Bobath?
A. Treatment should be active and dynamic, facilitating normal movement patterns
B. The patient learns diagonal patterns of movement
C. Encourage and assist the patient to use associated reactions
D. Facilitate dysfunctional motor patterns

325. You are performing an isokinetic test on a patient post 2 weeks of ankle rehabilitation. This is the first test you have performed on this patient to determine strength and endurance. Which of the following would make the test results inaccurate?
    A. Calibrating the equipment regularly
    B. Aligning the anatomical axis joint with the mechanical axis
    C. Following standard testing protocols
    D. Communicating with the patient softly when the patient is performing the trial reps and more loudly to encourage full participation during testing

326. A 60-year-old patient has an injury to the brachial plexus as a result of an automobile accident. Muscle testing shows the patient has a fair minus grade of rhomboids, levator scapulae, and serratus anterior. The physician has determined that the patient has injured the dorsal scapular and long thoracic nerves. Which of the following best describes the origin of injury to the brachial plexus?
    A. From the rami of the plexus
    B. From the trunks of the plexus
    C. From the lateral cord of the plexus
    D. From the medial cord of the plexus

327. Upon initial examination of a patient status post right ankle fracture, the physical therapist notices the patient is unable to perform toe raises. You determine that the patient has suffered significant weakness to the gastrocnemius muscle. The patient is placed on a program of strengthening and increasing range of motion. Of the following innervation levels, which one would involve injury to the gastrocnemius muscle?
    A. L4, L5
    B. L5, S1
    C. S1, S2
    D. L2, L4

328. A patient status post cerebrovascular injury is examined by the physical therapist and the chart reads as follows: "The patient has the following characteristics: paralysis and weakness on the right side, possible motor apraxia, and a decreased discrimination between left and right." You cannot read the diagnosis and the physician's history notes in the chart. Based on the information available in the chart, which of the following areas is the patient's injury?
    A. Right hemisphere injury
    B. Left hemisphere injury
    C. Cerebellar injury
    D. Brainstem injury

329. You are utilizing electrical stimulation to stimulate a denervated muscle of your patient. Which of the following types of electrical current would you most likely select to use on this patient to elicit a response from your patient?
    A. Alternating current
    B. High-volt current
    C. Direct current
    D. Interferential stimulation

330. You are treating a patient who twisted her left ankle while participating in a tennis competition over the weekend. There is effusion of the ankle joint with increased temperature. The patient injured the ankle as a result of an inversion sprain. Which of the following ligaments would not be emphasized in planning this patient's treatment program?
    A. Deltoid ligament
    B. Anterior talofibular ligament
    C. Calcaneofibular ligament
    D. Posterior talofibular ligament

331. You are treating a patient who sustained an injury at work from a fall. The patient has been attending all scheduled appointments for physical therapy and should be able to return to work in approximately 2 weeks. As a result of a workman's compensation claim, the patient has a registered nurse to monitor his case. You receive a call from his nurse inquiring about his attendance in physical therapy and when he will be able to return to work. The patient has signed the appropriate release forms for communication with the nurse. Based on this information, which of the following would be the most appropriate response to the nurse?
    A. Tell the nurse you cannot answer the question, and that she should contact the referring physician regarding his return to work date.
    B. Tell the nurse that the patient has attended physical therapy daily and should return to work in 2 weeks.
    C. Tell the nurse that the patient has attended all physical therapy sessions and she will need to call the physician for the patient's medical release to return to work.
    D. Copy the patient's chart and give it to the RN.

332. A physician has prescribed iontophoresis for a patient with acute inflammation. The chemical ion to be utilized in this case by direct current should be negative. Which of the following chemical ions listed below would be appropriate to use for a negative current?
    A. Hydrocortisone
    B. Lidocaine
    C. Magnesium
    D. Salicylate

333. A patient has a spinal cord injury. You are collecting data on what muscle movements this patient has available. You ask the patient to perform upper extremity extension so you can evaluate the triceps muscle. The patient is able to straighten the elbow with the arm free in space. Upon palpation, you find that the patient is not utilizing the triceps but is substituting with the supraspinatus, infraspinatus, and teres minor. Which of the following muscle groups is this patient utilizing for substitution of the triceps?
    A. Deltoid
    B. External rotators of the shoulder
    C. Internal rotators of the shoulder
    D. Serratus anterior

334. You have determined that treating a neurological patient with an exteroceptive stimulation technique would be quite effective in the inhibition of muscles that are extremely spastic. Which of the following techniques listed below would be best in utilizing exteroceptive stimulation treatment programs?
    A. Prolonged icing
    B. Quick icing
    C. Hot packs
    D. Quick stretch

335. The patient complains of hip pain beginning at the greater trochanter with radiating symptoms extending down below the knee. There are no physical signs of injury and the patient is slightly tender to palpation on the greater trochanter and has limited flexibility. You suspect the patient's problems may be a result of iliotibial band tightness. To evaluate the iliotibial band, which of the following tests would be the most appropriate to utilize?
    A. Thomas test
    B. Straight leg raise test
    C. Trendelenburg's test
    D. Ober's test

336. You are implementing a treatment program for a patient with a separated shoulder. The patient sustained the injury as a result of diving for a catch during a football game. In implementing this patient's treatment program you would need to monitor the separated shoulder over the course of the patient's treatment program. Which of the following areas would you be monitoring on this patient?
    A. Acromioclavicular joint
    B. Coracoclavicular joint
    C. Glenohumeral joint
    D. Sternoclavicular joint

337. A 26-year-old patient sustained a spinal cord injury as a result of a diving accident. The patient presents the following functional outcomes: vital capacity is 60% to 80%, patient is independent in bed mobility, patient is independent with pressure relief and a manual wheelchair, and the patient can assist with independent transfers. Based on the above listed outcomes, what would be the most likely level of lesion in this patient?
    A. C4
    B. C5
    C. C6
    D. C7, C8

338. A patient is sent to physical therapy complaining of back pain with symptoms intermittently radiating down the left lower extremity. Muscle testing reveals 4-/5 quadriceps strength, 4-/5 hamstring strength, tenderness to palpation in the PSIS region, and slouched sitting posture. Next you are collecting data on the sensory distribution of the cutaneous nerves on this patient. Dermatome distribution is not intact to sharp and dull touch along the area of the anterior thigh or on the inside of the medial aspect of the anterior thigh. In which level of dermatome distribution listed below does this patient have a deficit?
    A. L1
    B. L2
    C. L3
    D. L5

339. You are performing mobilization on a patient to increase knee flexion status post anterior cruciate ligament (ACL) reconstruction. Utilizing the concave-convex rule, which of the following techniques would be the most appropriate mobilization technique to use?
    A. Anterior glide of tibia
    B. Superior patella
    C. Posterior glide of tibia
    D. Inferior glide of tibia

340. A total hip replacement patient is sent to the rehabilitation department for physical therapy. The patient is 4 weeks status post total hip replacement and is able to progress from partial weightbearing to full weightbearing utilizing a walker. Which of the following gait patterns would be best to implement for a patient with full weightbearing status?
    A. Walker first, then the involved lower extremity, then the uninvolved extremity is advanced.
    B. Walker first, then one leg, then the other leg is advanced.
    C. Walker first, then the uninvolved lower extremity, then the involved lower extremity is advanced.
    D. Uninvolved extremity first, then the walker, then the involved lower extremity is advanced.

341. You are performing a manual muscle test on a patient to evaluate the posterior shoulder joint muscles. The patient is positioned prone with the shoulder at the edge of the table, his arm hanging down over the side. You place the scapula in a position of adduction with some lateral rotation of the inferior angle and elevation of the shoulder girdle. You then provide pressure against the weight of the suspended arm, which will exert a force that abducts the scapula. The patient's shoulder is placed in 90° of abduction with lateral rotation and the elbow is completely extended. Based on this information, which of the following muscles are you most likely testing?
    A. Lower trapezius
    B. Upper trapezius
    C. Middle trapezius
    D. Serratus anterior

342. You are treating a patient who was hit in the left hip during football practice. The physician is concerned that the iliofemoral ligament of the hip has been damaged. Which of the following statements would not be true regarding the iliofemoral ligament?
    A. This ligament prevents overextension, abduction, and lateral rotation of the hip
    B. It is also called the Y-ligament of the hip
    C. It attaches to the inferior superior iliac spine
    D. It is located anteriorly superior to the hip

343. You are treating a patient with a foot injury. The patient reports that his podiatrist thought the spring ligament became injured as a result of his fall. Which of the following best describes the spring ligament of the foot?
    A. It is also called the plantar calcaneocuboid ligament
    B. It is called the short plantar ligament
    C. It helps to maintain the medial arch of the foot by supporting the head of the talipes
    D. The spring ligament is not highly elastic

344. You are assisting in applying electrical stimulation to the low back of a patient secondary to muscle spasm. Which area would show the best conductivity of all tissue to the electrical current?
    A. Tendon
    B. Muscle
    C. Bone
    D. Skin

345. A patient comes to the clinic complaining of inflammation and pain. The physician diagnosed the patient as having bursitis and recommended iontophoresis for treatment. Which of the following is the most frequent location of bursitis?
    A. Subacromial area
    B. Knee
    C. Elbow
    D. Ischial tuberosity

346. You are studying the various types of arthritis, specifically rheumatoid arthritis versus osteoarthritis. Which of the following would best describe the etiology of rheumatoid arthritis?
    A. Acute joint trauma or injury
    B. Sodium urate crystal formation near the joint
    C. Degeneration caused by aging to the articular cartilage
    D. Degeneration caused by aging to the muscles

347. You are treating an 18-year-old male patient for rotator cuff tendonitis. The physical therapist suspects the patient actually has a dislocated shoulder. Which of the following would you not expect to find when treating the patient for acute shoulder dislocation?
    A. The head of the humerus can be easily palpated
    B. There is localized pain in the shoulder
    C. There is crepitus in the joint
    D. The patient is holding the shoulder in a flexed position

348. You are studying diabetes mellitus and diabetes insipidus in your clinical pathology course. Which of the following statements is not true about diabetes mellitus, but best describes diabetes insipidus?
    A. It is a disorder of carbohydrate metabolism
    B. It results from insulin deficiency
    C. It is associated with the pancreas
    D. It is associated with the pituitary gland

349. A PTA works as a part-time employee of an inpatient treatment facility as well as being a self-employed contractor to several group homes. Is it the responsibility of the PTA to obtain individual malpractice and liability insurance for the contracted work?
    A. Yes, it is the responsibility of the PTA working as an independent contractor to carry individual liability coverage unless previously negotiated with the group home to provide coverage
    B. No, liability coverage from the PTA's primary work setting provides comprehensive coverage and carries over to all other work settings
    C. No, it is assumed that the responsibility of the group homes to carry liability insurance for their contracted service providers
    D. Liability coverage is not necessary but membership in the APTA is necessary

350. You are performing manual muscle tests on a right shoulder of a patient with a rotator cuff injury. You are looking for the maximum strength of the posterior deltoid. When performing manual muscle test for maximum strength, which of the following statements best describes what the patient needs for maximum strength?
    A. High maximum consumption of 02 during testing
    B. An isometric contraction involving the muscle fibers
    C. Complete fatigue of the muscle prior to contraction
    D. The maximum number of motor units to fire under testing

351. Your patient is a 34-year-old female with calcified bursitis of the shoulder. Which of the following would be the proper or most beneficial setting for the ultrasound frequency and dosage?
    A. One milliHertz and .5 watts per cm²
    B. One milliHertz and 1.5 watts per cm²
    C. Three milliHertz and .5 watts per cm²
    D. Three milliHertz and 1.5 watts per cm²

352. You are having a patient exercise utilizing isokinetics for strengthening of the quadriceps and hamstring muscles. The patient is 8 weeks status post ACL reconstruction and requires strengthening of both quadriceps and hamstring muscles. Which of the following would be a normal ratio of quadriceps to hamstring strength?
    A. Two to one
    B. Three to one
    C. Three to two
    D. Three to three

353. You are performing ultrasound under water for a patient experiencing foot pain in the medial arch. When administering ultrasound under water, which of the following would be the best distance for the sound head in relationship to the medial arch?
    A. The sound head should be in direct contact with the medial arch of the foot.
    B. The sound head should be approximately 3 inches away from the medial arch of the foot.
    C. The sound head should be approximately 1 inch away from the medial arch of the foot.
    D. The sound head should be approximately 4 inches from the medial arch of the foot.

354. You are working as a team with a physical therapist and nurse in a cardiac rehabilitation program. A patient who is an inpatient is to be discharged from stage one cardiac rehabilitation to a stage two program. Which of the following would not be a physical therapy goal to expect this patient to accomplish at the end of stage one cardiac rehabilitation?
    A. Independent in activities of daily living
    B. Independent in dietary and nutritional education for a home program
    C. Increased maximal oxygen consumption
    D. Independent in patient and family education regarding risk factors

355. You are performing a leg length evaluation on a 16-year-old male. In order to properly measure leg length it is important to know the landmarks used to compare the actual leg lengths of both lower extremities on this individual. Which of the following landmarks would you be using for measurement to gain the most accurate test results?
    A. Anterior inferior iliac spine to the lateral malleolus
    B. Anterior inferior iliac spine to the medial malleolus
    C. Anterior superior iliac spine to the lateral malleolus
    D. Posterior superior iliac spine to the medial malleolus

356. You are walking down the hallway on the hospital's rehabilitation floor and witness a patient fall. He hits his head on the door. A physician has determined that he has suffered a concussion. Which of the following best defines a concussion?
    A. Any severe blow to the head
    B. A fracture of the skull
    C. Swelling of the brain as a result of trauma
    D. A temporary state of paralysis of the nervous function, including loss of consciousness

357. You are a physical therapist assistant providing ultraviolet radiation to a patient. Which of the following would you anticipate to be the most sensitive area of the patient to the ultraviolet radiation?
    A. Hands
    B. Feet
    C. Arms
    D. Face

358. You are treating a 42-year-old female patient for adhesive capsulitis of the right shoulder. You are performing muscle palpation to evaluate areas of tenderness. The patient is in a prone position and her arm is hanging over the edge of the table. The scapula has moved forward on the rib cage secondary to the weight of the arm being partially rotated upward. Upon palpation, you identify the spine of the scapulae and palpate above the spine. You perform abduction to the arm to feel the muscle contraction. You identify the muscle underneath the trapezius and deltoid. Of the muscles listed below, which is the most likely muscle that you are attempting to palpate?
    A. Supraspinatus
    B. Teres minor
    C. Teres major
    D. Subscapularis

359. The patient has a peripheral nerve injury affecting the wrist and hand. You notice that the wrist cannot be extended actively, the digits are partially extended due to the tendon action but not actively contracting, and the grasp is weak. The patient demonstrates a wrist drop secondary to paralysis of the extensors of the wrist and long extensors of all the digits; the flexors of the digits are intact. Based upon this information, what type of peripheral nerve injury does this patient have?
    A. Median nerve paralysis
    B. Ulnar nerve paralysis
    C. Radial nerve paralysis
    D. Ulnar/median nerve paralysis

360. A patient is a weightlifter who injured his quadriceps muscle during a maximal lift. You are interested in performing an eccentric contraction for strengthening. Which of the following exercises would be most appropriate for this patient?
    A. Lowering a weight during a hard press, performing a negative repetition
    B. Isokinetics
    C. Exercise bicycle
    D. Accelerating the lifting on initiation of movement

361. You are implementing a treatment program of pelvic traction for a patient with a back disorder. Which of the following percentages would cause distraction of the vertebral bodies with lumbar traction?
    A. 50% of the patient's body weight
    B. 35% of the patient's body weight
    C. 30% of the patient's body weight
    D. 25% of the patient's body weight

362. You are performing goniometric measurement of the shoulder for external rotation. How should the stationary arm of the goniometer be positioned to appropriately measure this patient?
    A. Longitudinally with the shaft of the ulna
    B. Longitudinally with the styloid process
    C. Parallel or perpendicular to the midline of the trunk
    D. Longitudinally over the shaft of the humerus

363. The patient is a 22-year-old tennis player with a shoulder injury. You are palpating the external rotators of the shoulder. You are palpating the muscle to determine if tenderness or edema exists. The ideal position for palpation of this muscle as it relates to the joint could best be described by which of the following?

A. Loose-packed position
B. Closed-packed position
C. 20° of movement
D. 90° of movement

364. A patient is sent to physical therapy with an ulnar nerve injury on the right hand. The patient works at a factory 8 hours a day sorting various parts. The patient is very motivated with rehabilitation and anxious to be aggressive in physical therapy. Which of the following muscles are you going to emphasize with this patient in physical therapy?
A. Flexor pollicis longus
B. Flexor carpi ulnaris
C. Flexor digitorum superficialis
D. Flexor carpi radialis

365. The PTA instructor in the physical therapist assistant program is explaining to you the various laws and how they relate to physical therapy. The instructor describes a law as follows: "prohibition against exclusion of people from jobs, services, or activities based solely on their disability." The major difference between this new law and the old law on the books is that the term "disability" is used instead of "handicap." Which of the following laws is the instructor describing to you?
A. Section 504 of the Rehabilitation Act of 1973
B. The Americans with Disabilities Act of 1990
C. Civil Rights Act of 1964
D. The Age Discrimination Act of 1975

366. A pediatric patient is referred to the clinic for physical therapy. You have no experience in pediatrics or a reasonable understanding of how to treat and progress this particular cerebral palsy child. Which of the following would be appropriate for you to perform ethically and legally with this particular patient?
A. Since you are not qualified to treat pediatrics, do not accept this patient and refuse the physical therapist's request for services.
B. Accept the patient but do not promise overoptimistic results to the patient and physical therapist.
C. Accept the patient; perform a thorough examination and attempt treatment to the best of your ability.
D. Report to the supervising physical therapist that you do not feel qualified or comfortable working with this patient and the patient should be referred to another certified staff member or outside center that treats pediatric patients.

367. A patient is sent from the psychiatric ward to physical therapy for aerobic exercise to alleviate his anxiety. When in the clinic the patient becomes withdrawn. The patient occasionally shifts from withdrawal into obscene language, and the patient demonstrates very bizarre behavior with several mood shifts. The patient is not antisocial and does not exhibit delusions of persecution. The patient seems to have problems cooperating with physical therapy. Based on these symptoms, which of the following most likely describes the condition of this patient?
A. Paranoia
B. Depression
C. Schizophrenia
D. Psychopathy

368. You are studying anatomy of the knee in anatomy and physiology class. In regard to the knee joint, which one of the following statements is true?
A. The lateral meniscus is larger than the medial meniscus. It is shaped like the letter "C."
B. The lateral collateral ligament of the knee is attached to the meniscus.
C. The medial meniscus is the smaller of the menisci and is shaped like the letter "O."
D. The posterior cruciate ligament has a distal attachment from the posterior intercondylar of the tibia.

369. Your patient is being discharged from the hospital to his home. To provide for continuity of care, the patient will continue to receive home physical therapy. As the physical therapist assistant, which of the following would be the appropriate action for you to take to assure the patient's continuity of care?

A. Refer the patient to a home health physical therapist assistant of whom you have heard good reports.

B. Report to the patient's home yourself and treat him on the side, away from the hospital.

C. Provide the social worker a report on the patient's status.

D. Telephone the physical therapist assistant who will be continuing to see the patient at home and give him an update on the patient, as well as a report on the appropriate exercises you have been performing, including any protocols.

370. A patient is a cross-country track runner who pulled a hamstring muscle. During which period of time during gait would the hamstring muscle be the most active?
    A. Midstance to heel-off
    B. Swing phase
    C. Acceleration to midswing
    D. Midswing to deceleration

371. You are performing ultrasound under water to a patient's left hand. In performing the ultrasound under water, which of the following would be the most important safety factor to be considered?
    A. Utilizing a plastic bucket instead of a metal whirlpool
    B. Keeping the ultrasound head moving
    C. Keeping the ultrasound under 1.0 watts per cm2
    D. Connecting the ultrasound to a ground fault interruption circuit

372. You have been called to report to the physical therapy department. There is a patient being brought into the emergency room with severe burns and open wounds on both posterior lower extremities. The physical therapist and physical therapist assistant are to begin working with this newly admitted burn patient. Which of the following would be the first priority of the physical therapist assistant?
    A. Examination of muscle strength and range of motion
    B. Splinting to control contractures and edema
    C. Closing the wound with dressing
    D. Beginning immediate wound cleaning, debridement, and sterile dressing

373. You are performing palpation on a patient with general lower back pain. Which of the following landmarks would be most helpful to isolate the L4 vertebral level upon palpation of this patient?
    A. Anterior superior iliac spine
    B. Posterior superior iliac spine
    C. Iliac crest
    D. Greater trochanter

374. A patient is a 43-year-old female who was injured when a pan of hot water spilled, scalding her left forearm. The patient suffered a second-degree, superficial burn. Which of the following would be the healing characteristics expected for this patient?
    A. Healing within 3 to 7 days, no scarring, no pigment changes
    B. Healing less than 3 weeks, minimal scarring, pigment changes
    C. Healing greater than 6 weeks, scar formation may occur, may need grafting
    D. Requires grafting

375. A 28-year-old male patient is sent to the clinic with low back pain. You perform modalities to reduce inflammation and pain. The physical therapist suggests that you include Williams' exercises to strengthen the patient secondary to poor posture. Upon postural evaluation, you notice an anterior tilt of the pelvis. Which of the following muscles would you be strengthening with Williams' exercises?
    A. Abdominal and gluteus maximus muscles
    B. Gluteus medius
    C. Gluteus medius and minimus muscles
    D. Erector spinae

376. When performing ultrasound on a patient, it is important to be aware of contraindications for its utilization. One contraindication is performing ultrasound over the epiphyseal or growth plate of a child. Which of the following statements is not true concerning the growth plate?
    A. It serves as a site of progressive lengthening that is needed in the long bones
    B. It lies between the epiphysis and diaphysis as a transverse disc
    C. It is formed of cartilage
    D. It is found in all bones

377. A patient is sent to physical therapy with an order for training with a cane. The patient suffered a sprained ankle and has progressed from crutch ambulation to requiring a cane along with an air cast. Which of the following would be proper utilization of a cane for this patient?
    A. Use it on the same side as the ankle injury
    B. Use it on the opposite side the ankle injury
    C. Use it during the stance phase
    D. Use it during the push-off phase

378. A 20-year-old patient hospitalized with a diagnosis of schizophrenia begins to hear voices and walks to the staircase to peer over. The patient says, "I want to kill the voices." The most appropriate response from the PTA would be to:
    A. Ask the patient to identify the voices.
    B. Talk to the patient while moving the patient from the staircase.
    C. Discuss the voices and why the patient wants to kill them.
    D. Tell the patient that the voices are not really there.

379. In studying physical therapy you are learning about the differences regarding various spina bifida disorders. You are specifically studying spina bifida myelocele. Which of the following would best describe this disorder?
    A. A soft tissue tumor in the meninges
    B. A soft tissue tumor in the spinal cord
    C. The most severe form of spina bifida
    D. A herniated sac contained within the spinal cord

380. A patient has been referred to your clinic after being evaluated at the Midwest Arthritis Spine Center. The patient has been diagnosed as having rheumatoid arthritis rather than osteoarthritis. Which of the following would you expect to observe in a rheumatoid arthritic patient?
    A. Involvement of the proximal interphalangeal joints
    B. Chronic inflammation
    C. Involvement of the distal interphalangeal joints
    D. Involvement of the weightbearing joints

381. Bursae may be found in most of the locations within the body. In which of the following anatomical areas would the bursae most likely not be found?
    A. Subtendinous
    B. Intramuscular
    C. Subcutaneous
    D. Subfacial

382. A patient in the clinic has been receiving hot pack, ultrasound, and massage to the cervical region for 1 month. Today after treatment, you record in his notes: no complications with treatment. One hour later the patient calls you complaining of a red spot under his ear. What should you do next?
    A. Have the patient come to the clinic so you can inspect the area and put a dressing on it.
    B. Have the patient come to the clinic so you can inspect the area, and notify your supervising physical therapist of the patient's complication.
    C. Ignore the patient since he always exaggerates his symptoms.
    D. Tell the patient to call back tomorrow if the red spot is still present.

383. You have a 42-year-old female status post removal of lymphatic system in the axillary region secondary to cancer. The physical therapist wants you to work on edema control through measurement for a pressure garment and massage 1 day post-surgery. How should the massage be performed for best results?
    A. You decide not to do massage but Jobst compression pump
    B. Massage the proximal segment first
    C. Massage the distal segment first
    D. Order a garment and check on the patient daily

384. A patient comes to the clinic for left elbow tendonitis. The treatment plan is friction massage, phonophoresis, and exercises followed by an ice massage. Which of the following physiological responses generally occurs from cold treatments?
    A. Increased respiratory rate, increased cardiac output.
    B. Increased stroke volume, increased tidal volume, increased intestinal blood flow to the organs.
    C. Decreased stroke volume, decreased intestinal blood flow to the internal organs.
    D. Decreased respiratory rate, decreased tidal volume.

385. You are treating a patient for psoriasis with ultraviolet lamps. You have performed a minimal erythemal dosage test for third-degree erythema. This is five times the minimal erythemal dosage. How many times will the patient be treated per week?
    A. Daily
    B. Twice a day
    C. Every other day
    D. Once weekly

386. A 3-year-old female comes to the clinic with the following symptoms: neck deformity that causes rotation and tilting of the head. The mother reports that it is a result of a motor vehicle accident (MVA) 2 weeks ago. What treatment would you recommend to the mother for a home program to obtain maximal results?
    A. No home program; treatment should only be performed by a physical therapist
    B. Ice packs and stretching
    C. Electrical stimulation
    D. Stretching exercises and proper positioning/postural instructions

387. You are performing a postural observation on a patient from the posterior view. You are specifically observing alignment for the hip, knee, and ankle joints. Which of the following is normal alignment?
    A. Hip joint neutral, knee neutral, slight out-toeing of feet
    B. Hip joint neutral, knee neutral, slight in-toeing of feet
    C. Hip joint slightly anterior, knee neutral, slight out-toeing of feet
    D. Hip joint slightly posterior, knee neutral, slight out-toeing of feet

388. Muscular contraction of the cardiac chambers is different from the electrical conduction system. The normal conduction pathway for muscular contraction of the heart to follow is which of the patterns listed below?
    A. Left atrium, right atrium, ventricles
    B. Right atrium, left atrium, ventricles
    C. Right ventricle, left ventricle, atrium
    D. Left ventricle, right ventricle, atrium

389. A patient enters the clinic with an injury in the brachioradialis muscle of the left forearm. The patient was injured when he was delivering a piano and the lid slammed down on his forearm. The patient now has limited action of the left forearm. With an injury to the brachioradialis muscle, which actions would now most likely be limited in this patient?
    A. Forearm supination
    B. Forearm supination, elbow flexion, wrist flexion
    C. Forearm pronation, elbow flexion
    D. Forearm pronation, supination, elbow flexion

390. You are performing physical therapy in a nursing home where orthostatic hypotension occasionally occurs in some of the elderly patients. Which of the following would not be true concerning orthostatic hypotension?
    A. Can occur as a result of a patient assuming an upright position
    B. Common after long periods of bedrest
    C. Common in elderly patients
    D. Lasts for only 24 hours

391. A patient begins participation in the cardiac rehabilitation program under supervision of a treatment team. You are carefully monitoring the patient's response to exercise during the exercise program. Which of the following would be a normal response to exercise?
    A. Cardiac output/heart rate increases in a linear relation with increase in workload.
    B. Cardiac output/heart rate decreases in a linear relation with increase in workload.
    C. As cardiac output increases, the heart rate decreases.
    D. Heart rate increases as cardiac output decreases.

392. A patient has an ankle sprain, which is healing well. The patient needs to increase range of motion to resume full activity. Of the following, which movement will take place in the ankle subtalar joint?
    A. Pronation/supination
    B. Eversion/inversion
    C. Adduction/abduction
    D. Dorsiflexion

393. In examination of a shoulder patient, the physical therapist requests that you pay particular attention to the supraspinatus, infraspinatus, and teres minor (SITS) muscles. Which of the following would best describe the SITS muscle action on the humeral head?
    A. Abduction of the humeral head
    B. Adduction of the humeral head
    C. Elevation of the humeral head
    D. Depression of the humeral head

394. Vertebral joints have characteristics that distinguish different levels. In studying anatomy, you learn of a vertebra that has a bifid spinous process. Which of the following vertebrae has a bifid spinous process?
    A. Cervical vertebra
    B. Thoracic vertebra
    C. Lumbar vertebra
    D. Sacral vertebra

395. A patient enters the clinic with what appears to be pinched nerves in the cervical spine area. The patient is reporting radiating symptoms into the left upper extremity that follow no particular dermatome pattern. The patient reports that he is going to have a test in which some type of electrodes are inserted into the muscle to test which nerves are injured. Based on this information, which of the following tests is the patient most likely having?
    A. Electromyogram
    B. Arthroscopy
    C. Electrocardiogram (EKG)
    D. Myelogram

396. In the anatomy lab, the physician instructs you to perform dissection of the femoral triangle. Which of the following muscles borders the femoral triangle?
    A. Sartorius, adductor longus
    B. Sartorius, adductor magnus
    C. Gracilis, adductor longus
    D. Gracilis, adductor magnus

397. A 21-year-old male comes to the clinic with a prescription for physical therapy. The diagnosis is a brachial plexus injury involving the left shoulder upper extremity. The patient was injured in an automobile accident when a drunk driver hit his car, driving the car into a telephone pole. The patient will need extensive rehabilitation for the brachial plexus injury. Particularly noted was that the lateral cord of the brachial plexus was injured. Which nerve arises from the lateral cord of the brachial plexus?
    A. Median nerve
    B. Ulnar nerve
    C. Axillary nerve
    D. Musculocutaneous nerve

398. You are in neurology class studying abnormal and normal reflexes. You are specifically concerned with the abnormal reflex called asymmetric tonic neck reflex, or ATNR. The integration level for this reflex is the brainstem. The stimulus would be for the therapist to turn the head to one side. Which of the following would be the correct response to the stimulus of turning the head to one side?
    A. Upper extremity extension and lower extremity flexion
    B. Upper extremity flexion and lower extremity extension
    C. Withdrawal of lower extremity from the stimulus
    D. Arm/leg extension on the side that the head is turned toward, flexion on opposite side

399. You have a patient in physical therapy that has been a secretary for 20 years. The patient reports pain in the mid-back as a result of working over a computer for marathon typing sessions. The curvature of the spine can best be described as the following: it is in the anterior-posterior direction in which the convexity is in the posterior direction. Which of the following would be a correct terminology for this curvature of the spine?
    A. Scoliosis
    B. Sway back
    C. Flat back
    D. Kyphosis

400. The physical therapist you are teamed with has performed an initial examination on a patient 2 weeks status post rotator cuff tendon repair. The orders are to begin general strengthening of the rotator cuff muscle with strengthening being limited to shoulder range of motion 90° or lower. Which of the following muscles would not be emphasized initially in this patient's treatment program?
    A. Infraspinatus
    B. Teres major
    C. Supraspinatus
    D. Subscapularis

401. A patient is referred to physical therapy with a diagnosis of Erb-Duchenne palsy/paralysis. The recommended treatment program would emphasize maintaining range of motion and preventing contractures. Erb-Duchenne paralysis is a result of damage to which of the following nerve roots?
    A. C4, C5
    B. C5, C6
    C. C7, C8
    D. T1, T2

402. A patient is referred to physical therapy with a burn on the elbow as a result of a gasoline flashback from a fire. The patient is currently in moderate pain and requires debridement and range of motion. Following treatment of whirlpool, debridement, and range of motion, which of the following would be the correct position in which to place the elbow?
    A. Extension, supination
    B. Flexion, pronation
    C. Extension, pronation
    D. Flexion

403. A patient is referred to physical therapy for range of motion and strengthening. The patient presents the following history: he reports that he has a collagen vascular disorder affecting the connective tissue. The patient reports that he is currently taking medication, and the doctor has recommended physical therapy for joint conservation techniques and maintaining range of motion. The patient presents the classic "butterfly rash." Which of the following diseases are you most likely dealing with?
     A. Scleroderma
     B. Dermatomyositis
     C. Lupus erythematosus
     D. Polynodosa

404. You are working with a cerebral palsy child. You notice that the child has great difficulty reaching for an object with one hand. The child prefers to reach for an object with both hands. What age would be considered normal for a child to be able to reach for an object with one hand?
     A. 6 months
     B. 12 months
     C. 15 months
     D. 18 months

405. You are studying the code of ethics and standards of ethical conduct for a physical therapist assistant. Which of the following would not be a standard of ethical conduct for the physical therapist assistant?
     A. PTA respects the rights and dignity of all individuals
     B. PTA provides services independently to patients
     C. PTA provides services within the limits of the law
     D. PTA makes those judgments that are commensurable with his or her qualifications

406. You are assisting the physical therapist in a case. The physical therapist informs you that she feels that the patient is pretending to be ill to arouse sympathy for his condition. The therapist suspects that the patient is slow to recuperate because he continues to receive benefits from the insurance company during a slow recovery. Which of the following most likely describes this individual?
     A. Patient is negligent
     B. Patient is a hypochondriac
     C. Patient is a malingerer
     D. Patient is paranoid

407. A patient is referred to physical therapy for a post cesarean exercise program. The physical therapist informs you that the patient is in day 3 post cesarean and needs to be started on an exercise program. Which of the following exercises would not be appropriate?
     A. Pelvic floor exercises
     B. Diaphragmatic breathing
     C. Leg slides
     D. Leg lifts

408. You are maintaining SOAP notes on a patient for physical therapy. The therapist has performed an initial examination and the physical therapist assistant is responsible for daily notes on the patient's condition. Which of the following would be the best reason for maintaining SOAP notes on a patient?
     A. Legal purposes
     B. Educational purposes
     C. Improvement of patient care
     D. Third-party payers

409. The physical therapist instructs you to set a patient up on a particular exercise program keeping in mind the metabolic equivalent (MET). This is a unit of the number of millimeters of oxygen consumed per gram of body weight. The physical therapist suggests that you work the patient at two METs. Two METs mean that the work requires twice the amount of oxygen. Which of the following activities would you have the patient performing for two METs?

A. Lifting light weights of 2 to 3 pounds
B. Walking 3.5 mph
C. Cycling 8 mph
D. Walking 4 mph

410. A patient is referred to physical therapy. Prior to receiving services, the patient's insurance is verified. The type of insurance that this patient has limits the total number of treatments or visits for the problem to six visits. The patient also pays a small fixed fee for each visit—$5.00 per visit. Your facility has signed up to participate with this patient's insurance; therefore you accept him for treatment. Which of the following does this patient most likely have?
A. HMO
B. Medicaid
C. Medicare
D. Workman's compensation

411. A muscle is known to have proximal and distal attachments. It is necessary to know the attachments for palpation and manual muscle tests. Which of the following is the proximal attachment of a limb muscle?
A. Tendon
B. Insertion
C. Belly of muscle
D. Origin

412. You are observing a patient walking in the parallel bars. Upon observation, you notice that the patient has anteversion of the hip. This would result in which of the following to the knee?
A. Hyperextension
B. Genu recurvatum
C. Genu valgus
D. Genu varus

413. The physical therapist suggests that you start to massage a patient with back pain to reduce muscle spasms and assist in alleviating pain. The physical therapist recommends that the massage you utilize consists of a series of brisk blows in alternating fashion. Which of the following massages has the physical therapist recommended?
A. Tapotement massage
B. Friction massage
C. Kneading massage
D. Vibration

414. Your patient is a 36-year-old factory worker who comes to physical therapy secondary to crushing injury of the right hand injured in a molding press. The patient reports to physical therapy for examination and treatment. You begin treatment to reduce edema and assist in alleviating pain while regaining range of motion. You palpate the distal row of the carpal bones to determine pain and edema. Which of the following would you not be palpating in the distal row of the carpal bones?
A. Trapezoid
B. Lunate
C. Capitate
D. Hamate

415. The nervous system is composed of a parasympathetic and sympathetic system. Which of the following would be an effect of sympathetic activity on the heart rate of a patient?
A. Increase
B. Decrease
C. Remain level
D. Decrease blood flow to the heart

416. A patient enters the clinic with a right shoulder injury sustained during a softball game. The physician sends a prescription to do an extensive strengthening program to the medial rotators of the right shoulder. The physical therapist requests that you begin treatment exercises to the medial rotators. Which of the following groups of muscles compose the medial rotators of the shoulder joint?
    A. Pectoralis major, anterior deltoid, subscapularis, teres major
    B. Infraspinatus, teres minor, anterior deltoid
    C. Infraspinatus, teres minor, posterior deltoid
    D. Teres major, posterior deltoid

417. You did not pass the first practical in gait laboratory so you are now studying to take the second test. You study the following question from a sample packet: "During the swing phase, acceleration stage, which muscle begins to contract just before push-off to assist in initiating the forward swing of the leg?"
    A. Gluteus maximus, semitendinosus, biceps femoris
    B. Gluteus medius, semitendinosus, biceps femoris
    C. Semimembranosus, semitendinosus, biceps femoris
    D. Quadriceps

418. A 37-year-old female executive fell when riding her mountain bicycle, resulting in a fractured right wrist. She comes to your clinic and wants to know what the normal range of motion for wrist flexion and extension would be for full recovery. Which of the following is the correct answer?
    A. Flexion 0 to 90°, extension 0 to 90°
    B. Flexion 0 to 90°, extension 0 to 70°
    C. Flexion 0 to 80°, extension 0 to 70°
    D. Flexion 0 to 70°, extension 0 to 90°

419. You are teaching a spinal cord patient proper pressure relief in the wheelchair. You explain that every 10 to 15 minutes he will need to provide pressure relief independently to prevent sores or ulcers. What is the minimal level of injury this patient can have in order to be able to provide independent care to himself?
    A. C4
    B. C5
    C. C6
    D. C8

420. In the hospital where you work the policy states that all notes must be written in the SOAP format. Your patient tells you that his chief concern is limited movement or loss of range of motion in the left shoulder. Where does this information go in the SOAP format?
    A. Subjective
    B. Objective
    C. Assessment
    D. Plan

421. You are treating a 28-year-old male with lateral epicondylitis secondary to work. His chief complaint is pain with weakness in the left elbow. The order is for ice pack, phonophoresis, and massage. What would be the best type of massage for this patient?
    A. General massage
    B. Friction, transverse massage
    C. Shiatsu massage
    D. Effleurage massage

422. You are treating a 63-year-old lawyer for back pain who is referred to an orthopedic surgeon 60 miles out of town. The orthopedic surgeon owns his private clinic and tells the patient he must have physical therapy at his clinic. The patient approaches you because driving 20 minutes or more increases pain. What should you tell the patient?

A. The physician is a fraud and trying to make more money for his own physical therapy practice.

B. The physician owns his clinic, which is illegal; find another physician.

C. Tell the patient he has the right to attend the clinic of his choice. If he has any concerns he should talk to his family physician who originally referred him to physical therapy.

D. Since the patient is a lawyer and interested in the physical therapy profession, discuss the legal and ethical information with him.

423. You have a 26-year-old female with a lacerated hand injury. The doctor orders paraffin treatments and range of motion. What should be the typical treatment temperature for paraffin?
    A. 50°C
    B. 30°C
    C. 40°C
    D. 126°C

424. You are performing a postural observation on a 16-year-old track and field star. Upon posture observation, you notice that the patient has pronated feet. Which of the following would best describe this?
    A. Lateral convexity of the Achilles' tendon due to a medial weight line.
    B. Eversion of the calcaneus with lateral convexity of the Achilles' tendon.
    C. Eversion of the calcaneus with a medial weight line.
    D. Inversion of the calcaneus with a medial weight line.

425. You are working at a hospital that has not approved the SOAP note format but instead uses the problem-oriented medical record (POMR) format. What are the four major components of the POMR format?
    A. Subjective, objective, assessment, plan
    B. Subjective, objective, progress, potential for rehabilitation
    C. Subjective, laboratory test with physician medical history, assessment, prognosis for rehabilitation
    D. Subjective, treatment plan, assessment, prognosis

426. A patient comes to the clinic with a swollen right thumb. The patient reports that he was at work operating the press machine when the press closed and caught his thumb. The patient will need joint immobilization to restore range of motion; otherwise he has escaped with minimal injury. The carpometacarpal joint of the thumb is classified as what type of joint?
    A. Uniaxial
    B. Biaxial
    C. Saddle
    D. Hinge

427. In determining a target heart rate for a 62-year-old patient, you would use the calculation for maximum heart rate. Which of the following best describes the calculation for maximum heart rate?
    A. Pulse rate for 60 seconds
    B. Count pulse for 15 seconds x 4, plus age
    C. 220 plus age
    D. 220 minus age

428. The physical therapist assistant may utilize physical or mechanical techniques, as well as manual therapy techniques. Which of the following is not an example of manual therapy techniques performed by a physical therapist assistant?
    A. Grade one mobilization
    B. Grade two mobilization
    C. Grade three mobilization
    D. Grade five mobilization

429. You have a patient reporting neck pain with a bulging disc at level C6, C7. The patient tells you that she suffers from temporomandibular joint (TMJ) problems on and off and is currently receiving treatment for this condition. The physician's order is for cervical traction. What would be best for this patient?

A. Do not perform cervical traction secondary to medical history
B. Sitting cervical traction
C. Supine cervical traction with cervical spine pillow
D. Saunders cervical traction device

430. You are given the description of a type of electrical stimulation as follows: medium-frequency current, approximately 4000 Hz, and utilizes four electrodes in a crossed pattern on the patient. What type of electrical stimulation is being described?
A. Low-volt electric stimulation
B. High-volt electric stimulation
C. Russian stimulation
D. Interferential current stimulation

431. You are assisting the physical therapist in teaching a four-point crutch gait pattern to a 16-year-old basketball player who fractured his left tibia. The patient is nonweightbearing on the left lower extremity. Which answer below describes this pattern?
A. (L) crutch, (R) foot, (R) crutch, (L) foot
B. (L) crutch, (R) crutch, swing through, (R) foot
C. (L) crutch, (R) foot, (L) foot, (R) crutch
D. (R) crutch, (R) foot, (L) crutch, (L) foot

432. Which of the following physics laws states that the intensity of radiation to a surface will fall off relative to the angle formed between the source and the patient? Clinical application of this law means the ultrasound should be perpendicular to the patient for best results.
A. Inverse square law
B. Ohm's law
C. Cosine law
D. Joule's law

433. While on the cardiopulmonary floor, the physical therapist asks you to consult on a case. You find a 36-year-old male whose breathing alternates between periods of deep breathing and apnea. Therefore, the pattern of breathing is hyperapnea and apnea, especially when sleeping. What is another term for this type of breathing or disorder in rate and rhythm?
A. Ataxic breathing
C. Biot's respiration
C. Cheyne-Stokes respiration
D. Sighing respiration

434. A 16-year-old female basketball player twisted her ankle, causing injury to the lateral ligaments. In physical therapy you are to begin rehabilitation to the lateral ligaments. Which lateral ligament/ligaments of the ankle joint will you be rehabilitating?
A. Deltoid
B. Anterior talofibular, posterior talofibular, calcaneofibular
C. Spring ligament, deltoid ligament
D. Anterior talofibular, spring ligament, calcaneofibular

435. There are typically three classifications of exercises utilized to rehabilitate a patient. These consist of isotonic, isokinetic, and isometric exercises. Which of the following is described by this phrase: "no change in muscle length but the muscle will develop tension"?
A. Isotonic
B. Isokinetic
C. Isometric
D. Passive/range of motion

436. You are measuring crutches for a patient with a knee sprain. The patient is to be nonweightbearing on the left lower extremity. What would be the proper measurement guidelines for fitting the crutches to this patient?
    A. 20° to 30° of elbow flexion and two fingers width between the axilla and the crutch.
    B. 20° to 30° of elbow flexion and one finger width between the axilla and the crutch.
    C. 25° to 40° of elbow flexion and two fingers width between the axilla and the crutch.
    D. 10° to 20° of elbow flexion and one finger width between the axilla and the crutch.

437. You have reevaluated a TMJ patient's ability to open and close the jaw. You measure the patient's ability to open the jaw after 2 weeks of treatment for pain and inflammation. The patient now closes the jaw. Which muscle listed below is responsible for closing the jaw?
    A. Masseter
    B. Pterygoideus lateralis
    C. Pterygoideus medialis
    D. Zygomaticus

438. You are observing the posture of a patient walking in and out of the parallel bars. You notice that the patient maintains an elevated pelvis on the right as it compares to the left side. Of the following, which muscle elevates the pelvis?
    A. Quadratus lumborum
    B. Pectineus
    C. Gemellus inferior
    D. Gemellus superior

439. You are collecting data on the flexor withdrawal reflex. You perform the stimulus on the sole of the foot with the lower extremity in extended position to start. Which of the following would be the normal response as a result of this stimulus?
    A. The leg will withdraw from the stimulus
    B. The leg will extend with the stimulus
    C. The leg on the opposite side will flex with the stimulus
    D. The leg on the opposite side will extend with the stimulus

440. While working in the burn unit, you decide to do a study of how patients respond to correct positioning as a result of a burn and how that directly relates to their decreased ability to develop a contracture. You perform a cross-sectional research study with the physical therapist. Which of the following would best describe a cross-sectional research study?
    A. Interviewing the same people over the same time period
    B. Interviewing different people through their lifespan
    C. Interviewing the same people through their lifespan
    D. Interviewing different people over the same time period

441. You are working in the burn unit and receive a patient with a burn of the axillary region of the right shoulder. You are instructed by the physical therapist to place this patient in a position to minimize the risk of developing a contracture. Which of the following would be the correct position?
    A. In a position of comfort
    B. Shoulder adduction
    C. Shoulder abduction, flexion
    D. Shoulder abduction, extension

442. A patient is in physical therapy to reduce muscle spasms and low back pain, which are interfering with his ability to work. The therapist instructs you to set the patient up on high volt galvanic stimulation. Which of the following is the most important choice to do first in the application procedure?
    A. Determine electrode choice, disposable or carbonized rubber
    B. Select the polarity to use and set dial
    C. Set machine intensity to zero
    D. Explain the procedure to the patient

443. You are treating a patient in a nursing home with a stage two ulcer of the greater trochanter. The patient's condition is deteriorating over a period of months with an increase of infection in the area. Which of the following would be a correct description of the body's first line of defense against bacterial infection?
    A. Phagocytes
    B. Macrophages
    C. Lymphocytes
    D. Neutrophils

444. The physical therapist instructs you to treat a patient for greater trochanter bursitis. You will be treating several muscles that insert into the greater trochanter. How many muscles insert into the greater trochanter?
    A. 4
    B. 5
    C. 6
    D. 7

445. An 8-year-old male enters the clinic with a diagnosis of fracture of the distal radius. The patient's mother reports that the patient was riding his bicycle down a steep hill when he fell off. The physician sends the patient to therapy for examination because he is concerned about possible nerve damage. A fracture of the distal radius will result in possible nerve damage to which nerve?
    A. Musculocutaneous
    B. Radial
    C. Ulnar
    D. Median

446. You are assisting in developing policy and procedure for the physical therapy department. You are responsible for setting up a written policy in regard to a nosocomial infection. Which of the following defines a nosocomial infection?
    A. Acute inflammatory response
    B. Allergic response to medications
    C. Infection acquired in the hospital by the patient
    D. Result of the body's rejection of blood type

447. You perform a manual muscle test on a 26-year-old hip patient. The patient can perform full range of motion in supine position for hip adduction/abduction. In sidelying, the patient cannot perform hip adduction/abduction. Using this information, what would you determine this patient's muscle grade to be?
    A. Poor
    B. Trace
    C. Fair
    D. Good

448. You perform manual muscle testing on a L3, L4 spinal cord patient, who is a 21-year-old male and uncooperative. Which of the following considerations is not correct to utilize in manual muscle testing?
    A. Informing the patient of what you will be doing
    B. Stabilizing the proximal part
    C. Lining up the origin and insertion
    D. Testing bilaterally starting with the injured side first

449. You start percussion on a 55-year-old male. The patient is in the intensive care unit secondary to severe angina. He is experiencing lung congestion and needs to clear his lungs. The patient is oriented, pleasant, and cooperative. How should you proceed in the treatment of this patient?
    A. Proceed with treatment as ordered by the physical therapist.
    B. Treatment is not appropriate; refer back to the physical therapist for advice.
    C. Treatment is not appropriate so do not evaluate the patient.
    D. The patient is not a physical therapy candidate and you should refer him to a respiratory therapist.

450. Your patient is a 16-year-old basketball player who fractured his left tibia. The patient is now nonweightbearing (NWB) left lower extremity and needs gait training. The patient has good strength and coordination. Which crutch gait pattern would be best to teach him?

A. Four point
B. Swing through
C. Three point
D. None, start the patient out with a cane first

451. Several types of contractions may take place with an individual muscle or muscle groups. These are classified in kinesiology with specific terms. Of the following, which is referred to as the muscle group whose contraction is considered to be the principal agent in producing a joint motion?
A. Antagonist
B. Concentric
C. Agonist
D. Eccentric

452. You are working in the gait analysis laboratory in physical therapist assistant school. The instructor is giving a lab practice test. She asks the following question: "During the push-off phase of gait during the stance phase, which muscles play an important role in providing a normal push-off?"
A. Quadriceps, anterior tibialis, flexor digitorum longus
B. Gluteus maximus, quadriceps, anterior tibialis
C. Anterior tibialis, peroneus brevis
D. Gastrocnemius, soleus, flexor hallucis longus

453. While in the neurointensive care unit you are asked to treat a patient who was involved in an auto accident. He is an 18-year-old male who is comatose. The following posture is observed when you turn the light on: lower extremities are plantar flexed and fully extended, upper extremity is positioned with shoulder adducted, elbow extended, forearm pronated, and wrist flexed. Which best describes the posture you observed?
A. Decerebrate rigidity
B. Decorticate rigidity
C. Decerebrate spasticity
D. Decorticate spasticity

454. An 86-year-old female falls down the stairs into her basement and breaks her hip. During the course of therapy, rehabilitation goes exceptionally well and the patient is completely healed except for the hip adductor muscle group, where nerves appear to have been permanently damaged and will not recover. Which nerve or nerves innervate the hip adductor muscles?
A. Obturator and sciatic
B. Sciatic
C. Obturator
D. Femoral and obturator

455. When palpating the spine of the scapula you notice a large muscle knot in your patient. For a point of reference in your progress notes you record that the patient has muscle spasms at the spine of the scapula. What vertebral level would you say corresponds with the spine of the scapula to further clarify your notes?
A. T5
B. T3
C. T7
D. T12

456. A patient enters the clinic after sustaining a whiplash injury in an automobile accident. While performing your evaluation, you observe active range of motion for the cervical spine. You ask the patient to perform cervical rotation to the opposite side. Which of the following groups would be responsible for performing cervical rotation to the opposite side?
A. Longus capitis, rectus capitis anterior and posterior
B. Splenius cervicis, splenius capitis
C. Sternocleidomastoid, scalenus anterior, upper trapezius
D. Sternocleidomastoid, scalenus anterior, rectus capitis anterior

CHAPTER 32

Sample Test Answers

1. B. The correct medical name for this inner ear disease is Meniere's disease. Meniere's disease is a disease of the inner ear characterized by episodes of vertigo, progressive unilateral nerve deafness, ringing in the ears, and a sense of pressure in the ears.

   Otitis media is an inflammation of the middle portion of the ear. Otitis externa is an inflammation of the external canal or auricle of the external ear.

2. C. A disorder characterized by the growth of cartilage in the epiphyses of the long bones resulting in the limbs remaining short, and transmitted as an autosomal dominant gene, is achondroplasia.

   Osteogenesis imperfecta is a genetic disorder involving defective development of the connective tissue. It is inherited as an autosomal dominant trait and characterized by abnormally brittle and fragile bones that are easily fractured by the slightest trauma. Typically, the patient presents with multiple fractures with minimal trauma. Fibrous dysplasia pertains to an abnormal condition characterized by fibrous displacement of the osseous tissue within the affected bones. Bone tumor is any abnormal growth of new tissue (benign or malignant).

3. D. Fibrous dysplasia is not another name for thyrotoxicosis as this pertains to an abnormal condition characterized by the fibrous displacement of the osseous tissue within the affected bones.

   Graves' disease, as well as primary and secondary hyperthyroidism, is also called thyrotoxicosis. The condition of hyperthyroidism is typically caused by secretions of the thyroid gland, which increase the basal metabolism rate, causing an increased demand for food to support the metabolic activities.

4. A. Cushing's syndrome is a metabolic disorder resulting from hypersecretion of the adrenal cortex or excessive production of glucocorticoid. It may be caused by a tumor of the adrenal glands or excessive stimulation of the gland that results in hyperfunctioning of the anterior pituitary.

   Adrenogenital syndrome is a condition characterized by hypersecretion of adrenocortical androgens, resulting in somatic masculinization. Addison's disease is a condition caused by partial or complete failure of the adrenocortical function. All three general functions of the adrenal cortex are lost (glucocorticoid, mineralocorticoid, and androgenic).

5. A. Transcutaneous electrical nerve stimulation (TENS) is the only type of stimulation that the patient can utilize 24 hours a day. The patient is set up for independent use of a TENS unit to assist in alleviating pain.

6. D. The femoral, obturator, and inferior gluteal nerves innervate the hip adductor muscles, which consist of the pectineus, gracilis, adductor longus, adductor brevis, and adductor magnus. Their innervation would include the inferior gluteal nerve for the gluteus maximus, the femoral nerve for the pectineus, and the obturator nerve for the adductor brevis, adductor longus, adductor magnus, and gracilis.

7. D. Evaporative coolants or sprays do not significantly lower tissue temperature below the surface. Evaporative coolants cause a chemical action that produces a cool feeling on the outside surface of the skin.

    Ice massage, cryopressure, and ice towels would all decrease swelling by decreasing tissue temperature.

8. C. Iontophoresis is a modality in which chemical substances are entered into the body with a direct current to decrease inflammation.

    Myoflex with ultrasound, phonophoresis, and ultrasound are treatments that may use anti-inflammatories but they are not chemical substances placed into the body with a direct current.

9. B. Convection is the transfer of heat energy by combining mechanisms of fluid and conduction (eg, diathermy, paraffin).

    Conversion does not exist. Conduction is heat transferred from one part of the body to another through molecular collision (eg, hot packs). Radiation is heat transferred in the form of electromagnetic waves without heating the intervening medium (eg, warming by the sun).

10. D. In performing treatment for a patient with left upper extremity edema secondary to a mastectomy it would not be appropriate to perform whirlpool. Whirlpool, by placing the arm in a dependent position, would only increase the fluid. You would want to emphasize reducing edema through isometric exercises, Jobst compression pump, and massage.

11. D. Intermittent mechanical traction is described as intermittent traction when there is typically a hold and rest period.

    Autotraction utilizes a special traction bench made up of two sections that can be individually angled and rotated. The patient applies traction by pulling with his or her own arms. With gravity lumbar traction, the lower border and circumference of the rib cage are anchored through a specially made vest secured to the top of the bed. The patient is placed on a bed, which is tilted vertically, putting the patient in a position in which the free weight of the legs and hips exerts a traction force on the lumbar spine by gravity. With manual traction the therapist grasps the patient and manually applies traction force either for a few seconds or by a sudden, quick thrust.

12. C. A patient with paranoia would exhibit psychotic behavior, appearing suspicious, resentful, and rigid.

    Hypochondria is a disorder characterized by a chronic, abnormal concern about health. Hysteria is a state of tension or excitement characterized by unmanageable fear and temporary loss of control over the emotions. Depression is an emotional state characterized by feelings of sadness, despair, emptiness, and hopelessness.

13. B. A patient with depression would appear pessimistic, irritable, lack self-confidence, and have a gloomy outlook on life.

    Hysteria is a general state of tension or excitement in a person, characterized by unmanageable fear and temporary loss of control over the emotions. A psychopath is a person who has an antisocial personality disorder. Schizophrenia is any one of a large group of psychotic disorders characterized by a gross distortion of reality, disturbances of communication, withdrawal from social interaction, and disorganized and fragmented thought, perception, and emotional reaction.

14. D. Premature labor is defined as labor that occurs between the 20th and 37th week of pregnancy.

15. C. Hypertonia is a condition characterized by excessive tone in the limbs, making them resistant to both active and passive movement.

    Flaccidity is characterized by weak, soft, and flabby muscles that lack normal muscle tone. Hypotonia is characterized by less than adequate muscle contractions and a state of decreased motor neuron excitability. Rigidity is a condition of hardness, stiffness, or inflexibility.

16. A. The minimal level a patient can have to perform self range of motion independently is C7.

    At C4 and C5, a patient can only direct range of motion. At C7 and C8, a patient would be independent in range of motion.

17. D. Autograft is the surgical transplant of skin from one part of the body to another location on the same individual. Grafting has been found to be effective for timely wound closure and to decrease scar tissue formation.

18. B. Sacral sparing occurs when the patient has paralysis and loss of sensation except in the sacral area.

Cauda equina injury involves the lower end of the spinal cord at the first lumbar vertebra and the bundle of lumbar, sacral, and coccygeal nerve roots that emerge from the spinal cord and descend through the spinal canal of the sacrum and coccyx. Central cord syndrome occurs when there is damage to the central portion of the cord and an incomplete lesion. Typically, greater deficits are found in the upper extremities than the lower extremities upon evaluation. Brown-Séquard's syndrome is a traumatic neurologic disorder resulting from compression of one side of the spinal cord, typically seen after a knife-type injury. There is also an incomplete lesion that typically results in loss of motor function on the same side as the lesion and loss of pain and temperature on the opposite side.

19. B. Central cord syndrome occurs when there is damage to the central portion of the cord and an incomplete lesion. Typically, greater deficits are found in the upper extremities than the lower extremities upon evaluation.

Anterior cord syndrome results in damage to the anterior part of the spinal cord. This is an incomplete lesion and sense of light touch proprioception and position are usually intact. Brown-Séquard's syndrome results in hemisection of the spinal cord. Sacral sparing occurs in the sacral area and is an incomplete lesion. Typically, sensation will be intact in the sacral area; however, paralysis and loss of sensation are complete in all other areas below the level of lesion.

20. B. Scleroderma is a relatively rare autoimmune disease affecting the blood vessels and connective tissue. It is characterized by fibrous degeneration of the connective tissue of the skin, lungs, and internal organs.

Chronic contractures are an abnormal condition of a joint, characterized by flexion and fixation. Fibrositis is an inflammation of fibrous connective tissue, usually characterized by a poorly defined set of symptoms, including pain and stiffness of the neck, shoulder, and trunk. Myositis is an inflammation of muscle tissue, usually of the voluntary muscles.

21. C. A patient with scleroderma typically would have contractures secondary to fibrosis where skin is bound down to the tissue. An appropriate treatment program would be stretching and flexibility to reduce muscle contractures and maintain range of motion.

Aerobic conditioning, strengthening, and isokinetic exercises would not be the primary treatment for this patient, as the initial goal would be to maintain or regain range of motion and prevent contractures. Strengthening may be added later, as well as isokinetic exercises, depending on the patient's condition.

22. B. The horizontal plane divides the body into upper and lower parts for the purpose of kinesiology study.

The sagittal plane divides the body into right and left sides. The frontal plane divides the front and the back. The rotary plane does not exist.

23. C. The sagittal plane divides the body into right and left sides.

24. C. Normal alignment of a patient from the lateral view would be the head in neutral position with the scapula flat against the upper back and the shoulder in neutral position with the plumb line falling through the shoulder joint.

Normal alignment from the posterior view would be the head in neutral position, scapula in neutral position, level alignment in comparison to each other, with the plumb line falling straight through the thoracic and lumbar spine.

25. B. Functional performance of the lower extremity requires that a patient have a muscle grade of fair plus.

26. C. Normal range of motion for distal interphalangeal joint flexion is 0 to 80°.

Normal range of motion for distal interphalangeal joint extension would be 80° to 0. Normal range of motion for proximal interphalangeal joint flexion would be 0 to 120°, and extension 120° to 0. Normal range of motion for metacarpophalangeal joint flexion would be 0 to 90°, and extension 0 to 30°.

27. A. Thirty-six degrees would be the correct temperature conversion from Fahrenheit to Celsius. This is performed by the following: Celsius = (temperature in Fahrenheit - 32) x 5/9 (98°F – 32) = 66 x 5 = 330/9 = 36°C.

28. C. Isokinetics would not be an appropriate treatment protocol for a patient 2 weeks status post ACL reconstruction surgery. This is because isokinetics is an aggressive form of exercise that should be instituted in ACL protocol only as recommended by a physician.

     Quad sets, isometrics, and straight leg raises would all be appropriate in developing the quad and also would not present any injury to the ACL surgery.

29. D. A TENS unit would be contraindicated for this patient with a history of chronic back pain. This is because the patient's history reveals that the patient has a pacemaker in place, type unknown.

     Hot packs, ultrasound, and pelvic traction would be appropriate treatment modalities to administer and would not be contraindicated secondary to the pacemaker.

30. A. Rheobase is defined as a minimum intensity of an electrical stimulus to elicit a minimal contraction.

     Chronaxie is the minimal time that a stimulus of twice rheobase stimulates a tissue (strength duration curve). Anode is a positive electrode. Cathode is a negative electrode.

31. D. Chronaxie is the minimal time that a stimulus of twice rheobase stimulates a tissue (strength duration curve).

     Galvanic current is steady and uninterrupted direct current and is unidirectional. Faradic current is low amplitude, long duration, and one direction.

32. C. Three degrees of freedom is the maximum number that any single joint in the body can possess. For example, for the glenohumeral joint, this would include flexion, extension, abduction, adduction, internal and external rotation.

33. A. Antagonist is defined as a muscle group that is noncontracting and passively elongates or shortens to permit the motion to occur.

34. C. Inverse square law states that the intensity of radiation from a light source varies inversely to the square of the distance from the source. Clinical application means the further the infrared light (eg, is moving from the patient), the greater the decrease in intensity will be.

35. B. A patient in a coma would show no voluntary movement, be unresponsive to stimulus, have no reflexes, and exhibit a positive Babinski response.

     The aftereffect of a cerebrovascular accident depends on the location and extent of ischemia. Paralysis, weakness, speech defect, aphasia, and even death may occur. Patients in a stupor would exhibit a state of lethargy and unresponsiveness in which they seem unaware of their surroundings.

36. A. A patient with posterior column deficit would exhibit the following: an unsteady gait with a wide base of support, a positive Romberg's sign, and watching the ground when ambulating. The patient would land with the heel first, then the toes, creating a double tapping sign. Also, the patient would have loss of position sense in the legs.

37. C. The hip joint has three degrees of freedom in flexion/extension, abduction/adduction, internal/external rotation.

38. A. A first-class lever has a fulcrum between the weight and the applied force. It is frequently used to monitor posture and balance. The atlantooccipital joint (axis) head (weight) is an example of a first-class lever.

     In a second-class lever, the force arm is longer than the weight arm. An example is the brachioradialis and wrist extensors on elbow flexion. In a third-class lever the weight arm is longer than the force arm, designed for producing speed or for moving a small weight a long distance. A third-class lever is situated at all the joints of the upper and lower extremities of the body. There is no fourth-class lever.

39. B. In a second-class lever, the force arm is longer than the weight arm. An example is the brachioradialis and wrist extensors on elbow flexion.

40. C. Tibialis anterior, peroneus tertius, and extensor hallucis longus are muscles that are active during the swing phase, acceleration stage. These muscles remain active throughout the entire stage to help shorten the extremity so it can clear the ground by holding the ankle in a neutral position.

41. C. During the swing phase, deceleration stage, the hamstring muscles contract to slow down the swing phase just prior to heel strike, thus permitting the heel to strike quietly in a controlled manner.

42. D. A greenstick fracture is an incomplete fracture in which the bone is bent but fractured only on the outer arc of the bend. Children are likely to have greenstick fractures.

    Open fracture (also called a compound fracture) is a fracture in which the broken end or ends of the bone have torn through the skin. In a closed fracture, the broken bones are contained within the skin. In a comminuted fracture, there are several breaks in the bone, thereby creating numerous fragments.

43. B. In an impacted fracture there is a bone break in which the adjacent fragmented ends of the fractured bone are wedged together.

    In a displaced fracture, a traumatic bone break takes place in which two ends of a fractured bone are separated from each other. An intraarticular fracture involves the articular surfaces of a joint.

44. C. Q wave is the first downward deflection you see when reading the EKG. It represents the first part of the QRS complex.

    T wave is the component of the cardiac cycle shown on an electrocardiogram as a short, inverted, U-shaped curve following the ST segment. P wave is the component of the cardiac cycle shown on an electrocardiogram as an inverted U-shaped curve that follows the end of the T wave and precedes the spike of the QRS complex. QRS complex is the components of the ventricular electric events of the cardiac cycle shown on an electrocardiogram as a sharp, angular complex normally less than 0.1 seconds in duration, reflecting the time it takes for the ventricular myocardium to depolarize.

45. C. The sinus node, which is an area of specialized heart tissue near the entrance of the superior vena cava that generates the cardiac electric impulse and is, in turn, controlled by the autonomic nervous system, discharges an impulse at the rate of 60 to 100 beats per minute.

46. A. The sinus node is located in the right atrium of the heart.

47. B. The valve between the left atrium and left ventricle is the mitral valve; the right atrioventricular valve is the tricuspid valve. Because of their position in the heart these valves are referred to as atrioventricular valves.

    The semilunar valve is a valve with half-moon shaped cusps (eg, aortic valve and pulmonary valve). Pulmonary valve is a cardiac structure composed of three semilunar cusps that close during each heartbeat to prevent blood from flowing back into the right ventricle from the pulmonary artery. Aortic valve is a valve in the heart between the left ventricle and the aorta, composed of three semilunar cusps that close in diastole to prevent blood from flowing back into the left ventricle from the aorta.

48. C. Pectus carinatum is best described as a sternum that is displaced anteriorly, increasing anterior-posterior diameter.

49. C. A patient in supine position with the lower extremities plantar flexed and internally rotated, and the upper extremities positioned in shoulder adduction, elbow flexion, and wrist flexion would best be described as exhibiting posture of decorticate rigidity.

    Hemiplegia is characterized by posture that is paralyzed on one side of the body. Decerebrate rigidity is posture of the lower extremities plantar flexed and fully extended, upper extremities positioned in shoulder adduction, elbow extension, forearm pronation, and wrist flexion. Spasticity extensor does not exist.

50. A. The description of this patient's injury shows that he had decorticate rigidity, which would typically be found in an injury of the corticospinal tracts.

51. B. Flexor carpi ulnaris, which functions to flex and adduct the hand, does not have dual innervation.

    Flexor digitorum profundus, flexor pollicis brevis, and the lumbricales all have dual innervation by the median nerve and the ulnar nerve.

52. D. With a patient who has an injury involving the tibialis muscles, you can expect to have a deep peroneal nerve involved, as that is what innervates the anterior tibialis muscle.

53. A. The medial collateral ligament provides the medial stability of the knee.

    Medial meniscus is a cushion or shock absorber between the bone and does not provide stability. The anterior cruciate ligament provides anterior stability. The medial meniscus does not provide stability.

54. C. The group of muscles that attach to the ischial tuberosity are as follows: semimembranosus, biceps femoris, and semitendinosus.

55. C. Teres major does not attach to the greater tuberosity of the humerus.

    Muscles that attach to the greater tuberosity of the humerus include supraspinatus, teres minor, and infraspinatus.

56. A. All of the wrist extensor muscles have a common origin at the lateral epicondyle of the elbow.

57. D. L2 is the vertebral level at which the spinal cord ends.

58. B. Amyotrophic lateral sclerosis is also called Lou Gehrig's disease. It is a degenerative disease of the motor neurons, characterized by atrophy of the muscles of the hands, forearms, and legs, spreading to involve most of the body.

    Parkinson's disease is a slowly progressive, degenerative, neurologic disorder characterized by resting tremor, pill rolling of the fingers, a masklike face, shuffled gait, forward flexion of the trunk, and muscle rigidity and weakness. Hodgkin's disease is a malignant disorder characterized by painless, progressive enlargement of lymphoid tissue. Marfan's syndrome is an abnormal condition characterized by elongation of the bones, often with associated abnormalities of the eyes and cardiovascular system.

59. D. Brown-Séquard's syndrome is a traumatic, neurologic disorder resulting from compression of one side of the spinal cord, above the 10th thoracic vertebrae. Brown-Séquard's syndrome results in hemisection of the spinal cord. It is typically seen after a knife-type injury. This also is an incomplete lesion that typically results in loss of motor function on the same side as the lesion and loss of pain and temperature on the opposite side.

60. C. The biceps correspond with the C5 reflex.
    The brachioradialis corresponds with C6. The triceps correspond with C7.

61. C. C7 corresponds with the triceps.
    C5 corresponds with the biceps. C6 corresponds with brachioradialis. C8 corresponds with finger flexion.

62. C. The facial nerve is the correct answer because the patient has a diagnosis of Bell's palsy. Bell's palsy is a condition that causes paralysis of the facial nerve.

63. D. Flexor carpi ulnaris does not assist in pronation of the radioulnar joint. Muscles active in pronation include brachioradialis, pronator teres, pronator quadratus, and flexor carpi radialis.

64. D. Subscapularis is the muscle that attaches to the lesser tuberosity of the humerus.
    Teres minor, infraspinatus, and supraspinatus attach to the greater tuberosity of the humerus.

65. C. The median and ulnar nerves innervate the flexor digitorum profundus.

66. A. If the patient could isolate and move only the levator scapulae and rhomboid muscles, the correct answer is medial rotation downward. Levator scapulae and rhomboid muscle actions are responsible for medial rotation downward on the scapulae.

67. B. The median nerve innervates the second and third digits of the hand.

    The ulnar nerve would be responsible for the fourth and fifth digits.

68. C. The origin for the tensor fasciae latae muscle is the iliac crest.

69. D. The Y-shaped ligament in the hip is referred to as the iliofemoral ligament.

70. B. The posterior tibialis is the muscle that attaches to the navicular tubercle of the foot.

71. A. The anterior cruciate ligament prevents anterior displacement of the tibia on the femur.

    The posterior cruciate ligament prevents posterior displacement of the tibia on the femur. The medial collateral ligament is responsible for medial stability of the knee. The lateral collateral ligament is responsible for lateral stability of the knee.

72. A. The trigeminal nerve, the largest pair of cranial nerves, is responsible for the act of chewing. The pterygoideus lateralis muscle assists in chewing and protrusion, as does the buccinator muscle.

    The facial nerve is responsible for innervating the scalp, forehead, eyelids, muscles of facial expression, cheeks, and jaw. The accessory nerve is responsible for movements of the head and shoulders. The vagus nerve is responsible for taste and swallowing.

73. A. A characteristic that is not typically seen with an upper motor neuron lesion is muscle atrophy. A patient with an upper motor neuron lesion typically has spasticity and hyperreflexia, and Babinski's sign is possible.

74. B. Lactic acid build-up following exercise will cause muscle fatigue.

    Glycogen and glucose are fuels used for exercise.

75. D. Residual volume is the amount of gas left over after maximum expiration. It helps prevent the lungs from collapsing.

    Dead air space is the area in which no gas exchange takes place. Forced inspiratory volume is the amount of air that can be forcibly inspired after maximum inspiration. Expiratory reserve volume is the maximum volume expired after normal expiration.

76. C. Bradycardia is described as an abnormal circulatory condition in which the myocardium contracts steadily but at a rate of 60 contractions a minute or less.

    Tachycardia is an abnormal condition in which the myocardium contracts regularly but at a rate greater than 100 beats per minute.

77. C. Tachycardia is an abnormal condition in which the myocardium contracts regularly but at a rate greater than 100 beats per minute.

78. C. Blood pressure readings above 140/90 are indicative of hypertension. Typically, hypertension is indicated when three different readings are all 140/90 or above.

79. D. A benefit not associated with aerobic exercise is a decrease in aerobic capacity.

    Decrease in serum lipid levels, increase in HDL levels, and an increase in aerobic capacity are benefits from an aerobic exercise program.

80. D. Pallor is not a cardinal sign of inflammation. Pallor is an unnatural paleness or absence of color in the skin.

Rubor is redness that accompanies inflammation. Calor, or heat, is generated by inflammation of tissues. Tumor is a swelling or enlargement occurring in inflammatory conditions.

81. A. The radial nerve, which is the largest branch of the brachial plexus, arising on each side as a continuation of the posterior cord, is the nerve that passes through the anatomical snuffbox of the wrist. Therefore, if you were evaluating a patient who might have suffered an injury to the nerve crossing the anatomical snuffbox, you would evaluate the radial nerve.

The median nerve is one of the terminal branches of the brachial plexus that extends along the radial portions of the forearm and hand and supplies various muscles and the skin of these parts. The ulnar nerve is one of the terminal branches of the brachial plexus that arises on each side from the medial cord of the plexus. The musculocutaneous nerve is one of the terminal branches of the brachial plexus.

82. A. The anterior talofibular ligament is the ligament most frequently injured when an inversion plantar flexion sprain occurs. As a whole, the lateral ligaments are more vulnerable.

83. D. The fibrogelantinous pulp in a disc is called the nucleus pulposus, which is the central portion of each intervertebral disc, consisting of a pulpy, elastic substance that loses some of its resiliency with age.

84. B. The midbrain, one of the three parts of the brainstem and lying below the cerebrum and just above the pons, is not considered one of the three major brain regions.

The three major divisions of the brain region are (1) brainstem, which is the portion of the brain comprising the medulla oblongata, the pons, and the mesencephalon; (2) cerebellum, the part of the brain located in the posterior cranial fossa behind the brainstem; (3) cerebrum, the largest and uppermost section of the brain divided by a central sulcus into the left and right cerebral hemispheres.

85. B. The parasympathetic nervous system is responsible for control of internal functions under quiet conditions.

The autonomic nervous system is the part of the nervous system that regulates involuntary vital functions.

86. A. In preparation for the fight or flight responses, the sympathetic system is activated.

87. C. The structure that controls body temperature and appetite in the body is the hypothalamus. It is a portion of the diencephalon of the brain.

Pons is any slip of tissue connecting two parts of a structure or an organ of the body. The medulla is the most internal part of a structure or organ. The adrenal gland is either of two secretory organs perched atop the kidneys.

88. D. A tendon is connective tissue surrounding a muscle that projects beyond the ends of the muscle fibers and becomes cordlike.

Aponeurosis is a strong sheet of fibrous connective tissue that serves as a tendon to attach muscles to bone. Fascia is the fibrous connective tissue of the body that may be separated from other specifically organized structures. Myofibril is a slender, striated strand of muscle tissue.

89. D. The patella or kneecap is classified as a sesamoid bone.

The long bones contribute to the height or length of an extremity. Short bones occur in clusters and usually permit movement of the extremities.

90. C. Respiration is the transfer of gases between body cells and the environment. The rate varies with the age and condition of the person.

91. A. The Valsalva's maneuver is a forced expiratory effort against a closed airway, as when an individual holds his or her breath and tightens the muscles in a strenuous effort to move a heavy object or to change position in bed. In pregnancy, Valsalva's maneuver both increases pressure on the pelvic diaphragm and causes fluctuations in venous return to the heart.

92. B. The synapse is the region surrounding the point of contact between two neurons, across which nerve impulses are transmitted through the action of a neurotransmitter.

 Ranvier's nodes are constrictions in the medullary substance of a nerve fiber at more or less regular intervals. Schwann cells are cells of ectodermal origin that comprise the neurilemma.

93. D. Mechanoreceptors are described as any sensory nerve endings that respond to mechanical deformation of tissue.

94. B. Myosin are thick filaments, called the I band.

 Actin are thin filaments attached to the Z line.

 Myofibrils are slender striated strands of muscle tissue.

95. C. The gluteus muscles are any of the three muscles that form the buttocks: (1) gluteus maximus, (2) gluteus medius, and (3) gluteus minimus. The origin for the gluteus muscles is the ilium. The ilium is one of the three bones (ilium, ischium, and pubis) that make up the hip bone.

 The pubis is one of a pair of pubic bones that form the hip bone and join the pubic bone from the opposite side at the pubic symphysis. The ischium, one of the three parts of the hip bone, joins the ilium and pubis to form the acetabulum.

96. C. The tibialis posterior muscle inserts into the navicular tuberosity.

 Sesamoid is any one of numerous small, round, bony masses embedded in certain tendons that may be subjected to compression and tension. Calcaneus is the heel bone. It is the largest of the tarsal bones. It articulates proximally with the talus and distally with the cuboid.

97. A. Trapezium is the correct carpal bone that you would be palpating since it articulates directly with the thumb, which is controlled by the thenar muscles.

98. A. Mitochondria, small rodlike or granular organelles within the cytoplasm, are the powerhouse of the cell where ATP is made.

 Cytoplasm is all of the substance of a cell other than the nucleus. Ribosome is a cytoplasmic organelle composed of ribonucleic acid and protein that functions in the synthesis of protein. Nucleus is the central controlling body within a living cell.

99. D. Seventy percent of the body consists of water (H_2O).

100. A. The ulnar nerve lies behind the medial epicondyle of the elbow. It can be easily palpated at the "funny bone" of the elbow, as it lies along the groove between the olecranon process and the medial epicondyle of the humerus.

101. A. The main function of erythrocytes, also known as the red blood cells, is to transport oxygen in the body. Erythrocytes are biconcave discs that contain hemoglobin confined within a lipoid membrane. Erythrocytes originate in the marrow of the long bones.

102. C. Leukocytes are the white blood cells of the body and their primary function is to protect the body against infection. There are five types of leukocytes, classified by the presence or absence of granules in the cytoplasm of the cell.

 Agglutinin is a specific kind of antibody whose interaction with antigens is manifested as agglutination. Agglutinin acts on insoluble antigens in stable suspension to form a cross-linking lattice that may clump. Erythrocytes are red blood cells.

103. B. The heel bone into which the Achilles' tendon inserts is called the calcaneus. It is the largest of the tarsal bones. It articulates proximally with the talus and distally with the cuboid.

The cuboid bone is on the lateral side of the foot, proximal to the fourth and fifth metatarsal bones. The talus is the second largest tarsal bone. It supports the tibia and rests on the calcaneus. The first metatarsal is one of five bones numbered one to five from the medial side of the foot.

104. B. You would not perform rehabilitation to the anterior tibiofibular since it is not a lateral ligament of the ankle.

Calcaneofibular, posterior talofibular, and anterior talofibular are lateral ligaments of the ankle. The purpose of the calcaneofibular is posterior displacement of the foot, dorsiflexion. The purpose of the posterior talofibular is posterior displacement of the foot. The purpose of the anterior talofibular is anterior displacement of the foot, medial tilting of the talus, and plantar flexion.

105. D. The platysma is one of a pair of wide muscles at the side of the neck. The platysma is innervated by the cervical branch of the facial nerve and serves to draw the angles of the mouth downward.

The levator anguli oris is responsible for elevation of the corners of the mouth. The buccinator is the main muscle of the cheek. The buccinator is innervated by buccal branches of the facial nerve, functioning to aid in chewing of food and compression of the cheeks. The orbicularis oris is the muscle surrounding the mouth. It is innervated by buccal branches of the facial nerve and serves to close and purse the lips.

106. A. The stimulus for testing flexor withdrawal is applied to the sole of the foot with the lower extremity in extended position to start.

107. B. The correct response to this stimulus would be upper extremity extension and lower extremity flexion.

108. B. In the prone position, the patient will show an increase in flexor tone.

Placed in supine, the patient will show an increase in extensor tone. If placed in sidelying, the patient will show an increase in extensor tone in the sidelying limbs and an increase in flexor tone on the nonweightbearing limb.

109. B. Having the patient bounce several times on the soles of the feet with weightbearing is the stimulus you would be using to test the positive support reaction. The response would be an increase in extensor tone in the lower extremity.

110. A. An increase in extensor tone occurs when the patient's positioned in supine for the tonic labyrinthine reflex. No specific stimulus is required and the response is dependent upon patient positioning. Prone increases flexor tone, sidelying increases extensor tone, the other sidelying limb increases flexor tone in the nonweightbearing limb.

111. C. A positive response to bouncing a patient several times on the soles of the feet but not allowing him to bear weight would be increased flexor tone in the lower extremities.

112. D. An increase in extensor tone in sidelying limbs and flexor tone in nonweightbearing limbs would occur when a patient is positioned sidelying when testing for tonic labyrinthine reflex.

113. D. Moro's reflex is a reflex that is performed with a stimulus of a sudden movement to cause a startle reaction. The time period to test this reflex is 3 to 6 months of age. The integration level is midbrain. The response is that startle reaction causes extension reaction of the extremities.

114. D. The grasp reflex has an integration level of the midbrain. The time period is from 3 to 6 months of age. The stimulus is placing an object in the palm of the hand and the response is the fingers would grasp the object. It is an incorrect statement that the grasp reflex occurs between 6 to 9 months of age.

115. C. An incorrect or untrue statement regarding a cerebral palsy child is that the child can hold or bring the head into a normal position. Typically, a cerebral palsy child cannot hold or bring the head into a normal position. Such children cannot support themselves. Typically, they will demonstrate a scissors gait pattern. They will usually have an exaggerated reflex response. They may be classified as either spastic, ataxic, or athetoid. They may be either passive or stiff and cannot adjust body position.

116. A. The posterior tibial nerve is the nerve that is compressed as a result of tarsal tunnel syndrome. Tarsal tunnel syndrome is an abnormal condition characterized by pain and numbness in the sole of the foot. The condition may be corrected by appropriate orthopedic therapy or surgery.

117. D. Calcaneus valgus refers to excessive eversion of the foot.

118. C. Congenital dysplasia of the hip is a congenital orthopedic defect in which the head of the femur does not articulate with the acetabulum because of an abnormal shallowness of the acetabulum. As a result, a patient with congenital dysplasia would show a limitation in hip abduction. Treatment consists of maintaining continuous abduction of the thigh so that the head of the femur presses into the center of the shallow cavity, causing it to deepen.

119. B. Coxa vara is the correct term to describe the disorder of the upper femur in which the angle of inclination is below 110°.

     Coxa valgus is a hip deformity in which the angle formed by the axis of the head and neck of the femur and the axis of its shaft is significantly increased. Transient synovitis is a temporary inflammatory condition of the synovial membrane of a joint as the result of an aseptic wound or traumatic injury. The knee is most commonly affected. Osteitis pubis is an inflammation of the hip bones caused by infection, degeneration, or trauma.

120. D. Spondylolisthesis is best described as gradual slipping of one vertebra over another, most commonly the fifth lumbar vertebra over the first sacral vertebra.

121. D. Torticollis is a deformity of the neck that causes rotation and tilting of the head in the opposite direction. Treatment may include surgery, heat, support, or immobilization, depending on the cause and severity of the condition.

122. B. Measurements will take place from the anterior superior iliac spine (the ASIS) to the medial malleolus of the ankle.

123. D. Myositis, which is a muscle inflammation, would not be contraindicated for a massage.

     Hematomas, herniated discs, and phlebitis are contraindicated for massages.

124. D. The patient's hip should be placed in extension and abduction to prevent a contracture.

125. D. The neck should be placed in hyperextension to best minimize the chances of having a neck flexion contracture. Neck flexion contracture would be typically seen in an anterior burn, as this would be a position of comfort for the patient.

126. D. In a double blind study, both the administrator and subjects are ignorant of experiment conditions.

     In a dependent study, a hypothetical effect is manipulated by the experiment. In an independent study, a hypothetical cause is manipulated by the experiment. In a blind study, the subjects are ignorant of actual experiment conditions.

127. C. Interrater reliability refers to testing consistency among raters.

     Test-retest refers to consistency over time. Validity refers to the reliability of the experiment and whether it accurately measures what it is supposed to measure.

128. D. An exercise prescription does not need to include the time of day for a patient to exercise.

     The intensity, duration, and frequency of exercise should all be included.

129. C. Polyneuropathy is an abnormal condition affecting the nerves.

     Neuropathy is any abnormal condition characterized by inflammation and degeneration of the peripheral nerves. Neurosis is any faulty or inefficient way of coping with anxiety or inner conflict. Neurorrhaphy is a surgical procedure to suture a severed nerve.

130. B. Scleroderma is a rare autoimmune disease affecting the blood vessels and connective tissue. There is a gradual hardening of the skin and swelling of the distal extremities.

    Dermatomyositis is a disease of the connective tissues. It is characterized by eczematous inflammation of the skin and tenderness and weakness of the muscles. Granulomatosis is a disease characterized by the development of granulomas.

131. C. Dyspnea is a shortness of breath or difficulty in breathing.

    Syncope is a brief lapse in consciousness caused by transient cerebral hypoxia. It is usually preceded by light-headedness. Hypoxia is an inadequate, reduced tension of cellular oxygen. Hypercapnia is greater than normal amounts of carbon dioxide in the blood.

132. D. Four-point gait pattern would be a slow, stable gait pattern of left crutch, right leg, right crutch, left leg.

    A three-point gait involves a nonweightbearing sequence— the crutch advances first, then the uninvolved leg, then the crutch. A two-point gait requires more balance—the opposite crutch and leg advance simultaneously. A swing-through is used when both lower extremities are involved and a patient swings the crutches, then hops on one leg.

133. A. Dorsi-plantar flexion assist ankle braces assist in plantar flexion of the ankle and during the push-off phase of gait.

    Dorsiflexion assist aids in dorsiflexion during the swing phase. Dorsiflexion stop restricts dorsiflexion and allows free range of motion in plantar flexion. With free motion ankle joint, there is no restriction on any ankle movement.

134. C. This is a stage-three ulcer. A stage-three ulcer involves full thickness of the dermis and undermining of the deeper tissues, and the muscle may be involved.

    Stage-one ulcer destruction is limited to the epidermis and redness may be noted. Stage-two involves the epidermis, dermis, and subcutaneous fat; there may be redness, edema, blistering, and hardening of the tissue. In stage four, full thickness is involved, penetrating to the fascia with possible muscle involvement, and there is usually bone destruction.

135. D. Approximation is used to promote stability.

    Traction is used to promote mobility. Contract-relax is used to increase range of motion. Slow reversal is used to strengthen weakened muscle.

136. C. Capillary hemorrhaging best describes a hemorrhage in which there is oozing and gradual seeping of blood from the wounded area. This type of hemorrhage can be controlled through elevation of the injured part and direct pressure applied over the wound.

    Arterial hemorrhage is a condition in which the artery has been damaged or severed. This results in a very rapid flow of bright red blood, which usually escapes in a rhythmical spurting with each heartbeat. Venous hemorrhage is characterized by a rapid state of infusion of dark blood from the wounded area. Internal hemorrhage is unexposed and can only be identified through x-ray or diagnostic techniques.

137. A. Standard deviation of the mean plus or minus one is graded based on the score of 68% of the students.

138. B. With a posterior knee burn, a knee flexion contracture would be common. Therefore, a posterior splint with an extension should be the first priority of the therapist to prevent knee flexion contracture.

139. A. For partial weightbearing, the walker should be advanced first, then the patient should advance the involved lower extremity, then the uninvolved.

140. D. Cheyne-Stokes will result in a breathing pattern that is gradually faster and deeper with alternating periods of apnea.

Biot's will result in slow rate, shallow depth, irregular rhythms, typically associated with a central nervous system disorder. Orthopnea describes an abnormal condition in which a person must sit or stand in order to breathe deeply or comfortably. This occurs in many disorders of the cardiac and respiratory systems. Apneusis will result in slow rate, deep inspiration followed by expiration, apnea associated with brainstem disorders. The rate of apneustic breathing is usually around 1.5 cycles per minute.

141. D. In order to perform an ethical research study, prior to starting the research a patient should sign an informed consent document.

    Informing the patient that he or she has the right to terminate the experiment at any time, debriefing the patient following the experiment, and explaining the end results of the experiment to the patient are necessary for a study to be ethical. However, an informed consent document must be signed first.

142. B. Cervical traction should be started with 16 lbs in an attempt to get some separation of the cervical vertebra and the intervertebral disc.

143. B. A muscle grade of poor would equal 20% muscle strength.

    Poor minus would equal 10%, poor plus would equal 30%, and trace would equal 5%.

144. C. The most appropriate exercise for a patient in early stages of rehabilitation after a nonsurgical operation would be closed-chain isokinetic exercise, such as a stair machine.

145. D. The patient should be checked frequently for red spots or the beginning stages of bedsores. Additionally, he or she should be turned frequently to different positions to prevent further aggravation of a sore. It is commonly recommended that the patient be turned every 2 hours.

146. D. The American Red Cross has recently recommended calling 911 (EMS) before instituting CPR, because if the adult has suffered cardiac arrest, he will need defibrillation immediately to increase his chances for survival.

147. A. Apley's compression test is designed to assist in the diagnosis of a torn meniscus.

    Anterior drawer test assists in the diagnosis of anterior cruciate ligament stability. Posterior drawer test assists in the diagnosis of the posterior cruciate ligament stability. Lachman's test determines the integrity of the anterior cruciate ligament.

148. B. The hamstring group is responsible for decelerating the unsupported limb and should be emphasized in the treatment of this patient.

149. C. A patient receiving nonsurgical rehabilitation should be able to participate in sports again, but only in light activities and with the assistance of a brace.

150. C. The stair machine would be the most appropriate choice to start with a patient who is to receive closed-chain kinetic exercise.

    Isokinetics with extension blocked minus 20°, straight leg raises in all planes, and short arc quads are examples of open-chain kinetic rehabilitation.

151. A. Bleeding should receive the first consideration if the patient has a wound. Direct pressure should be applied to stop the bleeding.

    With shock, body temperature should be kept normal; extreme variations of temperature will accentuate the condition. The correct body position should be arranged with the head and trunk level and the lower limbs elevated. Lastly, oxygen should be administered if available.

152. A. Strengthening for bed mobility for a C6 quadriplegic should emphasize the pectoralis major. The pectoralis major serves to flex, adduct, and medially rotate the arm in the shoulder joint.

153. D. You should contact the patient's physical therapist and relay all important information. This will ensure the best continuity of care for the patient, as the home therapist will be informed regarding the patient's progress and what procedures to follow.

154. A. Given the information provided in this question, the patient is most likely experiencing heat cramps. Heat cramps are caused by depletion in the body of both water and salt because of heat exhaustion. They usually occur after vigorous physical exertion in an extremely hot environment or under other conditions causing profuse sweating.

    Heat syncope results in weakness, fatigue and loss of motor tone. The patient will typically have blurred vision and an elevated body temperature. Heat exhaustion results in fatigue, weakness, incoordination, and elevated body temperature. With heat hyperpyrea, the patient becomes irrational, with muscle flaccidity and involuntary limb movements as well as seizures.

155. D. In acute impingement syndrome, it is important to initially keep exercise below 90° of range of motion. This is done to avoid aggravating the impingement syndrome while attempting to begin some general strengthening.

156. C. Traction would be the least likely treatment modality delegated to the aide because setting it up properly has clinical importance and damage could occur if the equipment is set up incorrectly.

157. A. When the stimulus is flexion of the head, the positive reaction will result in arm flexion and leg extension.

    If the test stimulus had been extending the patient's head, the positive response then would have been arm extension and leg flexion.

158. C. Utilizing the rule of nines, an anterior arm is assigned a value of 4.5% and an anterior leg a value of 9%. Therefore, the correct answer would be 13.5%.

159. C. A Knight Taylor spinal brace is utilized for fractures above the L3 region; it is a rigid, high-back brace.

    Lumbar corsets are made from a canvas or cloth and are not utilized with a fracture. A Taylor spinal brace is a semirigid brace that is used in thoracic and lumbar spine disease. A Jewett brace is a three-point brace that prevents hyperextension.

160. B. Utilizing the Rule of Nines, the percentage of burns listed for a child's arm is 9% and for the leg 14%, so the correct answer would be 23%.

161. D. Check the knee bolt alignment to make sure the placement is not too lateral for the patient, which would then result in a medial whip. Since the most common cause of medial whip is the knee bolt alignment, this is the most appropriate to check first. You may then want to check the other areas.

    Improper socket fit may result in the following gait deviations: vaulting, circumduction, and pistoning of the socket. Resistance on the plantar flexion bumper may result in the following gait deviations: instability of the knee, foot slap, and rotation of the foot at heel strike. Red spots may be an indication of an improper socket fit.

162. D. Pistoning of the socket would be a gait deviation as a result of poor socket fit, weak suspension, and overly soft knee friction.

    Lateral whip is generally caused by a knee bolt alignment that is too medial. Rotation of the foot at heel strike is usually a result of too much toe-out or resistance on the heel cushion or plantar flexion bumper. Instability of the knee is most commonly caused by a plantar flexion resistance that is too high.

163. C. An antalgic gait results when a patient will not bear weight on the injured lower extremity.

    Steppage gait results in the patient lifting the knee very high to clear the foot. Foot slap occurs when the patient has a weak or absent dorsiflexor when the foot slaps down on the ground. Abducted lurch occurs when the patient leans over the hip to place the center of gravity over the hip. It is a compensatory technique for a gluteus medius muscle weakness.

164. A. Since posture plays a very important role in correcting back pain disorders, even though the patient is short on time, posture should be emphasized on day 1.

165. D. To perform proper chest physical therapy on the right middle lobe the patient should be in the left sidelying position, rotated a half turn backward, with the bed elevated 14 inches. Pillows may be placed under the right hip, and percussion should be performed on the right side at nipple level.

166. C. When treating a wound patient, the least important to note in the progress notes would be the strength of the hip muscles since you are primarily focusing on the wound and rehabilitation of wound healing.

167. D. A correct example would be dressing and undressing. This is one of the activities of daily living that would help retrain the patient in a functional activity.

168. A. Disadvantages of isometric exercise are muscle strength is limited to the range of motion, during the exercise there is no improvement in muscle endurance, and no eccentric workload is created.

169. D. Isokinetics allows for variable velocity training and control of the velocity at selected speeds. Some common manufacturers of isokinetics include Cybex, Lido, and Biodex.

170. B. Pulmonary edema produces dull percussion sounds with wheezing and crackling upon auscultation.

   Atelectasis will produce dull percussion sounds and decreased breath sounds with auscultation. Pneumonia will produce dull percussion sounds, decreased breath sounds, and sounds of a pleural lung. Pneumothorax will result in hyperresonance and increased breath sounds.

171. A. When treating a patient 3 days postoperative, it would be appropriate for the patient to have monitored ambulation with no symptoms.

   Lower extremity ergometry for 15 or 30 minutes and upper extremity ergometry x 15 minutes would be too aggressive to start on a patient 3 days post cardiac surgery.

172. B. Proprioception tests the patient's ability to determine the direct position sense.

   Kinesthesia tests the patient's ability to determine movement sensation. Graphesthesia tests the ability of a patient to recognize letters and numbers written on the patient's skin. Barognosis is the ability to determine the weight of an object.

173. C. When a P wave is absent or abnormal, this can clinically be indicative of atrial or ventricular arrhythmia.

   An abnormal T wave would be indicative of ischemia. An abnormal Q wave would be indicative of a past history of a possible myocardial infarct. An abnormal ST segment would result in pericarditis.
   Normal results:
   ST—pulse in EKG time before ventricular repolarization
   QRS—ventricular depolarization
   T—ventricular repolarization

   Abnormal results:
   ST elevated—new infarct
   ST depressed—may indicate ischemia
   Inverted T wave—ischemia
   Q wave—seen in infection
   P wave absent—atrial/ventricular arrhythmia

174. D. Proper body mechanics for a post-cesarean patient would be to get up from a lying position by rolling over to the side, swinging the legs over the edge, and getting up slowly.

   When sitting, the patient should avoid soft chairs, as they are hard to get up from and have poor back support. When standing, the patient should keep the chin in and contract the abdominal muscles. When bending over, the patient should keep a curve in the low back with one foot in front of the other.

175. B. The upper abdominal reflex test involves thoracic 8, 9, 10.

The lower abdominal reflex test involves thoracic 10, 11, 12.

176. B. The immediate procedure would be to start performing CPR by opening the airway and tilting the head back.

177. B. Moist heat would be the most appropriate modality to be performed on this patient in a physical therapy setting.

Rest, which is not a modality but may be indicated, would be appropriate in the sidelying position, with pillows between the knees and under the abdomen for support, as well as a towel roll at the waist for support.

178. A. Bell's palsy is a paralysis of the facial nerve, resulting from trauma to the nerve, compression of the nerve by a tumor, or possibly an unknown infection. The typical treatment is direct current electrical stimulation to the motor points of the facial muscles.

179. C. Teaching proper body mechanics would be a psychomotor area that deals with motor skills.

Educational contacts are usually divided into three areas. First is cognitive, which deals with the information area; second is psychomotor, which deals with the motor skills; third is affective, which deals with feelings.

180. A. The glenohumeral joint's capsular pattern in a frozen adhesive capsulated shoulder starts with restriction of external rotation, then abduction, followed by internal rotation.

181. A. Strengthening considerations for a C4 quadriplegic would be limited to neck musculature and available movements pattern.

182. B. An appropriate treatment program for a pediatric patient with cystic fibrosis would include both breathing exercises and postural drainage. This would be the most aggressive form of treatment for this patient, which can be performed by a licensed physical therapist.

183. B. A patient with a capsular pattern of the hip will show first a decreased range of motion in flexion, then abduction, then internal rotation.

184. A. Observation of the patient's posture while the body is in motion is an example of dynamic balance equilibrium coordination testing.

Having the patient perform finger-to-nose and finger-to-finger tests to evaluate the quality of movement, testing the patient's ability to judge distance and speed of movement by drawing a circle, and evaluating the quality of movement control and speed with the patient pointing are examples of nonequilibrium coordination.

185. A. The most effective form of treatment for chondromalacia would involve performing quadriceps exercises in extension so no further degeneration of the patellar surface would occur.

186. D. The glenohumeral joint surfaces are the closest, with the muscles and ligaments maximally taut, when the joint is in a closed-packed position. The closed-packed position for the glenohumeral joint would be abduction and external rotation.

187. D. Light touch would be appropriate to perform on a patient to determine if the protective sensations are in place.

Deep pressure, proprioception, and two-point discrimination are examples of discriminative sensations.

188. D. Using a cottonball and rubbing lightly against the patient's skin would facilitate the sense of light touch.

Holding a hot or cold tube would develop temperature sensation, and sharp/dull test for pain sensation. The ability to determine the weight of an object would be best described as barognosis, which is a discriminative sensation.

189. A. Limb synergies are necessary for the intermediate stage of recovery and should be encouraged to assist the patient. Brunnstrom's suggestion for therapy emphasizes eliciting motor behavior in the sequence in which it would normally occur following stroke, which is not the same as the sequence of normal maturation.

190. C. Scaphoid pads can be used to support the longitudinal arch and to assist in correction of pes planus.

    A Thomas heel is a heel with an extended anterior medial border used to support the longitudinal arch and correct for flexible pes valgus. Rocker bottom builds up the sole over the metatarsal heads and allows additional push-off in weak or inflexible feet. Metatarsal bars take pressure off the metatarsal heads by building up the sole proximal to the metatarsal heads.

191. D. One of the disadvantages of a noncemented total hip replacement is that the patient must use an assistive gait device for up to 3 months.

192. B. Stage two is associated with redness, edema, blistering, and hardening of the tissue. In stage two there would also be an inflammation that extends into the fat layer with superficial necrosis.

    Stage one is associated with destruction limited to the epidermis; redness may be noted. Stage three involves full thickness of dermis and undermining of the deeper tissues, also the muscle may be involved. Stage four involves full thickness penetrating to the fascia with possible muscle involvement, and there is usually bone destruction.

193. B. The quadriceps group should be emphasized because it is actively involved just before toe-off to initiate the swing phase.

194. B. The most appropriate course of treatment for this patient would be contrast baths, electrical stimulation, and range of motion. The symptoms described by this patient characterize reflex sympathetic dystrophy. Most notably, this is characterized by persistent pain above the normal acceptable levels.

195. D. Leg slides would be the least appropriate exercise to begin on day 1 post cesarean.
    Diaphragmatic breathing, huffing, and pelvic floor exercises would all be appropriate to start on day 1.

196. B. Capsular end-feel is characterized by hard leather-like stoppage with slight give. This will occur in full normal range of motion.

    Bone-to-bone end-feel is defined by hard and abrupt stoppage to the joint motion. This typically occurs when performing passive range of motion and the bone contacts another bone. Empty end-feel is defined by a lack of stoppage to the joint. Springy block end-feel is defined by rebound movement felt at the end-range of passive range of motion. Two other end-feels include spasm end-feel and soft tissue approximation.

197. D. A cerebellar vascular injury will result in the symptoms of decreased balance, ataxia, decreased coordination, and a decreased ability for postural adjustment.

    A right hemisphere injury would result in paralysis of the left side. A left hemisphere injury would result in paralysis of the right side.

198. A. One gram of fat yields 9 calories.
    One gram of protein would yield 4 calories. One gram of carbohydrate would yield 4 calories.

199. C. Under no circumstances is a physical therapist assistant able to provide initial evaluations on inpatients or outpatients.

200. A. Strength duration curve is a test of excitability in which the intensity of the current required to produce a minimal contraction is measured.

    An electromyogram is a recording of the electrical potentials of a muscle. Nerve conduction velocity is a test that determines the time it takes for a muscle to respond after the nerve has been stimulated. Chronaxie is a test of electrical excitability of the peripheral nerves.

201. A. Forced expiratory volume is air that can be forcibly expired after maximum inspiration.

Forced expiratory volume is the amount that can be forcibly inspired after maximum inspiration. Inspiratory capacity is the maximum volume inspired from the resting expiratory level. Tidal volume is the amount of air inspired and expired during a single breath.

202. C. When implementing an exercise program of isokinetics after an ACL reconstruction, it would be appropriate to check with the referring physician's protocol prior to implementing isokinetics.

203. A. To initially reduce pain and maintain range of motion, grade-one mobilization would be indicated.

Grades three and four are more progressive and should be reserved for later, when the patient is out of acute pain. Grade five is a manipulation not performed by a physical therapist or physical therapist assistant.

204. D. Resting heart rate will decrease as a result of a cardiopulmonary training program that involves aerobic exercise.

205. D. Rhythmic stabilization, which is the simultaneous contraction of both the agonist and antagonist, is not an example of an exteroceptive stimulation technique.

Prolonged icing, quick stretch of the muscle belly and tendon, and high-frequency vibration are all examples of exteroceptive stimulation techniques.

206. C. Circumduction would be the gait deviation seen with the symptoms of the patient's prosthesis being too long and the socket too small. Also, there would be inadequate suspension.

Lateral trunk bending typically is a result of the prosthesis being too short. Medial whip occurs when the knee bolt alignment is too lateral. Lateral whip occurs when the knee bolt alignment is too medial.

207. B. A short-term goal should consist of something that is measurable and can be performed in a 1- to 2-week period. The patient's pain level decreasing from a 9 to 7 in a 1-week period is an example of a short-term goal.

The rest of the goals listed either do not have a timeframe or are considered long-term goals.

208. C. Hypermobility is a precaution but not an absolute contraindication.

Active inflammation, active infection, malignancy in the area of treatment and recent fracture are absolute contraindications to mobilization.

Precautions include: joint effusion, rheumatoid arthritis, osteoarthritis, presence of bony block.

Indications include: joint dysfunction, restriction of movement, pain.

209. D. In a prenatal care program, the patient is encouraged to avoid Valsalva's maneuver. Valsalva's maneuver both increases pressure on the pelvic diaphragm and causes fluctuations in venous return to the heart.

Kegel exercises are exercises for strengthening muscles of the pelvic floor. ADL modifications and relaxation training are all appropriate in a prenatal patient's program.

210. A. Moro's reflex is demonstrated when the infant has a startle response when his head suddenly drops backward unsupported.

A protective response occurs when the arms and legs extend to protect the body when falling or pushed. A Landau reflex occurs when the child is lifted under the thorax in a prone position and the spine and legs extend. An equilibrium reflex reaction is how the body adapts to maintain posture when there is change in the supporting surface.

211. A. Crutch ambulation with toe-touch weightbearing would be the most appropriate response for day 2 of a second-degree medial collateral ligament injury.

212. D. Physical therapist assistants may carry out only those procedures in which they have been trained; therefore this is not a code of ethics standard for the APTA.

213. C. Prior to isokinetic testing, a patient should be informed and educated regarding isokinetics.

   Next you should look up appropriate testing protocols. Choose a test that is reliable and reproducible. Have the patient warm up and test the uninvolved side first. Other factors to consider include regular calibration of equipment, stabilization of the patient, consistent verbal communication, and alignment of the anatomical axis with mechanical joint.

214. C. Partial curl-ups should not be performed secondary to not wanting to create a split of the rectus abdominis muscles that may develop before delivery.

   Diaphragmatic breathing, pelvic floor exercise, and postural instructions would be appropriate in a treatment program.

215. C. L4 represents anterior thigh below the knee level lateral aspect crossing the knee to the medial aspect into half of the great toe.

   L1 would involve the lower abdomen in the groin region. L3 would involve the anterior thigh above the knee level. S1 would involve the lateral calf anterior into the fifth toe.

216. B. A patient with a lesion of T9 to T12 should have the functional outcomes of vital capacity 80%, be independent with floor to wheelchair transfers, perform gait with bilateral KAFO and a walker.

   A patient with a lesion of T1 to T5 should have functional outcome of vital capacity 80%, be independent in bed mobility without special equipment, and possibly be independent with bilateral KAFO and parallel bars. A patient with a lesion of L4 to L5 should have functional outcomes of vital capacity 80%, be independent in bed mobility without special equipment, independent in transfers to and from the floor, and independent on all level surfaces. A patient with a lesion of T6 to T8 should have functional outcomes of vital capacity 80%, be independent in bed mobility without special equipment, independent in a manual wheelchair on all level surfaces.

217. B. Tibialis posterior adducts, inverts, and plantar flexes the foot.
   Tibialis anterior adducts, inverts, and dorsiflexes the foot.
   Peroneus longus abducts, everts, and plantar flexes the foot.
   Peroneus brevis abducts, everts, and dorsiflexes the foot.

218. A. A first-class lever is best described when the fulcrum is located between the weight and the applied force. Examples in the body would be atlantooccipital joint or the action of the triceps at the olecranon.

   An example of a second-class lever would be the pull of the brachioradialis muscle and wrist extensors on elbow flexion. With a third-class lever, the weight arm is longer than the force arm, designed for producing speed or for moving a small weight a long distance. An example of a third-class lever would be a deltoid or glenohumeral joint. No fourth-class lever classification exists.

   Definitions:
   Fulcrum: point of rotation
   Force arm: distance of the lever between the joint (fulcrum) and muscle attachment—affect force
   Weight: resistance arm—distance of the lever between fulcrum and weight

219. B. Since you can palpate a contraction but the patient cannot perform complete range of motion, the appropriate response would be trace.
   A muscle testing grade of zero: no palpable contraction.
   A muscle testing grade of poor: can produce movement in gravity-eliminated position only.
   A muscle testing grade of fair: can produce movement against gravity.

220. B. The dermis layer is composed largely of a fibrous connective tissue that will bind the epidermis to the underlying tissues. Contained within the dermis are blood vessels and nerves.

The epidermis is the outer layer of the skin. It contains striated squamous epithelium cells. The epidermis functions to protect the underlying tissue against water loss, effects of harmful chemicals, and mechanical injury. The subcutaneous tissue is composed of adipose tissue.

221. B. When skin is damaged by excessive exposure to heat, the first stage would be inflammation. Inflammation is a response to the injury or stress in which blood vessels dilate and become more permeable.

222. B. The pterygoideus lateralis muscle is responsible for opening the jaw.

All the other answers are incorrect because they are responsible for closing the jaw.

223. A. The radial carpal articulation of the wrist joint is classified as a condyloid joint and allows for motion in two planes—typically flexion/extension, abduction/adduction.

The hinge joint permits motion in one plane, typically flexion/extension (eg, elbow joint, ginglymus joint). The pivot joint movement is limited to rotation, (eg, atlantoaxial joint). The saddle joint permits no axial rotation but allows flexion, extension, adduction, and abduction (eg, carpometacarpal joint of the thumb).

224. D. As the patient stated that he had a fracture to the midshaft of the humerus, the radial nerve, which is the largest branch of the brachial plexus, would most likely be injured because it passes through the radial groove next to the bone. This occurs on the posterior aspect of the humerus.

225. C. The deltoid muscle is supplied by the axillary nerve, which originates from the posterior cord of the brachial plexus.

All other muscles are innervated by the terminal branches of the lateral cord of the brachial plexus.

226. C. Semimembranosus is the muscle that you would not be evaluating. The semimembranosus extends the thigh and flexes and medially rotates the leg.

The three muscles that insert into the pes anserinus are the gracilis, sartorius, and semitendinosus. The pes anserinus is located at the medial border of the tibial tuberosity. The gracilis adducts the thigh and flexes and rotates the leg medially. The semitendinosus extends the thigh and flexes and medially rotates the leg.

227. B. The peroneus tertius nerve would not be affected since it is supplied by the deep peroneal nerve.

228. D. The lateral collateral ligament assists in controlling knee rotation and adduction.

The anterior cruciate ligament prevents anterior displacement of the tibia on the femur. The posterior cruciate ligament prevents posterior displacement of the tibia on the femur. The medial collateral ligament assists in controlling knee rotation and abduction.

229. C. The deltoid ligament would need the least amount of rehabilitation since it is injured as a result of an eversion sprain.

This patient has an inversion sprain that would involve lateral ligaments, which are the anterior talofibular, calcaneofibular, and posterior talofibular.

230. C. These three pathologies together are best described as collagen vascular diseases.

Lupus erythematosus is a chronic inflammation disease of the connective tissue, affecting skin, joints, kidney, and nervous system. A butterfly rash is characteristic. Scleroderma is a chronic disease causing sclerosis of the skin and certain organs (eg, lungs, heart, and kidney). Skin is taut, edematous, firmly bound to subcutaneous tissue, and leathery. Dermatomycosis is a skin infection caused by certain fungi.

231. B. Thromboangiitis obliterans is a disease that involves arteries and veins of the lower extremity. It is characterized by excruciating pain in the leg or foot, which is worse at night, decreased sensation, and clamminess or coldness of the lower extremity.

Raynaud's disease involves the fingers. It is characterized by abnormal vasoconstriction of the extremities upon exposure to cold or stress. The attacks are characterized by severe blanching of the extremities, followed by cyanosis, then redness, usually with numbness, tingling, and burning. Thrombophlebitis involves a vein disorder, usually in conjunction with formation of a thrombus secondary to inflammation. Pitting edema is a symptom, not a disease.

232. B. The patient in balance skeletal traction of the lower extremity has most likely fractured the femur, since skeletal traction is used when there is a fracture in the long bone. Common traction can be used either for the distal part of the femur or tibia in treating fractures.

233. C. The superficial peroneal nerve innervates both the peroneus longus and peroneus brevis.

The deep peroneal nerve innervates the tibialis anterior, peroneus tertius, extensor hallucis longus, extensor digitorum longus, and extensor digitorum brevis.

234. D. Due to its structure and innervation, the cardiac muscle has both atrial and ventricular proportions.

235. C. Cardiac output refers to the amount of blood pumped by the heart in 60 seconds or 1 minute.

236. C. Sterling's law of the heart states that stretching the heart muscle will increase the vigor of contraction within physiological limits.

237. A. The period of relaxation is best described by diastole.

Systole is known as the period of contraction. Syncope is related to fainting. Tachycardia is related to heart rate of 100 beats per minute and above. Bradycardia is related to heart rate under 60 beats per minute.

238. C. A person with severe heart failure will not show higher than normal cardiac output.

239. B. Mitral stenosis would be a lesion in which both stroke volume and pulse pressure would be small.

Congestive heart failure is an abnormal condition characterized by circulatory congestion caused by cardiac disorders, especially myocardial infarction of the ventricles. Myocardial infarct is an occlusion of a coronary artery that causes myocardial ischemia.

240. B. Excessive fluid in the intercellular space would not be a characteristic of congestive heart failure. All other answers in these questions are signs and symptoms.

Stenosis is an abnormal condition characterized by the constriction or narrowing of an opening or passageway in a body structure. Orthopnea is an abnormal respiratory condition in which a person must sit or stand in order to breathe deeply or comfortably.

241. B. Myocardial infarctions most frequently occur in the left ventricle as a result of occlusion to the left coronary artery.

242. D. Thrombosis, or thrombi, is the most common cause of stroke in older adults because of sclerotic tissue/vessels.

Aneurysm is a localized dilation of the wall of a blood vessel, generally caused by atherosclerosis and hypertension. Hemorrhaging is bleeding externally or internally. Thrombosis is an abnormal vascular condition in which thrombus develops within a blood vessel of the body.

243. B. The P wave of the EKG corresponds to atrial depolarization.

Q wave would be indicative of a past history of a possible myocardial infarct. An abnormal ST segment would result in pericarditis.

244. A. The action of digitalis on a patient with congestive heart failure would be to decrease the heart rate and increase strength of the contraction.

245. B. Pulmonary edema is most often symptomatic of left ventricular failure.

246. C. In a patient with rheumatoid arthritis for a long duration, a common symptom would be ulnar deviation of the fingers.

    Rheumatoid arthritis is a systemic disease characterized by painful joints, tenderness, inflammation, swelling, redness, heat, fibrous adhesions, morning stiffness, and proliferation of granulation tissue known as pannus.

247. B. Given the type of fall and the symptoms described by the patient, she has most likely suffered a dislocated hip.

248. A. Osteoarthritis deals with changes in the bones rather than joint changes. It is not an acute inflammatory disease but a chronic disease that can often result in bony ankylosis.

249. B. The posterior cruciate ligament is most likely involved since the tibia can be displaced posteriorly on the femur with severe instability.

250. D. In order to perform inferior glide of the humeral head, the shoulder should be placed in abduction to 30°. This is necessary because otherwise it would not be possible to perform the inferior glide secondary to not being able to perform either anterior or posterior glide.

251. C. Popliteus is the muscle that attaches to the tibia and, through its actions, is responsible for unlocking the extended knee position.

252. C. Stage one wound healing is described as mobilization. This is the initial stage of wound repair.

    Stage two is migration, when the layer cells resurface the wound. Stage three is proliferation, when the cells along the edges of the wound are beginning the process of thickening the layer. Stage four is differentiation, when the epidermal cells take on the original cuboidal or rectangular shape.

253. C. Stage three involves full thickness of dermis and undermining of the deeper tissues; the muscles may be involved.

    Stage one is destruction limited to the epidermis; redness may be noted. Stage two is involvement of the epidermis, dermis, and subcutaneous fat, redness, edema, blistering and hardening of the tissue. With stage four, full thickness is involved penetrating to the fascia with possible muscle involvement, and there is usually bone destruction.

254. D. Reduction of nerve conduction velocity is not a process of aging.

255. D. Seventy percent of the weight of the human body is water.

256. B. Exercise with a low activity rate and long duration will help increase lipid metabolism, therefore assisting the patient in weight loss.

257. C. In regard to energy for muscle contractions, it is false that energy may be stored as cretin phosphate. All other statements are true.

258. C. All the above would take place except for a small decrease in maximum oxygen consumption capacity. Studies show that there is a decrease in maximum oxygen consumption capacity of approximately one third after a marked period of bed rest.

259. B. Increased blood glucose levels are the primary stimulus to insulin secretion.

260. C. The period between the 21st and 40th day is the time during prenatal development when the cardiovascular system is beginning its development and is most at risk.

261. B. A unit objective is something that will be completed by the end of the lecture. An objective is something that is quantifiable and time-delineated. A correct example of the unit objective would be demonstrating the three principles of body mechanics. Another example of an objective might be to list five physiological changes that occur during pregnancy, or to identify three possible sources of back pain during pregnancy.

The introduction, anatomy, physiology, and theories on labor are all part of the content of the lecture, but they are not an objective.

262. B. Disadvantages of isotonic exercise: loads muscle at the weakest point, momentum factor in lifting, does not develop accuracy at functional speeds.

263. B. The description in this question describes the Romberg's sign.

The labyrinthine righting is one of the five basic neuromuscular reactions involved in a change of body positions. The change stimulates cells in the canals of the inner ear, causing neck muscles to respond and adjust the head to the new position. The Babinski's sign involves the hallucis longus muscle.

264. C. The frontal lobe carries out the functions of personality and speech, as well as intelligence and motor activities. Vision is the responsibility of the occipital lobe. Sensory perception and interpretation are the responsibility of the parietal lobe. Hearing and speech are the responsibility of the temporal lobe.

265. B. The axillary nerve would most likely be injured since it is in the location of the shoulder. Some fibers of the nerve also supply the capsule of the shoulder joint.

The others would not be involved since they are located distally to the shoulder.

266. A. The median nerve is the nerve that innervates the thenar eminence. This would most likely be the nerve injured since you observed signs of atrophy.

267. A. With a lesion of the lateral cord brachial plexus, you would expect to find paralysis of the biceps, coracobrachialis, and the finger flexors.

Paralysis of the deltoid would most likely be a result of an axillary nerve lesion. Paralysis of wrist extension would be a result of the axillary nerve and the radial nerve. Paralysis of the intrinsic hand would involve the medial cord of the brachial plexus.

268. C. The only site on which you would be able to perform ultrasound would be over a healed scar on this patient. Fracture sites, over the spinal cord, and over the epiphyseal plate are all contraindications for ultrasound.

269. B. Most helpful for this patient would be to teach the patient rhythmic initiation. The patient would know how to initiate movement in using trunk control for transfers. This technique would help the patient to initiate movement from supine to sit or from left to right sidelying through using the trunk to roll.

270. A. Alveoli are the sites of gas exchange in the pulmonary system. Alveoli consist of small outpouching of walls of alveolar space through which gas exchange takes place between alveolar air and pulmonary capillary blood.

271. A. The diaphragm is the primary muscular force for respiration.

272. C. Moisture within epidermal cells does not tend to slow down invading pathogens.

273. B. Expiratory reserve volume describes the amount of air that can be forcibly exhaled at the end of a normal expiration.

274. C. Passive range of motion will affect pulmonary ventilation depending on the number of joints involved.

275. A. Pneumoconiosis is a condition that will result in pathological changes occurring in the lung tissue. These changes result from chronic inhalation of dust, usually mineral dusts of occupational or environmental origin.

276. A. Biot's would be the correct term to describe the breathing pattern in which the patient has a slow rate, shallow depth, apnea periods, and irregular rhythm. Biot's is typically associated with a central nervous system disorder, such as meningitis.

277. A. Paranoid patients use projection as a defense mechanism against others.

278. C. The maximum loose-packed position of the knee joint to perform mobilization would be 25° flexion.

279. C. Common pressure points in the sidelying position include the ears, shoulders, ribs, greater trochanter, medial and lateral condyles, and the ankles.

280. A. The prescription should include the diagnosis, date, precautions, treatment, and the physician's signature.

281. C. This patient most likely has talipes equinovarus, which is characterized by medial deviation and plantar flexion of the forefoot.

    Talipes calcaneovalgus is characterized by lateral deviation and dorsiflexion either outward from or inward toward the midline of the body.

282. A. Shoulder flexion is utilized in upper extremity amputees to assist in control of the prosthesis.

283. D. A Syme's amputation involves removal above the ankle joint, resulting in a bulbous end on the leg.

    A below-knee joint amputation is removal below the knee joint; the knee joint remains intact. A Chopart amputation is removal below the ankle joint. A metatarsal amputation is through the metatarsal heads.

284. D. Third-degree, full-thickness burns destroy the entire epidermis and dermis. The patient will experience no pain. There will be no blisters. There will be severe edema. The healing characteristics expected for this patient would require grafting.

285. C. Weak abductor muscles would be the possible anatomical cause.

    If the prosthesis is too short or in abduction, lateral trunk bending is caused by the prosthesis itself, not by an anatomical cause. If the prosthesis is too long, an abducted gait results, but again no anatomical cause is involved.

286. D. Low plantar flexion resistance would be the least likely prosthetic cause of instability of the knee. Instability of the knee can result if the knee joint is too anterior, plantar flexion resistance is too high, or dorsiflexion is unlimited.

287. C. The correct answer is questionnaire, which is sending out standardized forms for the therapists to answer and return.

    Cross-sectional describes interviewing a cross-section of different people over the same period of time. Developmental research is also known as historical research. It is a study over a long period of time. Survey pertains to one-on-one personal interviews.

288. A. An infection control policy of a hospital is set up to minimize the risk of nosocomial or community-acquired infections spreading to the patients or staff. To control infection, hand washing should occur prior to and after a patient's treatment.

289. D. If an individual has a lesion of the upper trapezius, it would be reasonable to expect the scapula to be rotated downward. If the scapula is rotated downward, this could cause subluxation of the sternoclavicular joint, which is the double gliding joint between the sternum and clavicle.

290. C. The annular ligament encircles the head of the radius and holds it in the radial notch of the ulna. Distal to the notch, the annular ligament forms a complete fibrous ring. Therefore, if the annular ligament were torn, the head of the radius would dislocate.

291. C. When the elbow joint is in midposition or semiprone, the joint will have the greatest advantage for optimum force output.

292. D. The combined action of the tendinous cuff muscles (SITS) would produce depression of the head of the humerus in the joint.

293. C. For a paraplegic, prolonged standing with braces in a lordotic position would result in stretching of the hip extensors and iliofemoral ligament.

294. C. T10 corresponds with impaired sensation of a dermatome pattern at the level of the umbilicus.
    T2—axillary region
    T4—nipple level
    T12—ASIS level

295. B. With symptoms of discoloration with mild atrophic changes in the nails, as well as mild swelling of the foot and ankle, you would most likely suspect chronic venous insufficiency. Venous insufficiency is an abnormal circulatory condition characterized by decreased return of the venous blood from the legs to the trunk of the body.

    Thrombophlebitis is an inflammation of a vein, often accompanied by formation of a clot. Lymphedema is a primary or secondary disorder characterized by the accumulation of lymph in soft tissue as well as swelling caused by inflammation, obstruction, or removal of lymph channels.

296. A. The appropriate treatment to recommend to this patient would be support hosiery, patient education in the principles of foot care, active exercise to the distal segment of the extremity, and elevation of the foot in bed.

297. D. The example given in this question would be that of dyssynergia. Dyssynergia describes any disturbance in muscular coordination.

    Dysmetria describes an abnormal condition that prevents the patient from properly measuring distances associated with muscular acts and also from controlling muscular action. It is typically characterized by over- or underestimating the range of motion needed to place the limbs correctly during voluntary movement. Dysdiadochokinesia is an inability to perform rapidly alternating movements, such as rhythmically tapping the fingers on the leg. Barognosis is the ability to perceive and evaluate weight.

298. C. The axis motion that the radial and ulnar deviation lies in would be the sagittal plane through the capitate. All other answers are incorrect.

299. B. Tensor fasciae latae would be the muscle responsible for tightness that would result in the hip joint remaining abducted and slightly flexed when lowered to the table. The tensor fasciae latae is one of the 10 muscles of the gluteal region arising from the outer lip of the iliac crest, the iliac spine, and the deep fasciae latae (also called tensor fasciae femoris).

    Psoas major acts to flex and laterally rotate the thigh and to flex and laterally bend the spine. Semitendinosus functions to flex the leg and rotate it medially after flexion and to extend the thigh. Rectus femoris functions to flex the leg.

300. C. The pattern of breathing for an upper chest breather would be for the patient to gasp for breath, and on occasion her shoulder and thorax would rise and her abdominal wall retract. This is because the patient is primarily breathing with her upper chest.

    Barrel chest is a large, rounded thorax. This is considered normal in some stocky individuals and some individuals who live in high-altitude areas who have developed increased vital capacities. Paradoxical breathing is a condition in which a part of the lung deflates during inspiration and inflates during expiration.

301. A. Normal expansion at the xiphoid process should measure approximately 5 to 10 cm.

302. C. Heberden's node is an abnormal cartilaginous or bony enlargement most frequently located in the distal interphalangeal joint of a finger, usually occurring in degenerative diseases of the joints.

303. D. During pregnancy, the presence of relaxin, which causes relaxation of connective tissue, can lead to abnormal movement and cause pain in the sacroiliac joint.

304. B. You would expect weakness in the motor activities of wrist flexion, finger extension, and elbow extension. You would not expect weakness in finger flexion because with a C7 nerve root impingement you would expect finger flexion motor activities to be intact and not involved.

305. A. Hip flexion would not be an emphasis in a geriatric program as typically this is not a limited range of motion seen in that age group. All other areas would be emphasized to reduce the limitations experienced by patients.

306. D. Continue the exercise program as previously outlined by you and the physical therapist.

307. A. A minimal erythemal dosage would be described as first degree and is barely noticeable. It produces slight redness 6 to 8 hours post-treatment with no peeling, blistering, or inflammation. Second-degree erythemal dosage would produce reddening of the skin 4 to 6 hours after treatment, mild sunburn, slight peeling, no blisters, and mild itch. Third-degree erythemal dosage produces intense reddening 3 to 4 hours post-treatment, marked peeling, severe itching, burning, slight edema, and second-degree burn. Fourth-degree erythemal dosage produces blistering, open sores, and intense reddening 2 hours post-treatment.

308. D. Prior to leaving, you should provide a thorough assessment of each patient's condition and the type of treatment to be administered. It would also be appropriate to call in during the day, early if possible, to see if any questions exist.

309. B. The most important treatment technique to start with this patient would be McKenzie exercises, since repeated flexion upon range of motion testing increases the low back pain. McKenzie exercises emphasize the "extension principle" to reduce back pain. Increased pain upon repeated flexion indicates that the patient should be treated with back extension exercises to reduce symptoms. Next you should review proper posture and body mechanics instruction.

310. D. If the patient has a script that is over 30 days old, it may not be valid according to the regulations in the state you are working. Medicare requires an update every 30 days. You should call the patient's physician to request a verbal approval so you can get the patient's therapy started immediately and request that a written prescription follows.

311. C. The most appropriate response would be to contact the supervising physical therapist and inform him or her that the current treatment technique is not producing significant change in the patient. Request a change of treatment in an attempt to gain progress with this patient.

312. C. A long-term goal would be to increase range of motion to 125° of flexion. Increase strength from 3+/5 to 4/5 for knee extension and increase strength from 3-/5 to 3+/5 for knee flexion are examples of short-term goals that could be accomplished in 2 weeks.

313. A. Following is the correct method for performing chest physical therapy on a patient's left lingular lobe: the patient should be in a right sidelying position, rotated backward one-quarter of a turn with the bed elevated 14 to 18 inches. It would be appropriate to perform percussion on this patient on the left side at the nipple level.

314. A. The first step in performing an educational program to a company with repetitive motion injuries would be to instruct the personnel in proper warm-up and stretching exercises as a prevention technique.

315. D. Typically juvenile arthritis, or Still's disease, is treated through aspirin in high doses, depending on the size of the child. Aspirin treatment is by physician implementation. The best choice for physical therapy implementation would be range of motion exercises and family education. Once range of motion is decreased, it is difficult for the patient to regain.

316. C. The most appropriate immediate treatment for a burn patient is passive range of motion in extension, as well as emphasizing position of the elbow in full extension. This is done to prevent flexion contractures. Whirlpool may be ordered, depending on the extent of the burn, for debridement. An active exercise program may be started tomorrow but it is critical to properly position the elbow until the next treatment to prevent further contracture or loss of movement.

317. A. Inferior glide is the correct mobilization technique to perform to increase abduction of the glenohumeral joint. Posterior glide would increase flexion, anterior glide would increase extension, and anterior glide—mobilization level 4 would increase extension and be too aggressive for this patient.

318. C. Cerebellar artery occlusion most likely results in coordination problems, as well as ataxia. A middle cerebral artery lesion would result in motor and sensory aphasia, as well as hemiplegia. A posterior cerebral artery lesion would result in loss of superficial touch and deep sensation, as well as contralateral hemiparesis. A vertebral artery lesion would result in loss of consciousness or coma.

319. D. Removal of less bone tissue is incorrect. In fact, a cemented hip requires more bone tissue removal. Advantages of a cemented hip would be that it allows for early weightbearing, surgeons' report a 90% success rate, and there is less postoperative pain.

320. A. You should contact the patient's family and request that they come to the hospital. It is important for the patient to have support personnel while being instructed in transfers into and out of a vehicle. If possible, use the actual vehicle in which the patient will be transported.

321. C. Adson's test is performed to determine the status of the subclavian artery and the presence of thoracic outlet syndrome. Drop arm test is performed to determine if there is a tear in the rotator cuff. Apprehension test is performed for chronic acute shoulder dislocation. Tinel's test is designed to elicit tenderness over a neuroma within a nerve, typically in the elbow joint region or for carpal tunnel syndrome.

322. C. The low-pressure mercury vapor lamp, otherwise known as cold mercury lamp, is applied against the skin to kill bacteria. The hot mercury lamp is a high-pressure mercury vapor lamp, used most commonly for psoriasis skin conditions. It cannot be placed against the skin. The ultraviolet lamp is used for dermatological disorders such as psoriasis and infection.

323. B. Prior to speaking with a patient's vocational rehabilitation counselor or RN, you should check that the appropriate releases are in order. The policy and procedure manual in your clinic should also have a statement on verbal information over the phone and consent to release information that you should review.

324. A. According to Bobath, treatment should be active and dynamic for the patient. Bobath's approach to treatment of a neurologic patient is based extensively on the importance of developing normal muscle tone as a preparation for normal movement patterns. One of Bobath's primary treatment goals is the use of postures and movement patterns to inhibit maladaptive and dysfunctional motor behavior and to release normal motor patterns.

325. D. Verbal communication with the patient should be consistent regardless of whether he or she is performing trial repetitions or test repetitions, so inconsistent communication would interfere with the accuracy of the test results. Calibrating equipment regularly, aligning the anatomical axis joint with the mechanical axis, and following standard testing protocols would increase the accuracy of test results.

326. A. The dorsal scapular and long thoracic nerves originate from the rami of the plexus. The subclavian nerve originates from the trunk of the plexus. The lateral pectoral and musculocutaneous nerves originate from the lateral cord. The medial pectoral and ulnar nerves originate from the medial cord.

327. B. The gastrocnemius innervation level involving injury to the gastrocnemius muscle is L5, S1. The innervation level of L4, L5 involves the anterior tibialis; S1, S2 involves flexor hallucis longus; L2, L4 involves the quadriceps muscle.

328. B. A left hemisphere cerebrovascular injury will result in symptoms of paralysis and weakness on the right side, possible motor apraxia, and a decreased discrimination between left and right.

329. C. Direct current is the only type of current that could be utilized to stimulate a denervated muscle. Direct current is necessary when stimulating a denervated muscle to get a response from the muscle.

330. A. The deltoid ligament, which is the medial ligament, would not be emphasized since injury to that area results in an eversion sprain. This case study emphasized that the injury was an inversion sprain, which includes the anterior talofibular, calcaneofibular, and posterior talofibular ligaments.

331. C. Tell the nurse the information regarding the patient's attendance as the proper release form is in the chart. However, have her call the physician for a medical release to return to work.

332. D. Salicylate is an anti-inflammatory drug that utilizes a negative chemical ion. Hydrocortisone, lidocaine, and salicylate are positive chemical ions.

333. B. External rotators of the shoulder, supraspinatus, infraspinatus, and teres minor would most likely be utilized in substitution for the triceps. The deltoid would typically substitute for the long head of the biceps. Internal rotators and serratus anterior would typically substitute for the pectoralis minor and coracobrachialis.

334. A. Prolonged icing is utilized for the inhibition of muscles, while quick icing and quick stretching would facilitate muscles.

335. D. Ober's test is used to test for iliotibial band tightness. The physical therapist performs the test by having the patient lie on the unaffected side with involved leg uppermost. The therapist abducts the leg and flexes the knee to 90°, the hip joint should remain in neutral position. The test is positive if the thigh remains abducted when the leg is released. Normally, the leg would adduct when released. Thomas test is used to test for hip flexor tightness or contracture. Straight leg raise test evaluates hamstring tightness. Trendelenburg's test evaluates the strength of the gluteus muscle.

336. A. The acromioclavicular joint is most commonly referred to when diagnosing an injury as a separated shoulder. The acromioclavicular is the gliding joint between the acromial end of the clavicle and the medial margin of the acromion of the scapula.

337. C. A patient with a C6 level of lesion would have functional outcomes of vital capacity of 60% to 80%, be independent in bed mobility, independent with pressure relief, independent in a manual wheelchair, and able to assist with independent transfers. A C4 level of lesion would have functional outcomes of vital capacity of 30% to 50%, be able to direct bed mobility and give occasional minimal assist, able to direct pressure relief activities, independent using a motorized wheelchair without hand controls on level surfaces, and able to direct all transfers. A C5 level of lesion would have functional outcomes of vital capacity of 40% to 60%, be able to give minimal assist with bed mobility, able to assist in a manual wheelchair, independent utilizing a motorized wheelchair with hand controls, and able to direct transfers. A C7, C8 level of lesion would have functional outcomes of vital capacity of 60% to 80%, be independent in bed mobility and pressure relief (including wheelchair push-ups), able to give moderate assist with transfers, independent on a level surface with a wheelchair.

338. B. L2 distribution is involved with the anterior thigh and the inside of the medial aspect of the anterior thigh. L1 distribution is involved with the lower abdomen and groin region. L3 distribution is involved with the anterior thigh above knee level, outside or lateral aspect crossing the medial border of the knee into the medial aspect of the calf. L5 distribution is involved with the anterior thigh laterally above the knee, down the lower extremity into half the great toe, 2nd, 3rd, and 4th toes.

339. C. Utilizing the concave-convex rule, the most appropriate mobilization technique to use would be the posterior glide of the tibia. The rule states that when a convex surface moves on a stable concave surface, the sliding of the convex surface occurs in the opposite direction of movement. When a concave surface moves on a stable convex surface, the sliding occurs in the same direction of movement.

340. B. If a patient has full weightbearing, the best gait pattern is to advance the walker first, then one leg, then the other leg. There is no specific pattern for full weightbearing as per uninvolved and involved, since they can equally bear weight.

341. C. The middle trapezius muscle is being tested in this question. When the lower trapezius is tested, the patient is prone with the arm over the side of the table. The arm is placed diagonally overhead so that the shoulder laterally rotates. Upper trapezius testing is done against the shoulder in the direction of depression by having the patient sit and bring the shoulder up toward the ear. Serratus anterior typically is tested with the patient standing, placing the arm in approximately 120° to 130° in flexion.

342. C. The iliofemoral ligament of the hip does not attach to the inferior superior iliac spine. It attaches to the anterior inferior iliac spine.

343. C. The spring ligament of the foot supports the head of the talipes, which helps to maintain the medial arch of the foot. All other statements regarding the spring ligament are false. The long plantar ligament supports the lateral longitudinal arch.

344. B. The muscle would be the only area to show conductivity of the electrical current.

345. A. The most frequent location in which bursitis is diagnosed is in the subacromial area. Bursitis is an inflammation of the bursa, the connective tissue structure surrounding a joint. The chief symptom is severe pain of the affected joint, particularly on movement. Treatment goals for bursitis include the control of pain and the maintenance of joint motion.

346. C. The etiology of rheumatoid arthritis is degeneration caused by aging; it is degenerative joint disease of articular cartilage. Gout is a form of arthritis in which sodium urate crystals are deposited near or in the joint, commonly in the great toe.

347. C. You would not expect to find crepitus in an acute shoulder dislocation. This is because crepitus is a sign of a chronic condition that typically would not be found in an 18-year-old male as a result of an acute shoulder dislocation.

348. D. The most distinctive feature of diabetes mellitus versus diabetes insipidus is that diabetes insipidus is associated with a pituitary disease, typically a tumor in the pituitary, while diabetes mellitus is associated with the pancreas.

349. A. It is the responsibility of the PTA working as an independent contractor to carry individual liability coverage. Liability coverage for a PTA working in any kind of treatment facility extends only to the patients/clients treated under the auspices of that facility.

350. D. When performing a manual muscle test, you are looking for the maximum strength of a particular muscle or the maximum number of motor units to fire.

351. B. The most beneficial and proper application of the ultrasound would be a frequency of 1 milliHertz and a dosage of 1.5 watts per cm^2 to gain the most therapeutic results for calcified bursitis of the shoulder.

352. C. A normal ratio for quadriceps to hamstring strength would be three to two.

353. C. When administering ultrasound under water, the sound head should be placed approximately 1 inch from the area to be treated, which in this case is the medial arch of the foot.

354. C. You would not expect a patient to show an increase in maximal oxygen consumption at the end of the stage one. All the other answers would be appropriate goals and the patient should have accomplished them through physical therapy and nurse education/instruction.

355. C. The proper landmarks to use to compare actual leg lengths of both lower extremities would be the anterior superior iliac spine to the lateral malleolus. The following is stated in Scully & Barnes, Physical Therapy: "Determining real leg length involves a measurement from one of the ASIS to either the lateral or medial malleolus of the same side. The most accurate method of real leg length measurement is to use a tape measure to measure the distance from the ASIS to the lateral malleolus. This method was shown to be more accurate than a measurement to the medial malleolus because differences in thigh girth do not affect this method of measurement as much (Woerman, 1984)." Although apparently not as accurate as the previous methods, probably the most common method of measuring real leg length is to perform a measurement from the ASIS to the medial malleolus of the same side.

356. D. A concussion may best be defined as a temporary state of paralysis of the nervous function. This will usually result in loss of consciousness following a blow to the head or head trauma.

357. D. The face would be the most sensitive area to ultraviolet radiation. Since the cornea absorbs all wavelengths beyond 295 nm, special care should be taken when radiating in the vicinity of the eyes. The eyes should be covered at all times. Treatments should be timed to the second. It is important to wear protective goggles for both the patient and the treatment provider.

358. A. Supraspinatus is the muscle you are palpating. The proximal attachment of this muscle is the supraspinatus fossa of the scapula and the distal attachment is the uppermost facet of the greater tubercle of the humerus. The deepest portion of supraspinatus lies underneath the trapezius muscle. Palpation would be felt during contraction of the muscle through a quick abduction movement to the arm.

359. C. A radial nerve paralysis would result in the extensors of the wrist and the long extensors of the digits being paralyzed. Medial nerve paralysis typically involves the flexors of the digit. In an ulnar nerve paralysis, basically the fourth and fifth digits of the hands are the ones most affected.

360. A. To perform an eccentric contraction, the muscle must lengthen as it develops tension. This is done through a negative repetition; lowering a weight during a hard press would be an example.

361. A. One needs 40% to 50% of the body's weight to cause distraction to the vertebral bodies.

362. C. In performing goniometric measurement of the internal or external rotators of the shoulder, the stationary arm should be parallel or perpendicular to the midline of the trunk. The moveable arm then will be longitudinally aligned with the shaft of the ulna and the styloid process. The axis for measurement is over the olecranon process.

363. A. The best position for a joint in order to palpate the muscle would be a loose-packed position. Loose-packed joint position is a point in the range of motion at which articulating surfaces are the least congruent and the supporting structures are the most lax.

364. B. The patient has an ulnar nerve injury and therefore the flexor carpi ulnaris, which is innervated by the ulnar nerve, would be emphasized. The median nerve innervates the flexor pollicis longus, flexor digitorum superficialis, and flexor carpi radialis.

365. B. The Americans with Disabilities Act of 1990, commonly referred to as the ADA. It prohibits the exclusion of people from jobs, services, or activities based on their disability. The major difference between this law and Section 504 of the Rehabilitation Act of 1973 is that the term "disability" is used rather than "handicap." The Civil Rights Act of 1964 prevents discrimination of job position or promotion based upon race, color, sex, religion or national origin. The Age Discrimination Act of 1975 prohibits discrimination against those between the ages of 40 and 70.

366. D. You should never take on work for which you are not qualified, as it may expose you to liability malpractice and would provide poor quality care to the patient. Discuss with the supervising physical therapist if any of the personnel at your facility are trained in pediatrics. It would be ethical to refer this patient to a facility that specializes in this type of care. However, you should check the policy and procedure manual in your department for referrals outside the hospital/clinic.

367. C. Schizophrenia is a psychotic disorder in which the patient often has fragmented thoughts, bizarre ideas, and becomes withdrawn. Responses are usually inappropriate and demonstrate severe mood shifts. Paranoia is a psychotic disorder in which the patient has delusions of persecution or grandiosity and is typically suspicious in all situations with all people. Depression is characterized by a feeling of sadness or helplessness. The patient typically has little drive for activity or achievement. Psychopathy is an antisocial personality disorder characterized by behavior patterns that lack moral and ethical standards.

368. D. The posterior cruciate ligament has a distal attachment from the posterior intercondylar of the tibia. The posterior cruciate proximal attachment is in the lateral side of the medial condylar of the femur. All of the other statements are false. The medial meniscus is larger than the lateral meniscus and is shaped like the letter "C." The lateral meniscus is smaller and shaped like the letter "O." Lastly, the lateral ligament of the knee is not attached to the lateral meniscus.

369. D. You should contact the patient's physical therapist assistant and relay all important information. This will ensure the best continuity of care to the patient, as the assistant will be informed of the patient's progress and what treatment programs are working successfully with the patient.

370. D. The hamstring is the most active during midswing to deceleration.

371. D. In performing ultrasound under water, the most important safety feature would be to have a ground fault interruption circuit so that the patient could not be accidentally electrocuted.

372. D. The first priority in dealing with a newly admitted burn patient would be to begin wound cleaning, debridement, and sterile dressing. Sterile whirlpool would be used in order to promote healing, control infection, and aid in loosening the necrotic tissue, making debridement easier. Sterile towels and dressing must also be used postwhirlpool. It is extremely important to maintain a sterile technique so that no cross infections occur. Next, you would proceed with splinting as necessary to prevent contractures.

373. C. Iliac crest is the landmark to use in palpation of the L4 region.

374. B. Second-degree burns affect the epidermis and possibly the superficial part of the dermis. The patient will experience severe pain. There will be considerable edema, mottled appearance, and blister formation. The healing characteristics expected for this patient would be less than 3 weeks, minimal scarring, and pigment changes.

375. A. When a patient exhibits poor posture, especially in the anterior tilt of the pelvis, you would utilize Williams' exercises to strengthen the abdominal and the gluteus maximus muscles.

376. D. It is found in all bones is an incorrect statement. The epiphyseal or growth plate may only be found in long bones after growth has been completed. It is then replaced by a dense calcified formation known as an epiphyseal line.

377. B. When utilizing a cane, the patient should always use it opposite the injured side; this is necessary for balance during ambulation.

378. B. Talk to the patient while moving the patient from the staircase. By talking with the patient, the therapist is acknowledging the patient's behavior and thought process, while at the same time ensuring increased safety for the patient.

379. C. Spina bifida myelocele is the most severe form of spina bifida. Soft tissue contained in the meninges describes spina bifida meningocele. Soft tissue contained in the spinal cord describes spina bifida myelomeningocele. A herniated sac contained in the spinal cord describes spina bifida syringomyelocele. Spina bifida occulta is a defective closure of the laminae of the vertebral column in the lumbosacral region without hernial protrusion of the spinal cord or meninges.

380. A. Rheumatoid arthritis involves the proximal interphalangeal joints. It is also noted for acute inflammatory signs and symptoms and is a systemic disease.

381. B. The bursae are not found in intramuscular locations. Bursae are most likely found where friction is possible (eg, between tendons, ligaments, and bones).

382. B. Any time a patient calls with a complication following treatment it is appropriate to have the patient come back to the clinic so you can inspect the area and accurately record the patient's injury or complication in your notes. It is also appropriate to notify the supervising physical therapist.

383. B. For the massage to be most effective, you would massage the proximal segment first. The Jobst garment would be measured and ordered to also assist with edema control.

384. B. Cold treatments will produce the following results: increased stroke volume, increased tidal volume, and increased intestinal blood flow to the organs.

385. D. This patient should receive treatment once a week with five times the minimal erythemal dosage. A patient with a third-degree erythemal burn would have tissue damage, peeling and itching, and he or she should receive treatment once a week. The minimal erythemal dosage treatment should be done daily for first degree. For second degree, a patient would be seen every day, two to five times minimal erythemal dosage. For fourth degree, a patient would be seen once every 3 to 4 months.

386. D. The case study emphasizes that the patient has a neck deformity that causes rotation and tilting of the head, more commonly described as torticollis. The appropriate treatment program for this clinical case would be stretching exercises and proper positioning and postural instruction. This would assist in reducing the neck rotation and tilting of the head at home.

387. A. When observing posture from the posterior view, the normal alignment would consist of the hip joint neutral, knee neutral, and slight out-toeing of the feet. Normal alignment from the side view would consist of the hip joint in the neutral position with the plumb line falling in the center of the joint. The knee joint should be in the neutral position with a plumb line slightly anterior to the joint but posterior to the patella. The ankle should be in neutral position with the plumb line slightly anterior to the lateral malleolus.

388. B. The normal conduction pathway for muscular contraction of the heart to follow is the right atrium, to the left atrium, to the ventricles.

389. D. The brachioradialis is responsible for forearm pronation, supination, and elbow flexion. These movements may now be limited due to the injury.

390. D. Orthostatic hypotension is an abnormally low blood pressure occurring when an individual assumes the standing posture. It can last for more than 24 hours, so this is a false statement.

391. A. The following would be considered a normal response to exercise: cardiac output/heart rate would increase in a linear relationship with the increase in workload. Some benefits from a patient exercising regularly may include a decrease in serum lipid levels, improvement in maximum oxygen consumption, increase in HDL levels, decrease in blood pressure, improved tolerance for activity/exercise, improved or relieved angina, improved aerobic capacity or decreased depression following a myocardial infarction.

392. B. Eversion and inversion movements take place at the subtalar joint of the ankle.

393. D. The SITS muscles (supraspinatus, infraspinatus, and teres minor) of the glenohumeral joint assist with depression of the humeral head.

394. A. The cervical vertebra, one of the first seven segments of the vertebral column, is the only vertebra in the body that has a bifid spinous process.

395. A. Electromyogram helps in diagnosing neuromuscular problems by applying surface electrodes or by inserting a needle electrode into the muscle and observing electric activity with an oscilloscope and a loudspeaker. Arthroscopy is the examination of the interior of a joint, performed by inserting a specially designed endoscope through a small incision. An EKG is a graphic record produced by an electrocardiograph. A myelogram is an x-ray film taken after injection of a radiopaque medium into the subarachnoid space to demonstrate any distortions of the spinal cord, spinal nerve roots, and subarachnoid space.

396. A. The femoral triangle is bordered by the following two muscles: sartorius and adductor longus.

397. D. The musculocutaneous nerve arises from the lateral cord of the brachial plexus. It is formed on each side by division of the lateral cord and the plexus into two branches. The median nerve is one of the terminal branches of the brachial plexus that extends along the radial portion of the forearm and the hand and supplies various muscles and the skin of these parts. The ulnar nerve is one of the terminal branches of the brachial plexus that arises on each side from the medial cord of the plexus. The axillary nerve is one of the last two branches of the posterior cord of the brachial plexus before the posterior cord becomes the radial nerve.

398. D. In the asymmetric tonic neck reflex, the correct response would be arm/leg extension on the side that the head is turned toward, and arm/leg flexion on the opposite side.

399. D. Kyphosis, an abnormal condition of the vertebral column and can be described as a curvature of the spine where the anterior-posterior direction in which the convexity is in the posterior direction. Conservative treatment consists of spine stretching exercises and sleeping without a pillow and with a board under the mattress. For severe kyphosis, a modified Milwaukee brace may be used. Scoliosis is a lateral curvature of the spine, a common abnormality of childhood. Treatment includes braces, casts, exercises, and corrective surgery.

400. B. Teres major is not a rotator cuff muscle. Therefore, it would not be emphasized in an initial treatment program of strengthening of the rotator cuff muscle. The infraspinatus, supraspinatus, and subscapularis, which are rotator cuff muscles, would be emphasized in a gentle strengthening program.

401. B. Erb's palsy is a result of damage to the C5, C6 nerve root. Signs of Erb's palsy include loss of sensation in the arm and paralysis and atrophy of the deltoid, biceps, and brachialis muscles. The typical position commonly seen in the affected extremity is adducted and internally rotated arm, elbow extended and forearm pronated. Treatment emphasizes preventing contractures and range of motion.

402. A. The elbow should be placed in extension with supination. This is done to assist in preventing flexion contracture.

403. C. A patient with a collagen vascular disorder, as well as the classic butterfly rash, would most likely have lupus erythematosus. Systemic lupus erythematosus is a chronic inflammatory disease affecting many systems of the body. Another characteristic of lupus erythematosus is the butterfly rash, which is an erythematous, scaling eruption of both cheeks joined by a narrow band of rash across the nose. Scleroderma is a rare autoimmune disease affecting the blood vessels and connective tissue. There is a gradual hardening of the skin and swelling of the distal extremities. Dermatomyositis is a disease of the connective tissues, characterized by eczematous inflammation of the skin and tenderness and weakness of the muscles.

404. A. At 6 months, a child should be able to reach for an object utilizing only one hand.

405. B. A physical therapist assistant provides services independently is an incorrect standard of conduct. The correct standard of conduct would be that physical therapist assistants provide services under the supervision of the physical therapist.

406. C. A malingerer is one who pretends to be ill to arouse sympathy or who intentionally slows the recuperation from a disorder to continue to receive insurance benefits or other emotional or social benefits from the disorder. If the physical therapist or physical therapist assistant suspects the patient is a malingerer, he or she should discuss the

case in a teamwork approach and notify the physician. Negligence is failure to do what another reasonable practitioner would have done under similar circumstances. A hypochondriac is a person with a chronic abnormal concern about the health of his or her body. A paranoid patient has a mental disorder characterized by an impaired sense of reality and persistent delusions.

407. D. Leg lifts would not be started on day 3 post cesarean. Leg lifts would be brought in possibly at day 5, 6, and beyond.

408. C. The primary reason for keeping records of a physical therapy patient is for the improvement of patient care. This would be the best choice. The other reasons given are also appropriate requirements (third-party payers for malpractice, legal purposes, and educational purposes). However, the single best reason for keeping patient records is for the improvement of patient care.

409. A. Lifting light weights of 2 to 3 pounds would be an example of 2 METs. Walking 2 miles, doing light woodwork, and playing an instrument would be other examples. Walking 3.5 mph would be an example of 3 to 4 METs. Cycling 8 mph and walking 4 mph would be an example of 4 to 5 METs.

410. A. HMO is a health maintenance organization with a policy that typically limits the number of visits and the patient's copay to a set fee. Typically, the patient is referred to a participating facility by a specific physician. Medicaid is a state-funded program designed for recipients that are financially needy. Medicare is a federally funded program designed for people over 65 years of age. Workman's compensation will cover a patient injured on the job. The amount of coverage and reimbursement varies according to the state.

411. D. Origin is the proximal attachment of a limb muscle. A tendon, one of many white glistening fibrous bands of tissue that attaches muscle to bone, refers to the tendinous structure. Insertion is the distal attachment of the muscle. Belly is the belly part of the muscle.

412. B. Anteversion of the hip would result in genu recurvatum to the knee. Hyperextension involves overextension beyond the normal limits of the hip. Genu valgus is a deformity in which the legs are curved inward so that the knees are close together, also called knock-knee. Genu varus is a deformity in which one or both legs are bending outward at the knee, also called bowleg.

413. A. Tapotement is a massage that consists of brisk blows in an alternating fashion. Friction massage is a type of massage in which deeper tissues are stroked or rubbed, usually through strong circular movements. Kneading massage is a grasping, rolling, and pressing movement. Vibration is not a massage.

414. B. You would not be palpating the lunate bone because it is not included in the distal row of the carpal bones. The carpal bones include the trapezoid, capitate, and hamate. The trapezoid is the smallest carpal bone, located in the distal row of carpal bones between the trapezium and the capitate. The capitate bone is one of the largest carpal bones, located at the center of the wrist and having a rounded head that fits the concavity of the scaphoid and lunate bones. The hamate bone is a carpal bone that rests on the fourth and fifth metacarpal bones and projects a hooklike process from its palmar surface.

415. A. The sympathetic nervous system activity will cause the heart rate to increase. In the flight response the sympathetic system would be activated. The parasympathetic nervous system is responsible for control of the internal functions under quiet conditions.

416. A. The medial rotators of the shoulders are the pectoralis major, anterior deltoid, subscapularis, and teres major. The lateral rotators of the shoulders are the infraspinatus, teres minor, and posterior deltoid.

417. D. During the swing phase, acceleration stage, the quadriceps muscle begins to contract just before push-off to assist in initiating the forward swing of the leg.

418. B. Normal range of motion for wrist joint flexion is 0 to 90°, and for extension, 0 to 70°. Normal range of motion for ulnar deviation is 0 to 30°. Normal range of motion for radial deviation is 0 to 20°.

419. C. At the C6 level, a patient can provide independent pressure relief. This is the minimal level of injury a patient can have in order to be able to provide independent care. At level C4, a patient is only able to direct pressure relief activities. At level C5, a patient is able to assist in manual wheelchair pressure relief. At level C8, a patient would be independent in pressure relief, including wheelchair push-ups.

420. A. Subjective data collection is the process in which data relating to the patient's problem is elicited from the patient. A patient who states that his chief concern is limited movement or loss of range of motion in the left shoulder is stating his own perception versus something that may be evaluated by objective standards. Therefore, this information should be placed under subjective in the SOAP note format.

421. B. Lateral epicondylitis is an inflammation commonly referred to as tennis elbow. Therefore, the best type of massage would be friction, transverse massage. Friction massage would be the most appropriate to assist in decreasing inflammation and healing of the tendons/muscles.

422. C. Tell the patient he has the right to attend the clinic of his choice. If he has any concerns he should talk to his family physician who originally referred him for physical therapy. It is important when talking that you be honest and upfront about the patient's options to choose where to go for physical therapy.

423. A. The typical treatment temperature for paraffin would be 50°C. The conversion to Fahrenheit is as follows: Fahrenheit = (temperature in Celsius x 9 ÷ 5 + 32). Therefore, temperature in Fahrenheit would be 50 x 9 = 450, divided by 5, which would be 90 + 32 = 122°F.

424. C. A patient with pronated feet would demonstrate eversion of the calcaneus with a medial weight line.

425. A. The major components of a problem-oriented medical record are subjective, objective, assessment, and plan.

426. C. The carpometacarpal joint in the thumb is unique in that it is classified as a saddle joint. A saddle joint permits no axial rotation but allows flexion, extension, adduction, and abduction. The uniaxial joint is a synovial joint in which movement is only in one axis, as with a pivot or hinge joint. A hinge joint is a synovial joint providing a connection in which articular surfaces are closely molded together in a manner that permits extension motion in one plane.

427. D. Maximum heart rate is calculated by 220 minus age. This number can be used to help determine target heart rate at which you want the patient to exercise, when it is multiplied by 60% to 90%, for example, depending on the level of exercise desired.

428. D. Grade five mobilization is an example of a manual therapy technique that could not be performed by a physical therapist assistant. Typically, it is performed by a physician with a patient under anesthesia. It is a manipulation of such force that it breaks the entire joint from being frozen. Grade five mobilization is defined as a thrusting movement done at the anatomical limits of the joint.

429. D. Saunders cervical traction device is recommended for a patient with temporomandibular joint (TMJ) dysfunction. The Saunders cervical traction device does not contact the jaw, thereby reducing further aggravation of the temporomandibular joints.

430. D. Interferential current stimulation is best described as a medium-frequency current, approximately 4000 Hz, and typically utilizes four electrodes in a crossed pattern on the patient. It is primarily used for pain relief and muscle spasms. Russian stimulation involves stimulation in the midrange frequency, typically 2400 to 2500 Hz. High-volt electric stimulation is typically set up with a rate of 50 to 120 Hz per 10 to 30 minute periods for acute pain. Low-volt electric stimulation operates with less than 150 V. Lower frequencies would not provide a smooth tetanic contraction.

431. A. A four-point crutch gait pattern for a patient who is nonweightbearing on the left lower extremity would be (L) crutch, (R) foot, (R) crutch, (L) foot.

432. C. Cosine law states that the intensity of radiation to a surface will fall off relative to the angle at which the radiation strikes the surface of the target. Clinically, this means the source (eg, ultrasound) should be perpendicular to the patient for best results. Inverse square law states that the intensity of radiation from a light source varies inversely to the square of the distance from the source. Clinical application means the further the infrared light (eg, is moving from the patient), the greater the decrease in intensity will be. Ohm's law states that the strength of an electrical current in a circuit is directly proportional to the applied electromotive force and inversely proportional to the resistance of the current. Joule's law states the amount of heat produced is proportional to the square of the current, the resistance, and the time that the current flows.

433. C. Cheyne-Stokes respiration is an abnormal pattern of respiration characterized by alternating periods of apnea and deep, rapid breathing. Ataxic breathing is a type of breathing associated with a lesion in the medullary respiratory centers characterized by a series of inspirations and expirations. Biot's respiration is an abnormal respiratory pattern characterized by irregular breathing, often accompanied with a sigh with periods of apnea. Sighing respiration is periodic deep forced inspiration of compressed gas or air in controlled ventilation.

434. B. Lateral ligaments of the ankle are the anterior talofibular, posterior talofibular, and calcaneofibular. The medial ligament of the ankle consists of the deltoid ligament.

435. C. Isometric is defined as "no change in muscle length but the muscle will develop tension." Isometric exercise is a form of active exercise that increases muscle tension by applying pressure against stable resistance. Isotonic is described as "speed is variable, the muscle shortens to develop tension." Isokinetic pertains to a concentric or eccentric contraction that occurs at a set speed against a force of maximal resistance produced at all points in the range of motion. Passive range of motion is a reference to a therapist's taking an extremity through a range of motion where the therapist performs all the work.

436. A. When measuring crutches, it is proper to have 20° to 30° of elbow flexion and a two-finger width between the axilla and the crutch. This allows the patient proper positioning to prevent axillary nerve damage. The patient should also be instructed not to lean on the crutches.

437. A. The masseter muscle is the thick, rectangular muscle in the cheek that functions to close the jaw. The pterygoideus lateralis assists in chewing and protrusion. The pterygoideus medialis functions for elevation and protraction of the lower jaw and assists in chewing. The zygomaticus causes the mouth's angles to draw upward and backward.

438. A. Quadratus lumborum is the muscle whose function is to elevate the pelvis. The quadratus lumborum helps maintain the pelvis in a neutral position during gait and assists with lateral trunk flexion. The pectineus muscle, the most anterior of the five medial femoral muscles, functions to flex and adduct the thigh and to rotate it medially. Gemellus inferior and gemellus superior are responsible for hip abduction.

439. A. The leg will withdraw from the stimulus on the same side in the flexor withdrawal reflex.

440. D. A cross-sectional research study is described as interviewing different people over the same time period.

441. C. A patient with a burn in the axillary region of the right shoulder should be placed in abduction and flexion to minimize the risk of developing a contracture.

442. D. In utilization of a therapeutic modality the most important choice is to explain the procedure to the patient. The patient needs to know what to expect from the application of the modality, where the safety switch is to turn the machine off, and expected results over the course of the treatments.

443. D. Neutrophils are the body's first line of defense against bacterial infection. Neutrophils are the circulating white blood cells essential for phagocytosis and proteolysis in which bacteria, cellular debris, and solid particles are removed and destroyed. Phagocyte is a cell that is able to surround, engulf, and digest microorganisms and cellular debris. Macrophage is any phagocytic cell of the reticuloendothelial system. Lymphocyte is one of two kinds of small leukocytes originating from fetal stem cells and developing in the bone marrow.

444. C. The greater trochanter is a large projection of the femur into which six muscles insert.

445. B. The radial nerve would most likely be injured, as it is in the closest proximity to the distal radius.

446. C. Nosocomial infection is acquired in the hospital by the patient. It is also called hospital-acquired infection.

447. A. A muscle grade of poor is defined as a production of movement only in a gravity-eliminated position.

448. D. Testing bilaterally, starting with the injured side, would be an incorrect method of performing manual muscle test. When performing manual muscle testing, it is appropriate to test bilaterally starting on the non-injured side and then comparing to the injured side. All other answers listed would be important in performing manual muscle testing. The following considerations should be followed when performing manual muscle testing: (1) test bilaterally starting with the noninjured side, (2) isolate the muscle you are testing, line up the origin and insertion, (3) palpate the muscle tested for contraction, (4) stabilize the proximal part; you need to know proper hand position to isolate the muscle you are testing, (5) apply the correct amount of resistance for testing strength and, to receive maximum cooperation from the patient, inform him of the treatment you are performing.

449. B. The treatment for this patient is not appropriate and you should refer back to the physical therapist for advice. This is because you have been instructed to start percussion on a patient who has severe angina. Angina is a contraindication to percussion.

450. B. A swing-through gait pattern would be the most appropriate for a nonweightbearing patient on the left lower extremity. The four-point gait pattern would involve left crutch, right foot, and right crutch, then left foot. The three-point gait pattern would involve using one crutch, lower extremity, and then right crutch. The easiest and best gait pattern would be a swing-through, using both crutches and hopping and swinging the leg through.

451. C. Agonist is defined as a muscle group whose contraction is considered to be the principal agent in producing a joint motion. Antagonist is defined as a muscle group that is noncontracting and passively elongates or shortens to permit the motion to occur. Concentric refers to a shortening in the contraction. Eccentric refers to elongation of the muscle during contraction.

452. D. Gastrocnemius, soleus, and flexor hallucis longus are muscles that are active during the push-off phase of gait to provide a normal push-off.

453. A. Decerebrate rigidity is posture of the lower extremities plantar flexed and fully extended, upper extremity with shoulder adducted, elbow extended, forearm pronated, and wrist flexed. Decerebrate rigidity would most likely have occurred if the patient had an injury to the diencephalon, pons, or midbrain.

454. A. The hip adductor muscles are innervated by the obturator and sciatic nerves. The muscles consist of adductor brevis, adductor longus, and adductor magnus.

455. B. T3 is the vertebral level to which the spine of the scapula corresponds.

456. C. Cervical rotation to the opposite side is the responsibility of the sternocleidomastoid, scalenus anterior, and upper trapezius.

Bibliography

Baxter R. *Pocket Guide to Musculoskeletal Assessment*. Philadelphia, Pa: WB Saunders; 1998.

Behrens BJ, Michlovitz SL. *Physical Agents in Theory and Practice for the Physical Therapy Assistant*. Philadelphia, Pa: FA Davis; 1996.

Bottomley J. *Quick Reference Dictionary for Physical Therapy*. Thorofare, NJ: SLACK Incorporated; 2000.

Curtis, K. *The Physical Therapist's Guide to Health Care*. Thorofare, NJ: SLACK Incorporated; 1999.

DeFranco J, Meyer T. *Outpatient Rehabilitation Certification Manual*. Hermann, Mo: Midwest Hi-Tech Publishers; 1998.

Fischback F. *Common Laboratory Diagnostics Test*. 2nd ed. Philadelphia, Pa: Lippincott; 1998.

Gogia P. *Clinical Wound Management*. Thorofare, NJ: SLACK Incorporated; 1995.

Goodman CC, Boissonnault WG. *Pathological Implications for the Physical Therapist*. Philadelphia, Pa: WB Saunders; 1998.

Guide to Physical Therapy Practice Act. Alexandria, Va: American Physical Therapy Association; 1999.

Hoppenfield S. *Physical Examination of the Spine and Extremities*. Norwalk, Conn: Appleton-Century Crofts; 1982.

Irwin S, Tecklin JS. *Cardiopulmonary Physical Therapy*. St. Louis, Mo: CV Mosby Co; 1995.

Kaufmann T. *Geriatric Rehabilitation Manual*. Philadelphia, Pa: Churchill Livingstone; 1999.

Kendall F, McCreary E. *Muscle Testing and Function*. 4th ed. Philadelphia, Pa: Lippincott, Williams & Wilkins; 1999.

Liebman M. *Neuroanatomy Made Easy and Understandable*. Gaithersburg, Md: Aspen; 1996.

Littell EH. *Basic Neuroscience for the Health Professions*. Thorofare, NJ: SLACK Incorporated; 1990.

Magee DJ. *Orthopedic Physical Assessment*. Philadelphia, Pa: WB Saunders Co; 1992.

Malone T, McPoil T, Nite A. *Orthopedic and Sports Physical Therapy*. 3rd ed. St. Louis, Mo: Mosby; 1997.

Merck Manual. Whitehouse Station, NJ: Merck Reseacrh Laboratories; 1996.

Michlovitz SL. *Thermal Agents in Rehabilitation*. 2nd ed. Philadelphia, Pa:FA Davis; 1990.

Molick, MH, Carr JA. *Manual on Management of Burn Patients*. Pittsburgh, Pa: Harmarville Rehab Center.

Monorkin CC, Levangie PK. *Joint Structure & Function: A Comprehensive Analysis*. Philadelphia, Pa: FA Davis Co; 1992.

Mosby's Medical Dictionary. 5th ed. St Louis, Mo: Mosby; 1998.

Normative Model of Physical Therapy Assistant Education. Version 99. Alexandria, Va: American Physical Therapy Association; 1999.

O'Connor LJ, Gourley RJ. *Obstetric and Gynecologic Care*. 2nd ed. Thorofare, NJ: SLACK Incorporated; 1999.

O'Sullivan S, Schmitz T. *Physical Rehabilitation Assessment and Treatment*. Philadelphia, Pa: FA Davis Co; 1994.

Perry J. *Gait Analysis: Normal and Pathological Function*. Thorofare, NJ: SLACK Incorporated; 1992.

Rothstein J, Wolfs RS. *The Rehabilitation Specialist Handbook*. Philadelphia, Pa: FA Davis Co; 1998.

Scanlon V, Saunders T. *Essentials of Anatomy*. Philadelphia, Pa: FA Davis; 1994.

Scully R, Barnes M. *Physical Therapy*. Philadelphia, Pa: JB Lippincott Company; 1989.

Shannon M, Wilson BA, Stang CL. *Health Professionals Drug Guide 2000*. Stamford, Conn: Appleton and Lange; 2000.

Sullivan, Markos. *Clinical Decision Making in Therapeutic Exercise*. 1995.

Tabors Encyclopedia Medical Dictionary. 18th ed. Philadelphia, Pa: FA Davis; 1997.

Tecklin JS. *Pediatric Physical Therapy*. 3rd ed. Philadelphia. Pa: Lippincott; 1999.

Test Answer Form

A B C D
1 ① ② ③ ④

A B C D
2 ① ② ③ ④

A B C D
3 ① ② ③ ④

A B C D
4 ① ② ③ ④

A B C D
5 ① ② ③ ④

A B C D
6 ① ② ③ ④

A B C D
7 ① ② ③ ④

A B C D
8 ① ② ③ ④

A B C D
9 ① ② ③ ④

A B C D
10 ① ② ③ ④

A B C D
11 ① ② ③ ④

A B C D
12 ① ② ③ ④

A B C D
13 ① ② ③ ④

A B C D
14 ① ② ③ ④

A B C D
15 ① ② ③ ④

A B C D
16 ① ② ③ ④

A B C D
17 ① ② ③ ④

A B C D
18 ① ② ③ ④

A B C D
19 ① ② ③ ④

A B C D
20 ① ② ③ ④

A B C D
21 ① ② ③ ④

A B C D
22 ① ② ③ ④

A B C D
23 ① ② ③ ④

A B C D
24 ① ② ③ ④

A B C D
25 ① ② ③ ④

A B C D
26 ① ② ③ ④

A B C D
27 ① ② ③ ④

A B C D
28 ① ② ③ ④

A B C D
29 ① ② ③ ④

A B C D
30 ① ② ③ ④

A B C D
31 ① ② ③ ④

A B C D
32 ① ② ③ ④

A B C D
33 ① ② ③ ④

A B C D
34 ① ② ③ ④

A B C D
35 ① ② ③ ④

A B C D
36 ① ② ③ ④

A B C D
37 ① ② ③ ④

A B C D
38 ① ② ③ ④

A B C D
39 ① ② ③ ④

A B C D
40 ① ② ③ ④

A B C D
41 ① ② ③ ④

A B C D
42 ① ② ③ ④

A B C D
43 ① ② ③ ④

A B C D
44 ① ② ③ ④

A B C D
45 ① ② ③ ④

A B C D
46 ① ② ③ ④

A B C D
47 ① ② ③ ④

A B C D
48 ① ② ③ ④

A B C D
49 ① ② ③ ④

A B C D
50 ① ② ③ ④

A B C D
51 ① ② ③ ④

A B C D
52 ① ② ③ ④

A B C D
53 ① ② ③ ④

A B C D
54 ① ② ③ ④

A B C D
55 ① ② ③ ④

A B C D
56 ① ② ③ ④

A B C D
57 ① ② ③ ④

A B C D
58 ① ② ③ ④

A B C D
59 ① ② ③ ④

A B C D
60 ① ② ③ ④

A B C D
61 ① ② ③ ④

A B C D
62 ① ② ③ ④

A B C D
63 ① ② ③ ④

A B C D
64 ① ② ③ ④

A B C D
65 ① ② ③ ④

A B C D
66 ① ② ③ ④

A B C D
67 ① ② ③ ④

A B C D
68 ① ② ③ ④

A B C D
69 ① ② ③ ④

A B C D
70 ① ② ③ ④

A B C D
71 ① ② ③ ④

A B C D
72 ① ② ③ ④

A B C D
73 ① ② ③ ④

A B C D
74 ① ② ③ ④

A B C D
75 ① ② ③ ④

A B C D
76 ① ② ③ ④

	A B C D		A B C D		A B C D		A B C D
77	① ② ③ ④	96	① ② ③ ④	115	① ② ③ ④	134	① ② ③ ④
78	① ② ③ ④	97	① ② ③ ④	116	① ② ③ ④	135	① ② ③ ④
79	① ② ③ ④	98	① ② ③ ④	117	① ② ③ ④	136	① ② ③ ④
80	① ② ③ ④	99	① ② ③ ④	118	① ② ③ ④	137	① ② ③ ④
81	① ② ③ ④	100	① ② ③ ④	119	① ② ③ ④	138	① ② ③ ④
82	① ② ③ ④	101	① ② ③ ④	120	① ② ③ ④	139	① ② ③ ④
83	① ② ③ ④	102	① ② ③ ④	121	① ② ③ ④	140	① ② ③ ④
84	① ② ③ ④	103	① ② ③ ④	122	① ② ③ ④	141	① ② ③ ④
85	① ② ③ ④	104	① ② ③ ④	123	① ② ③ ④	142	① ② ③ ④
86	① ② ③ ④	105	① ② ③ ④	124	① ② ③ ④	143	① ② ③ ④
87	① ② ③ ④	106	① ② ③ ④	125	① ② ③ ④	144	① ② ③ ④
88	① ② ③ ④	107	① ② ③ ④	126	① ② ③ ④	145	① ② ③ ④
89	① ② ③ ④	108	① ② ③ ④	127	① ② ③ ④	146	① ② ③ ④
90	① ② ③ ④	109	① ② ③ ④	128	① ② ③ ④	147	① ② ③ ④
91	① ② ③ ④	110	① ② ③ ④	129	① ② ③ ④	148	① ② ③ ④
92	① ② ③ ④	111	① ② ③ ④	130	① ② ③ ④	149	① ② ③ ④
93	① ② ③ ④	112	① ② ③ ④	131	① ② ③ ④	150	① ② ③ ④
94	① ② ③ ④	113	① ② ③ ④	132	① ② ③ ④	151	① ② ③ ④
95	① ② ③ ④	114	① ② ③ ④	133	① ② ③ ④	152	① ② ③ ④

153 A① B② C③ D④	172 A① B② C③ D④	191 A① B② C③ D④	210 A① B② C③ D④
154 A① B② C③ D④	173 A① B② C③ D④	192 A① B② C③ D④	211 A① B② C③ D④
155 A① B② C③ D④	174 A① B② C③ D④	193 A① B② C③ D④	212 A① B② C③ D④
156 A① B② C③ D④	175 A① B② C③ D④	194 A① B② C③ D④	213 A① B② C③ D④
157 A① B② C③ D④	176 A① B② C③ D④	195 A① B② C③ D④	214 A① B② C③ D④
158 A① B② C③ D④	177 A① B② C③ D④	196 A① B② C③ D④	215 A① B② C③ D④
159 A① B② C③ D④	178 A① B② C③ D④	197 A① B② C③ D④	216 A① B② C③ D④
160 A① B② C③ D④	179 A① B② C③ D④	198 A① B② C③ D④	217 A① B② C③ D④
161 A① B② C③ D④	180 A① B② C③ D④	199 A① B② C③ D④	218 A① B② C③ D④
162 A① B② C③ D④	181 A① B② C③ D④	200 A① B② C③ D④	219 A① B② C③ D④
163 A① B② C③ D④	182 A① B② C③ D④	201 A① B② C③ D④	220 A① B② C③ D④
164 A① B② C③ D④	183 A① B② C③ D④	202 A① B② C③ D④	221 A① B② C③ D④
165 A① B② C③ D④	184 A① B② C③ D④	203 A① B② C③ D④	222 A① B② C③ D④
166 A① B② C③ D④	185 A① B② C③ D④	204 A① B② C③ D④	223 A① B② C③ D④
167 A① B② C③ D④	186 A① B② C③ D④	205 A① B② C③ D④	224 A① B② C③ D④
168 A① B② C③ D④	187 A① B② C③ D④	206 A① B② C③ D④	225 A① B② C③ D④
169 A① B② C③ D④	188 A① B② C③ D④	207 A① B② C③ D④	226 A① B② C③ D④
170 A① B② C③ D④	189 A① B② C③ D④	208 A① B② C③ D④	227 A① B② C③ D④
171 A① B② C③ D④	190 A① B② C③ D④	209 A① B② C③ D④	228 A① B② C③ D④

	A B C D 229 ① ② ③ ④		A B C D 248 ① ② ③ ④		A B C D 267 ① ② ③ ④		A B C D 286 ① ② ③ ④
	A B C D 230 ① ② ③ ④		A B C D 249 ① ② ③ ④		A B C D 268 ① ② ③ ④		A B C D 287 ① ② ③ ④
	A B C D 231 ① ② ③ ④		A B C D 250 ① ② ③ ④		A B C D 269 ① ② ③ ④		A B C D 288 ① ② ③ ④
	A B C D 232 ① ② ③ ④		A B C D 251 ① ② ③ ④		A B C D 270 ① ② ③ ④		A B C D 289 ① ② ③ ④
	A B C D 233 ① ② ③ ④		A B C D 252 ① ② ③ ④		A B C D 271 ① ② ③ ④		A B C D 290 ① ② ③ ④
	A B C D 234 ① ② ③ ④		A B C D 253 ① ② ③ ④		A B C D 272 ① ② ③ ④		A B C D 291 ① ② ③ ④
	A B C D 235 ① ② ③ ④		A B C D 254 ① ② ③ ④		A B C D 273 ① ② ③ ④		A B C D 292 ① ② ③ ④
	A B C D 236 ① ② ③ ④		A B C D 255 ① ② ③ ④		A B C D 274 ① ② ③ ④		A B C D 293 ① ② ③ ④
	A B C D 237 ① ② ③ ④		A B C D 256 ① ② ③ ④		A B C D 275 ① ② ③ ④		A B C D 294 ① ② ③ ④
	A B C D 238 ① ② ③ ④		A B C D 257 ① ② ③ ④		A B C D 276 ① ② ③ ④		A B C D 295 ① ② ③ ④
	A B C D 239 ① ② ③ ④		A B C D 258 ① ② ③ ④		A B C D 277 ① ② ③ ④		A B C D 296 ① ② ③ ④
	A B C D 240 ① ② ③ ④		A B C D 259 ① ② ③ ④		A B C D 278 ① ② ③ ④		A B C D 297 ① ② ③ ④
	A B C D 241 ① ② ③ ④		A B C D 260 ① ② ③ ④		A B C D 279 ① ② ③ ④		A B C D 298 ① ② ③ ④
	A B C D 242 ① ② ③ ④		A B C D 261 ① ② ③ ④		A B C D 280 ① ② ③ ④		A B C D 299 ① ② ③ ④
	A B C D 243 ① ② ③ ④		A B C D 262 ① ② ③ ④		A B C D 281 ① ② ③ ④		A B C D 300 ① ② ③ ④
	A B C D 244 ① ② ③ ④		A B C D 263 ① ② ③ ④		A B C D 282 ① ② ③ ④		A B C D 301 ① ② ③ ④
	A B C D 245 ① ② ③ ④		A B C D 264 ① ② ③ ④		A B C D 283 ① ② ③ ④		A B C D 302 ① ② ③ ④
	A B C D 246 ① ② ③ ④		A B C D 265 ① ② ③ ④		A B C D 284 ① ② ③ ④		A B C D 303 ① ② ③ ④
	A B C D 247 ① ② ③ ④		A B C D 266 ① ② ③ ④		A B C D 285 ① ② ③ ④		A B C D 304 ① ② ③ ④

A B C D 305 ① ② ③ ④	**A B C D** 324 ① ② ③ ④	**A B C D** 343 ① ② ③ ④	**A B C D** 362 ① ② ③ ④
A B C D 306 ① ② ③ ④	**A B C D** 325 ① ② ③ ④	**A B C D** 344 ① ② ③ ④	**A B C D** 363 ① ② ③ ④
A B C D 307 ① ② ③ ④	**A B C D** 326 ① ② ③ ④	**A B C D** 345 ① ② ③ ④	**A B C D** 364 ① ② ③ ④
A B C D 308 ① ② ③ ④	**A B C D** 327 ① ② ③ ④	**A B C D** 346 ① ② ③ ④	**A B C D** 365 ① ② ③ ④
A B C D 309 ① ② ③ ④	**A B C D** 328 ① ② ③ ④	**A B C D** 347 ① ② ③ ④	**A B C D** 366 ① ② ③ ④
A B C D 310 ① ② ③ ④	**A B C D** 329 ① ② ③ ④	**A B C D** 348 ① ② ③ ④	**A B C D** 367 ① ② ③ ④
A B C D 311 ① ② ③ ④	**A B C D** 330 ① ② ③ ④	**A B C D** 349 ① ② ③ ④	**A B C D** 368 ① ② ③ ④
A B C D 312 ① ② ③ ④	**A B C D** 331 ① ② ③ ④	**A B C D** 350 ① ② ③ ④	**A B C D** 369 ① ② ③ ④
A B C D 313 ① ② ③ ④	**A B C D** 332 ① ② ③ ④	**A B C D** 351 ① ② ③ ④	**A B C D** 370 ① ② ③ ④
A B C D 314 ① ② ③ ④	**A B C D** 333 ① ② ③ ④	**A B C D** 352 ① ② ③ ④	**A B C D** 371 ① ② ③ ④
A B C D 315 ① ② ③ ④	**A B C D** 334 ① ② ③ ④	**A B C D** 353 ① ② ③ ④	**A B C D** 372 ① ② ③ ④
A B C D 316 ① ② ③ ④	**A B C D** 335 ① ② ③ ④	**A B C D** 354 ① ② ③ ④	**A B C D** 373 ① ② ③ ④
A B C D 317 ① ② ③ ④	**A B C D** 336 ① ② ③ ④	**A B C D** 355 ① ② ③ ④	**A B C D** 374 ① ② ③ ④
A B C D 318 ① ② ③ ④	**A B C D** 337 ① ② ③ ④	**A B C D** 356 ① ② ③ ④	**A B C D** 375 ① ② ③ ④
A B C D 319 ① ② ③ ④	**A B C D** 338 ① ② ③ ④	**A B C D** 357 ① ② ③ ④	**A B C D** 376 ① ② ③ ④
A B C D 320 ① ② ③ ④	**A B C D** 339 ① ② ③ ④	**A B C D** 358 ① ② ③ ④	**A B C D** 377 ① ② ③ ④
A B C D 321 ① ② ③ ④	**A B C D** 340 ① ② ③ ④	**A B C D** 359 ① ② ③ ④	**A B C D** 378 ① ② ③ ④
A B C D 322 ① ② ③ ④	**A B C D** 341 ① ② ③ ④	**A B C D** 360 ① ② ③ ④	**A B C D** 379 ① ② ③ ④
A B C D 323 ① ② ③ ④	**A B C D** 342 ① ② ③ ④	**A B C D** 361 ① ② ③ ④	**A B C D** 380 ① ② ③ ④

	A B C D		A B C D		A B C D		A B C D
381	① ② ③ ④	400	① ② ③ ④	419	① ② ③ ④	438	① ② ③ ④
382	① ② ③ ④	401	① ② ③ ④	420	① ② ③ ④	439	① ② ③ ④
383	① ② ③ ④	402	① ② ③ ④	421	① ② ③ ④	440	① ② ③ ④
384	① ② ③ ④	403	① ② ③ ④	422	① ② ③ ④	441	① ② ③ ④
385	① ② ③ ④	404	① ② ③ ④	423	① ② ③ ④	442	① ② ③ ④
386	① ② ③ ④	405	① ② ③ ④	424	① ② ③ ④	443	① ② ③ ④
387	① ② ③ ④	406	① ② ③ ④	425	① ② ③ ④	444	① ② ③ ④
388	① ② ③ ④	407	① ② ③ ④	426	① ② ③ ④	445	① ② ③ ④
389	① ② ③ ④	408	① ② ③ ④	427	① ② ③ ④	446	① ② ③ ④
390	① ② ③ ④	409	① ② ③ ④	428	① ② ③ ④	447	① ② ③ ④
391	① ② ③ ④	410	① ② ③ ④	429	① ② ③ ④	448	① ② ③ ④
392	① ② ③ ④	411	① ② ③ ④	430	① ② ③ ④	449	① ② ③ ④
393	① ② ③ ④	412	① ② ③ ④	431	① ② ③ ④	450	① ② ③ ④
394	① ② ③ ④	413	① ② ③ ④	432	① ② ③ ④	451	① ② ③ ④
395	① ② ③ ④	414	① ② ③ ④	433	① ② ③ ④	452	① ② ③ ④
396	① ② ③ ④	415	① ② ③ ④	434	① ② ③ ④	453	① ② ③ ④
397	① ② ③ ④	416	① ② ③ ④	435	① ② ③ ④	454	① ② ③ ④
398	① ② ③ ④	417	① ② ③ ④	436	① ② ③ ④	455	① ② ③ ④
399	① ② ③ ④	418	① ② ③ ④	437	① ② ③ ④	456	① ② ③ ④

Fri - 3 pm
wed 10^{30} — 10^{00}
9^{00}
6-7 —
7:45 8^{30}
8^{30}